1993

Pocket Book of Infectious Disease Therapy

1993

Pocket Book of Infectious Disease Therapy

John G. Bartlett, M.D.

Chief, Division of Infectious Diseases
The Johns Hopkins University School of Medicine
and The Johns Hopkins Hospital
Baltimore, Maryland

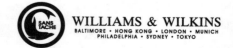

WILLIAMS & WILKINS
BALTIMORE · HONG KONG · LONDON · MUNICH
PHILADELPHIA · SYDNEY · TOKYO

Editor: Jonathan Pine
Associate Editor: Molly Mullen
Copy Editor: Susan S. Vaupel
Designer: Wilma Rosenberger
Illustration Planner: Ray Lowman
Production Coordinator: Kim Nawrozki

Accurate indications, adverse reactions, and dosage schedules for drugs are provided in
this book, but it is possible that they may change. The reader is urged to review the package
information data of the manufacturers of the medications mentioned.

Printed in the United States of America

First Edition 1990
ISBN 0-683-00443-3

93 94 95 96
1 2 3 4 5 6 7 8 9 10

PREFACE

The *1993 Pocket Book of Infectious Disease Therapy* is intended for physicians and other care providers who manage adult patients with infectious diseases. These include internists, generalists, surgeons, obstetricians, gynecologists, medical subspecialists and surgical subspecialists.

This book has the same lofty goals as the first three books: to provide standards of care with particular emphasis on antimicrobial agents, their selection and dosing regimens. As with prior editions there is extensive use of recommendations from various authoritative sources such as the Centers for Disease Control (CDC), the *Medical Letter on Drugs and Therapeutics,* the American Hospital Formulary Service, AMA Drug Evaluations and learned societies such as official statements of the American Heart Association (AHA), the American Thoracic Society and the Infectious Diseases Society of America (IDSA).

This book has extensive changes in terms of additions, deletions and revisions. Nearly all the tabular material has been updated to account for newly approved antibiotics, newly detected microbes and new recommendations for management. Extensive revisions have been made in the sections dealing with drug interactions, vaccinations, treatment of viral infection, tuberculosis, meningitis, hepatitis and urinary tract infections and HIV infection. New sections include the sepsis syndrome and a guide to the use of corticosteroids in infectious diseases and telephone numbers. New antibiotics included in tabular data include azithromycin, cefpodoxime, cefprozil, clarithromycin, dideoxycytidine (ddC), dideoxyinosine (ddI), itraconazole, ofloxacin, lomefloxacin, loracarbef, oxamniquine and teicoplanin.

The reader is encouraged to notify the author [Ross Research Building, Room 1159, The Johns Hopkins University School of Medicine, Baltimore, MD 21205; (410) 955-3150] if there are errors, differences of opinion or suggested additions.

CONTENTS

ANTIMICROBIAL AGENTS
  PREPARATIONS AND RECOMMENDED DOSING REGIMENS FOR
    ANTIMICROBIAL AGENTS..1-12
  COST OF ANTIMICROBIAL AGENTS 13-14
  PREFERRED ANTIMICROBIAL AGENTS FOR SPECIFIC PATHOGENS.................15-33
  ANTIMICROBIAL DOSING REGIMENS IN RENAL FAILURE 34-47
  ANTIMICROBIAL DOSING REGIMENS DURING DIALYSIS 48-51
  USE OF ANTIMICROBIAL AGENTS IN HEPATIC DISEASE 52
  ADVERSE REACTIONS TO ANTIMICROBIAL AGENTS 53-66
  USE OF ANTIBIOTICS IN PREGNANCY 67-73
  DRUG INTERACTIONS..74-81

PREVENTATIVE TREATMENT
  GUIDE FOR ADULT IMMUNIZATION...82-97
  PROPHYLACTIC ANTIBIOTICS IN SURGERY 98-102
  PROPHYLACTIC ANTIBIOTICS TO PREVENT ENDOCARDITIS IN THE
    SUSCEPTIBLE HOST 103-105
  TRAVELERS' CONDITIONS 106-110

NONBACTERIAL INFECTIONS
  TREATMENT OF FUNGAL INFECTIONS 111-118
  TREATMENT OF VIRAL INFECTIONS..119-125
  TREATMENT AND PREVENTION OF TUBERCULOSIS...................................126-134
  TREATMENT OF PARASITIC INFECTIONS 135-146

SPECIFIC TYPES OF INFECTIONS
  AIDS/HIV INFECTION 147-167
  SEPSIS SYNDROME..168-169
  GUIDELINES FOR USE OF STEROIDS...170-172
  COMPROMISED HOST..173-176
  TOXIC SHOCK SYNDROME 176
  ANAEROBIC INFECTIONS 177
  FEVER OF UNKNOWN ORIGIN 178
  LYME DISEASE 179-180
  SKIN AND SOFT TISSUE INFECTIONS 181-185
  BONE AND JOINT INFECTIONS..186-188
  OCULAR AND PERICULAR INFECTIONS 189-191
  CNS INFECTIONS...192-198
  UPPER RESPIRATORY TRACT INFECTIONS 199-203
  PULMONARY INFECTIONS..204-208
  ENDOCARDITIS..209-214

Intra-abdominal sepsis 215-217
Hepatitis...218-221
Infectious diarrhea...222-228
Urinary tract infections 229-233
Sexually transmitted diseases 234-243
Duration of treatment...244-245
INDEX...247-262

PREPARATIONS AND RECOMMENDED DOSING REGIMENS FOR
ANTIMICROBIAL AGENTS (ADAPTED FROM DRUG INFORMATION 92,
AMERICAN HOSPITAL FORMULARY SERVICE, 1992 pp 33-481)

Agent	Trade Names	Dosage Form	Usual Adult Regimen: Daily Dose, Route & Dose Interval
Acyclovir	Zovirax	5% ointment 3 & 15 gm tubes	Topical q3h
		200 mg caps	200 mg po; x3-5/day
		800 mg tabs	800 mg po; x5/day
		200 mg/5 ml susp	200-800 mg po; x3-5/day
		500;1000 mg vials (IV)	15-36 mg/kg/day IV over 1hr q8h
Amantadine	Symmetrel	100 mg cap & tabs 50 mg/5 ml syrup	100-200 mg/day po q12-24h
Amdinocillin	Coactin	0.5; 1 gm vial	40-60 mg/kg/day IM or IV q4-6h
Amikacin	Amikin	0.1;0.5;1 gm vials	15 mg/kg/day IV q8-12h
Aminosalicylic acid	PAS	0.5 gm tabs	150 mg/kg/day po q6-12h
Amoxicillin	Amoxil, Polymox, Trimox, Utimox, Wymox, Larotid	250;500 mg caps 125;250 mg/5 ml syrup	.75-2 gm/day po q6-8h
Amoxicillin + K clavulanate	Augmentin	125/31 mg/5 ml susp 250/62 mg/5 ml susp 125/31 mg tabs 250/125 mg tabs 500/125 mg tabs	.75-1.5 gm/day (amoxicillin) po q8h
Amphotericin B	Fungizone	50 mg vial	0.3-1 mg/kg/day IV over 4-8 hr q 1-2 days
Ampicillin	Omnipen, Amcill, Penamp, Polycillin, Principen, Totacillin	250;500 mg caps 125;250;500 mg/ 5 ml susp 3.5 gm + probenecid, 1 gm (for GC)	1-2 gm/day po q6h
Ampicillin sodium	Omnipen-N, Polycillin-N, Totacillin-N	0.125;0.25;0.5; 1; 2; 10 gm vials	2-8 gm/day IV q4-6h
Ampicillin + sulbactam	Unasyn	1:0.5 gm + 2:1.0 gm vials (Amp:sulbactam)	4-8 gm ampicillin/ day IV or IM q6h

(continued)

1

Agent	Trade Names	Dosage Form	Usual Adult Regimen: Daily Dose, Route & Dose Interval
Atovaquone	Mepron	250 mg tabs	750 mg po 3x/day w/food
Azithromycin	Zithromax	250 mg tabs	500 mg po first day, then 250 mg q24h x 5
Azlocillin	Azlin	2; 3; 4 gm vials	8-24 gm/day IV q6-8h
AZT	(see zidovudine)		
Aztreonam	Azactam	0.5; 1; 2 gm vials	1.5-6 gm/day IV or IM q6-8h
Bacampicillin	Spectrobid	400 mg tabs (equivalent to 280 mg ampicillin) 125 mg/5 ml syrup (equiv to 87 mg amp)	.8-1.6 gm/day po q12h
Bacitracin	Baci-IM	50,000 unit vials	10,000-25,000 units IM q6h; 25,000 units po q6h
Capreomycin	Capastat	1 gm vial	1 gm/day IM
Carbenicillin indanyl sodium	Geocillin	382 mg tabs	382-764 mg po q6h
Cefaclor	Ceclor	250;500 mg caps 125;187;250 & 375 mg/5 ml susp	1-2 gm/day po q8h
Cefadroxil	Duricef, Ultracef	500 mg caps; 1 gm tab; 125; 250; 500 mg/5 ml susp	1-2 gm/day po 1-2 x/day
Cefamandole nafate	Mandol	0.5;1;2;10 gm vials	2-18 gm/day IM or IV q4-6h
Cefazolin	Ancef, Kefzol, Zolicef	0.25;0.5;1;5;10;20 gm vials	2-6 gm/day IV or IM q8h
Cefixime	Suprax	200;400 mg tabs; 100 mg/5 ml susp	400 mg/day po, 1-2 x/day
Cefmetazole	Zefazone	1;2 gm vials	4-8 gm/day IV q6-12h
Cefonicid	Monocid	0.5;1;10 gm vials	1-2 gm/day IV or IM in 1 dose/day
Cefoperazone	Cefobid	1;2;10 gm vials	2-8 gm/day IM or IV q8-12h
Ceforanide lysine	Precef	0.5;1 gm vials	1-3 gm/day IV or IM q12h

(continued)

Agent	Trade Names	Dosage Form	Usual Adult Regimen: Daily Dose, Route & Dose Interval
Cefotaxime sodium	Claforan	0.5;1;2;10 gm vials	2-12 gm/day IV or IM q6h
Cefotetan	Cefotan	1;2;10 gm vials	2-4 gm/day IV or IM q12h
Cefoxitin sodium	Mefoxin	1;2;10 gm vials	2-18 gm/day IV or IM q4-6h
Cefpodoxime proxetil	Vantin	100;200 mg tabs 50 mg/5 ml; 100 mg/5 ml susp	200-800 mg/day po, q12h
Cefprozil	Cefzil	250;500 mg tabs 125;250 mg/5 ml susp	0.5-2 gm/day po, q12-24h usually 500 mg qd or bid
Ceftazidime	Fortaz, Tazidime, Tazicef, Ceptaz	0.5;1;2;6 gm vials	3-6 gm/day IV or IM q8-12h
Ceftizoxime sodium	Cefizox	1;2;10 gm vials	2-12 gm/day IV or IM q6-8h
Ceftriaxone	Rocephin	0.25;0.5;1;2;10 gm vial	1-2 gm IV or IM q12-24h
Cefuroxime	Zinacef	0.75;1.5 gm vial	2.25-4.5 gm/day IV or IM q6-8h
Cefuroxime axetil	Ceftin	0.125;0.25;0.5 gm tabs	0.5-1.0 gm/day po q12h
Cephalexin monohydrate	Keflex, Keftab, Cefanex, Keflet	0.25;0.5 gm caps 0.25;0.5 gm tabs 125;250 mg/5 ml susp	1-2 gm/day po q6h
Cephalothin sodium	Keflin	1;2;20 gm vials	2-12 gm/day IV q4-6h
Cephapirin sodium	Cefadyl	0.5;1;2;4 gm vials	2-4 gm/day IV q6h
Cephradine	Anspor	250;500 mg caps 125;250 mg/5 ml susp	1-2 gm/day po q6h
	Velosef	0.25;0.5;1;2 gm vials	2-8 gm/day IV or IM q6h
Chloramphenicol	Chloromycetin	250 mg caps	1-2 gm/day po q6h

(continued)

Agent	Trade Names	Dosage Form	Usual Adult Regimen: Daily Dose, Route & Dose Interval
Chloramphenicol palmitate	Chloromycetin	150 mg/5 ml syrup	1-2 gm/day po q6h
Chloramphenicol Na succinate	Chloromycetin sodium succinate	1 gm vial	2-4 gm/day IV q6h
Chloroquine HCl	Aralen HCl	250 mg amp (150 mg base)	200-250 mg base q6h IM or IV
Chloroquine PO₄	Aralen PO₄	500 mg tabs (300 mg base) 250 mg tabs (150 mg base)	300-600 mg (base) qd - q week
Chloroquine hydroxy	Plaquenil	200 mg tabs (155 mg base)	10 mg/kg/day po q24h
Cinoxacin	Cinobac	250;500 mg cap	1 gm/day po q6-12h
Ciprofloxacin	Cipro Cipro IV	250;500;750 mg tabs 200;400 mg vials	0.5-1.5 gm/day po q12h 800 mg/day IV q12h
Clarithromycin	Biaxin	250;500 mg tabs	500 mg/day po q12h
Clindamycin HCl	Cleocin HCl	75;150;300 mg cap	0.6-1.8 gm/day po q6-8h
Clindamycin PO₄	Cleocin PO₄	150 mg/ml in vials (2,4,6 ml)	1.8-2.7 gm/day IV q6-8h
Clindamycin palmitate HCl	Cleocin pediatric	75 mg/5 ml solution	0.6-1.8 gm/day po q6-8h
Clindamycin vaginal cream	Cleocin VC	2% 40 gm tube	Topical: 1/day x 7 days
Clofazimine	Lamprene	50;100 mg caps	50-300 mg/day po q8-24h
Cloxacillin	Tegopen Cloxapen	250;500 mg caps 125 mg/5 ml solution	1-2 gm/day po q6h
Colistin	Coly-Mycin S Coly-Mycin M	25 mg/5 ml susp 150 mg vial (IV)	2.5-5.0 mg/kg/day IV q6-12h
Cyclacillin	Cyclapen-W	250;500 mg cap 125;250 mg/5 ml susp	1-2 gm/day po q6h
Cycloserine	Seromycin	250 mg caps	0.5-1 gm/day po in 2 doses
Dapsone		25;100 mg tabs	25-100 mg/day po q24h

(continued)

Agent	Trade Names	Dosage Form	Usual Adult Regimen: Daily Dose, Route & Dose Interval
Demeclocycline	Declomycin	150;300 mg caps	600 mg/day po q6-12h
Dicloxacillin	Dycill, Dynapen Pathocil	125;250;500 mg cap 62.5 mg/5 ml susp	1-2 gm/day po q6h
Didanosine (Dideoxyinosine) (ddI)	Videx	25;50;100;150 mg tabs and 100;167;250;375 mg packets	>60 kg:200 mg (tabs) bid <60 kg:125 mg (tabs) bid
Dideoxycytidine (ddC)	HIVID	0.375;0.75 mg tabs	0.75 mg po tid
Diethylcarba-mazine	Hetrazan	50 mg tabs	6-13 mg/kg/day, 1-3 doses
Diloxanide	Furamide		500 mg po q8h
Doxycycline	Vibramycin Doxy caps, Doxy tabs Vibra-tabs Doxy-100,200	50 mg/5 ml susp 100 mg tabs 50;100 mg caps 100;200 mg vial	100-200 mg/day po q12-24h 200 mg/day IV q12h
Eflornithine	Ornidyl		400 mg/kg/day IV; 100 mg/kg po q8h
Emetine HCl		65 mg/ml (1 ml vial)	1-1.5 mg/kg/day up to 90 mg/day; IM or deep SC injection
Enoxacin	Penetrex	200;400 mg tabs	400-800 mg/day po q12h
Erythromycin	E-mycin;ERYC; Ery-Tab; E-Base Erythromycin Base Ilotycin, PCE, RP-Mycin, Robimycin	250 mg caps 250;333;500 mg tabs 2% topical	1-2 gm/day po q6h (topical for acne)
Erythromycin estolate	Ilosone	250 mg caps, 500 mg tabs 125;250 mg/5 ml susp	1-2 gm/day po q6h
Erythromycin ethylsuccinate	E.E.S. EryPed	200;400 mg tabs 200;400 mg/5 ml susp	1.6-3.2 gm/day po q6h
Erythromycin gluceptate	Ilotycin gluceptate	1 gm vial	2-4 gm/day IV q6h
Erythromycin lactobionate	Erythrocin lactobionate	0.5;1 gm vial	1-4 gm/day IV q6h

(continued)

Agent	Trade Names	Dosage Form	Usual Adult Regimen: Daily Dose, Route & Dose Interval
Erythromycin stearate	Eramycin Erypar; Erythrocin stearate; Ethril; Wyamycin S SK-erythromycin	250;500 mg tabs	1-2 gm/day po q6h
Ethambutol	Myambutol	100;400 mg tabs	15 mg/kg/day po q24h
Ethionamide	Trecator-SC	250 mg tabs	0.5-1 gm/day po in 1-3 daily doses
Fluconazole	Diflucan	50;100;200 mg tabs 100;200 mg vials	100-200 mg/day po or IV q24h
Flucytosine	Ancobon	250;500 mg cap	50-150 mg/kg/day po q6h
Foscarnet	Foscavir	24 mg/ml, 500 ml	90-180 mg/kg/day IV qd or tid
Furazolidone	Furoxone	100 mg tabs 50 mg/15 ml susp	100 mg po q6h
Ganciclovir	Cytovene	0.5 gm vial	5 mg/kg IV bid (induction) or qd (maintenance)
Gentamicin	Garamycin Gentamicin SO₄ Injection Isotonic (NaCl) Gentamicin SO₄ ADD-Vantage Gentamicin SO₄ in 5% dextrose piggyback	40;60;70;80;90; 100;120 mg vials 2 mg/ml for intrathecal use	3-5 mg/kg/day IV or IM q8h
Griseofulvin	Grisactin Fulvicin Grifulvin V Gris-PEG Grisactin Ultra Fulvicin P/G	microsize: 250 caps, 250;500 mg tabs 125 mg/5 ml susp ultramicrosize: 125; 165;250;330 mg tabs	500 mg - 1 gm po/day 330-750 mg po/day
Imipenem/ Cilastatin	Primaxin	0.25;0.5;0.75 gm vials (Imipenem: cilastatin is 1:1)	1-4 gm/day IV q6h
Interferon Alfa 2a	Roferon-A	3,18,36 mil unit vials	3 mil units 3x/wk (HCV) 30-35 mil units/wk (HBV) 30 mil units/m2 3x/wk (Kaposi Sarcoma) 1 mil units intralesion (condylomata)

(continued)

Agent	Trade Names	Dosage Form	Usual Adult Regimen: Daily Dose, Route & Dose Interval
Interferon (continued) Alfa 2b	Intron A	3,5,10,25,50 mil unit vials	As above
Iodoquinol	Yodoxin Diquinol Yodoquinol	210 mg tabs 650 mg tabs	650 mg/day po q8h
Isoniazid	Laniazid Tubizid	50;100;300 mg tabs 50 mg/5 ml (oral solu)	300 mg/day po q24h
	Nydrazid	1 gm vial (IM)	300 mg/day IM q12-24h
Itraconazole	Sporanox	100 mg caps	200-400 mg/day po q12-24h
Kanamycin	Kantrex Klebcil	.075;0.5; 1 gm vial 500 mg caps	15 mg/kg/day IV q8h
Ketoconazole	Nizoral	200 mg tabs	200-400 mg/day po q12-24h up to 1.6 gm/day
Lincomycin	Lincocin	250;500 mg caps 300 mg/ml (2,10 ml)	1.5-2.0 gm/d po q6-8h 1.8-8 gm/d IV q8-12h
Loracarbef	Lorabid	200 mg parvule	400-800 mg/day po q12h
Lomefloxacin	Maxaquin	400 mg caps	400 mg/day po q24h
Mefloquine	Lariam	250 mg tabs	1250 mg po x 1 (treatment); 250 mg po q wk (prophylaxis)
Mebendazole	Vermox	100 mg tabs	100 mg po x 1-2 up to 2 gm/day
Methacycline	Rondomycin	150;300 mg caps	600 mg/d po
Methenamine hippurate	Hiprex	1 gm tabs	1-2 gm/day po q12h
Methenamine mandelate	Mandelamine	0.35;0.5;1 gm tabs 250;500 mg/5 ml syrup 0.5; 1 gm granules	1-4 gm/day po q6h
Methicillin	Staphcillin	1;4;6;10 gm vial	4-12 gm/day IV or IM q6h
Metronidazole	Flagyl, Metryl Metizol, Protostat	250;500 mg tabs	0.75-2 gm/day po q12h
	Metric 21, Satric	500 mg vial	0.75-2 gm/day IV q6-12h

(continued)

Agent	Trade Names	Dosage Form	Usual Adult Regimen: Daily Dose, Route & Dose Interval
Mezlocillin Na	Mezlin	1;2;3;4 gm vial	6-24 gm/day IV q 4-6h
Miconazole	Monistat	200 mg amp 200 mg vaginal supp	0.6-3.6 gm/day IV q8h qd x 3
Minocycline	Minocin	50;100 mg caps & tabs 50 mg/5 ml syrup 100 mg vial	200 mg/day po q6-12h 200 mg/day IV q6-12h
Moxalactam	Moxam	1 gm vial	2-8 gm/day IV q6-8h
Nafcillin	Unipen Nafcil, Nallpen, Unipen	250 mg caps; 500 mg tabs 0.5;1;2;10 gm vial	1-2 gm/day po q6h 2-12 gm/day IV or IM q4-6h
Nalidixic acid	NegGram	0.25;0.5;1 gm tabs 250 mg/5 ml susp	4 gm/day po q6h
Neomycin	Mycifradin	500 mg tabs 125 mg/5 ml solu	3-12 gm po/day
Netilmicin	Netromycin	100 mg/ml vials	4-6.5 mg/kg/day IV or IM q8h
Niclosamide	Niclocide	500 mg tabs	2 gm (single dose)
Nitrofurantoin	Macrodantin Furadantin Furaton Furalan Faran	macrocrystals: 25;50;100 mg caps microcrystals: 50;100 caps/tabs 25 mg/5 ml susp	50-100 mg po q6h Suppressive treatment: 50-100 mg qd
Norfloxacin	Noroxin	400 mg tabs	400 mg po bid
Novobiocin	Albamycin	250 mg caps	1-2 gm/day po q6-12h
Nystatin	Mycostatin Nystex Nilstat	100,000 units/ml 500,000 unit tab 0.05;0.15;0.25;0.5;1;2; 5;10 billion units powder	5 ml swish, swallow or 5-10 ml po 3-5 x daily
Ofloxacin	Floxin	200;300;400 mg tabs	200-400 mg po q12h
Oxacillin	Bactocill, Prostaphlin	250; 500 mg caps 250 mg/5 ml solu 0.25;0.5;1;2;4;10 gm vials	2-4 gm/day po q12h 2-12 gm/day IV or IM q4-6h

(continued)

Agent	Trade Names	Dosage Form	Usual Adult Regimen: Daily Dose, Route & Dose Interval
Oxamniquine	Vansil	250 mg caps	12-15 mg/kg x 1 15 mg/kg q12h x 4
Paromomycin	Humatin	250 mg caps	2-4 gm/day po q6-12h
Penicillin G and V Crystalline G potassium	Pentids	(1 unit = 0.6 mcg) 0.2;0.25;0.4;0.8 million unit tabs 0.4 million units/5ml	1-2 gm po/day q6h
	Penicillin G for injection Pfizerpen	1;2;3;5;10;20 million unit vials	2-20 million units/day IV q4-6h
Crystalline G sodium	Penicillin G sodium for injection	5 million unit vial	2-20 million units IV/day q4-6h
Benzathine	Bicillin Bicillin L-A Permapen	200,000 unit tabs 3 million unit vial; 600,000 units/ml vial (1,2,4,10 ml vials)	Not recommended po 1.2-2.4 mil units IM
Benzathine+ procaine	Bicillin C-R	Benzathine: procaine/ml 150,000:150,000 units (10 ml) 300,000:150,000 (1,2,4 ml) 450,000:150,000 units (2 ml)	1.2-2.4 mil units IM
Procaine	Crysticillin Pfizerpen Wycillin	300,000 units (10 ml) 500,000 units (12 ml) 600,000 units (1,2,4 ml syringe)	0.6-4.8 mil units/day IM q6-12h
Phenoxyethyl penicillin (V)	Beepen VK, Betapen VK, Pen-Vee K, V-Cillin K, Veetids, Ledercillin VK, Robicillin VK	125;250;500 mg tabs 125;250 ml/5 ml susp	1-2 gm/day po q6h
Pentamidine	Pentam 300 NebuPent	300 mg vial 300 mg aerosol	4 mg/kg/day IV qd 300 mg/day/mo (prophylaxis)
Piperacillin	Pipracil	2;3;4;40 gm vials	6-24 gm/day IV q4-6h
Piperazine		250 mg tabs 500 mg/5 ml	3.5-5 gm/day

(continued)

9

Agent	Trade Names	Dosage Form	Usual Adult Regimen: Daily Dose, Route & Dose Interval
Polymyxin B	Aerosporin	500,000 unit vials 1 mg = 1,000 units 200,000 units + 40 mg neomycin	1.5-2.5 mg/kg/day IM or IV q4-6h
Praziquantel	Biltricide	600 mg tabs	20-75 mg/kg/day po in 3 doses
Primaquine		15 mg (base) tabs	15 mg po qd
Pyrantel	Antiminth	50 mg/ml susp	11 mg/kg x 1
Pyrazinamide		500 mg tabs	15-30 mg/kg/day po in 6-8 doses
Pyrimethamine	Daraprim	25 mg tabs	25 mg po q wk or daily up to 200 mg/day
Pyrimethamine + sulfadoxine	Fansidar	Sulfa-500 mg plus pyrimeth-25 mg	1 tab/wk 3 tabs (1 dose)
Quinacrine	Atabrine	100 mg	300-800 mg po/day
Quinine	Legatrin Quine 200,300 Quin-260 etc	130;200;300;325 mg caps 260;325 mg tabs	325 mg bid 650 mg q8h po
Quinine dihydrochloride		IV available from CDC	600 mg IV q8h
Rifabutin	Mycobutin	150 mg caps	600 mg/day po
Rifampin	Rifadin Rifamate	150;300 mg caps 300 mg cap with 150 mg INH 600 mg vials	600 mg/day po (TB) 600-1200 mg/day po (other indications) 600 mg/day IV
Spectinomycin	Trobicin	2;4 gm vials	2 gm IM x 1
Streptomycin		1 & 5 gm vial	1-2 gm IM/day

Sulfonamides
  Trisulfa-
  pyrimidines
	Triple sulfa
	Neotrizine
	Terfonyl
		Sulfadiazine,
		Sulfamerazine
		& Sulfamethazine,
		167 mg (each) tabs and
		167 mg (each) 5 ml susp
			2-4 gm/day po q4-8h

Sulfadiazine	Microsulfon	0.5 gm tabs	2-4 gm/day po q4-8h

(continued)

Agent	Trade Names	Dosage Form	Usual Adult Regimen: Daily Dose, Route & Dose Interval
Sulfamethox-azole	Gantanol	0.5; 1 gm tabs	2-4 gm/day po q8-12h
Sulfapyridine		0.5 gm tabs	1-4 gm/day po q6h
Sulfasalazine	Azulfidine	0.5 gm tabs 0.25 mg/5 ml susp	3-4 gm/day po q6h
Sulfisoxazole	Gantrisin	0.5 gm tabs	4-8 gm/day po q4-6h
Teicoplanin	Targocid	400 mg vials	6-12 mg/kg/day IV q24h
Tetracyclines Demeclocycline	Declomycin	150 mg cap 150;300 mg tab	600 mg/day po q6-12h
Doxycycline	Vibramycin	50;100 mg tabs 50;100 mg caps 50 mg/5 ml susp 100 mg vials	100-200 mg/day po q12-24h 200 mg/day IV q12-24h
Minocycline	Minocin	50;100 mg caps 50;100 mg tabs 100 mg vials	200 mg/day po or IV q12h
Oxytetracycline	Terramycin Uri-Tet	250 mg cap 50;125 mg/ml with lidocaine (IM)	1-2 gm/day po q6h 0.5-1 gm/day IM q12h
Tetracycline	Achromycin; Tetralan Brodspec; Panmycin Robitet; Sumycin, etc.	100;250;500 mg caps 250;500 mg tabs 125 mg/5 ml susp	1-2 gm/day po q6h
Thiabendazole	Mintezol	500 mg tabs 500 mg/5 ml susp	1-3 gm po/day
Ticarcillin	Ticar	1;3;6;20;30 gm vials	4-24 gm/day IV q4-6h
Ticarcillin + clavulanic acid	Timentin	3 gm ticarcillin + 100 mg CA vials	4-24 gm/day (ticarcillin) IV q4-6h
Tobramycin	Nebcin	20;60;80 & 1200 mg vials	3-5 mg/kg/day IV or IM q8h
Trimethoprim	Proloprim; Trimpex	100;200 mg tabs	200 mg/day po q12-24h

(continued)

11

Agent	Trade Names	Dosage Form	Usual Adult Regimen: Daily Dose, Route & Dose Interval
Trimethoprim-sulfamethoxa-zole	Bactrim, Septra Cotrim	Trimethoprim:sulfa 40 mg:200 mg/5 ml susp 80 mg:400 mg tabs 160 mg:800 mg DS tabs 16 mg:80 mg/ml (IV) (5,10,20 ml vials)	2-20 mg/kg/day (trimethoprim) po or IV q6-8h
Vancomycin	Vancocin pulvules Vancocin HCl (oral solu) Vancocin HCl IV Lyphocin	125;250 mg caps 1;10 gm vials 0.5;1 gm vials (IV)	0.5-2 gm/day po q6h 1-2 gm/day IV q6-12h
Vidarabine	Vira-A, Ara-A	200 mg/ml	15 mg/kg/day IV
Zidovudine	Retrovir, AZT	100 mg caps; 50 mg/ 5 ml syrup 240 ml Infusion - 10 mg/ml (20 ml)	500-600 mg/day po q4-8h 1-2 mg/kg IV q4h

COST OF ANTIMICROBIAL AGENTS

Acyclovir	200 mg cap	$ 0.82	Chloroquine	500 mg tab	$ 2.40
	800 mg cap**	$ 3.32	Plaquenil	200 mg tab	$ 0.95
	500 mg vial**	$ 44.02	Ciprofloxacin	750 mg tab	$ 4.97
Amantadine	100 mg tab	$ 0.72		400 mg vial**	$ 28.80
Amikacin	1 gm vial**	$119.42	Clarithromycin	250 mg tab	$ 2.50
Amoxicillin	250 mg cap	$ 0.82		500 mg tab	$ 2.50
Amoxil	250 mg cap	$ 0.21	Clindamycin	300 mg vial**	$ 7.04
Amoxicillin +			Cleocin	300 mg cap	$ 2.14
clavulanate	250 mg cap	$ 1.70	Clofazimine	100 mg cap	$ 0.20
Amphotericin B	50 mg vial**	$ 38.60	Clotrimazole	10 mg tab	$ 0.68
Ampicillin	250 mg cap	$ 0.07	Cloxacillin	500 mg tab	$ 0.38
Omnipen	250 mg cap	$ 0.62	Cycloserine	250 mg pulv	$ 3.14
Ampicillin	2 gm vial**	$ 12.64	Dapsone	100 mg tab	$ 0.18
Ampicillin +			ddC	0.75 mg	$ 2.13
sulbactam	1.5 gm vial**	$ 5.80	ddI	100 mg	$ 1.43
Atovaquone	250 mg tab	$ 2.13	Dicloxacillin	500 mg cap	$ 0.11
Azithromycin	250 mg tab	$ 8.12	Vibramycin	100 mg tab	$ 3.15
Aztreonam	1 gm vial**	$ 14.54		100 mg vial**	$ 16.15
Azulfidine	500 mg tab	$ 0.18	Erythromycin	250 mg tab	$ 0.11
Bacitracin	50,000 unit vial	$ 8.51	E-mycin	250 mg tab	$ 0.24
Bicillin	2.4 mil units**	$ 20.97	Erythromycin	1 gm vial**	$ 21.50
Cefaclor	250 mg pulv	$ 1.83	Erythropoietin	3000 unit vial	$ 36.00
Cefadroxil	500 mg cap	$ 2.70	Ethambutol	400 mg tab	$ 1.18
Cefamandole	2 mg vial**	$ 18.80	Fluconazole	50 mg	$ 4.37
Cefazolin	500 mg cap	$ 3.00		100 mg tab	$ 6.87
Cefixime	200 mg tab	$ 2.56		200 mg vial**	$119.00
Cefmetazole	2 gm vial**	$ 14.33	Flucytosine	500 mg cap	$ 1.66
Cefonicid	1 gm vial**	$ 27.11	Foscarnet	6 gm vial**	$ 73.25
Cefoperazone	2 gm vial**	$ 31.69	Gamimmune	250 ml vial**	$714.00
Ceforanide	1 gm vial**	$ 12.54	Ganciclovir	0.5 gam vial**	$ 34.80
Cefotaxime	2 gm vial**	$ 21.00	G-CSF	300 mcg vial**	$135.00
Cefotetan	1 gm vial**	$ 10.84	GM-CSF	350 mcg vial**	$135.00
Cefoxitin	2 gm vial**	$ 17.71	Gentamicin	80 mg vial**	$ 1.04
Cefprozil	250 mg tab	$ 2.63	Garamycin	80 mg vial**	$ 3.44
Ceftazidime	1 gm vial**	$ 14.60	Griseofulvin	500 mg tab	$ 0.93
	2 gm vial**	$ 20.73	ultramicro	250 mg tab	$ 0.68
Ceftriaxone	250 mg vial**	$ 10.24	Imipenem	500 mg vial**	$ 23.59
	1 gm vial**	$ 30.46	Interferon alpha	3 MU vial**	$ 26.96
Cefuroxime	750 mg vial**	$ 7.10	Isoniazid	300 mg tab	$ 0.02
Cefuroxime axeil	250 mg tab	$ 2.79	Itraconazole	100 mg cap	$ 4.10
Cephalexin	500 mg tab	$ 0.28	Ketoconazole	200 mg tab	$ 2.32
Keflex	500 mg tab	$ 2.30	Leukovorin	5 mg tab	$ 2.71
Cephalothin			Lomefloxin	400 mg	$ 4.47
Keflin	2 gm vial**	$ 6.55	Methenamine	1 gm tab	$ 0.33
Cephapirin	1 gm vial**	$ 3.98	Metronidazole	500 mg tab	$ 0.07
Cephradine	500 mg cap	$ 1.62	Flagyl	500 mg tab	$ 2.09
	500 mg vial**	$ 4.13		500 mg vial**	$ 7.81
	500 mg vial**	$ 5.20	Flagyl	500 mg vial**	$ 15.53
Chloramphenicol	1 gm vial**	$ 5.20	Mezlocillin	3 gm vial**	$ 11.90
Chloromycetin	250 mg cap	$ 1.05			

(continued)

Miconazole	200 mg vial**	$ 38.05	Rifampin	300 mg cap	$ 1.97
vag supp	200 mg	$ 7.05	Streptomycin	1 gm vial**	$ 3.95
2% creme	30 mg	$ 18.00	Sulfamethoxazole	500 mg tab	$ 0.06
Minocycline	100 mg cap	$ 1.90	Gantanol	500 mg tab	$ 0.47
Nafcillin	250 mg tab	$ 0.87	Sulfisoxazole	500 mg tab	$ 0.03
	2 gm vial**	$ 16.00	Gantrisin	500 mg tab	$ 0.21
Nalidixic acid	500 mg tab	$ 0.97	Tetracycline	500 mg tab	$ 0.05
Netilmicin	100 mg vial**	$ 10.11	Acromycin	500 mg tab	$ 0.06
Nitrofurantoin	50 mg tab	$ 0.60	Ticarcillin	3 gm vial**	$ 9.30
Macrodantin	50 mg tab	$ 0.59	Ticarcillin +		
Norfloxacin	400 mg tab	$ 2.25	clavulanate	3 gm vial**	$ 12.85
Nystatin tab	100,000 units	$ 0.15	Tobramycin	80 mg vial**	$ 7.88
Mycostatin tab	100,000 units	$ 0.90	Trimethoprim	100 mg tab	$ 0.14
susp 100,000			Trimethoprim-	DS tab	$ 0.07
units/ml	60 ml	$ 6.00	sulfamethoxazole	160 mg vial**	$ 5.80
Ofloxacin	400 mg tab	$ 3.38	Bactrim	DS tab	$ 1.05
	200 mg tab	$ 2.70	Septra	DS tab	$ 0.99
Oxacillin	500 mg caps	$ 1.30	Vancomycin	1 gm vial**	$ 37.00
	2 gm vial**	$ 21.74		125 mg parv	$ 4.73
Penicillin G	1 million unit vial**	$ 1.30	Vivonex TEN	1 packet	$ 5.39
	20 million unit vial**	$ 10.11	Zidovudine (AZT)	100 mg	$ 1.44
	500 mg tab	$ 0.07			
Penicillin V	250 mg tab	$ 0.04			
Pen-Vee-K	500 mg tab	$ 0.12			
Pentamidine	300 mg vial**	$ 98.75			
Piperacillin	3 gm vial**	$ 16.75			
Podofilox	3.5 ml bottle	$ 48.00			
Praziquantel	600 mg tab	$ 9.48			
Pyrazinamide	500 mg tab	$ 1.01			
Pyrimethamine	25 mg tab	$ 0.33			
Pyrimethamine +					
sulfadoxine	25/500 mg tab	$ 3.04			
Quinacrine	100 mg tab	$ 0.32			
Quinine	325 mg pulv	$ 0.38			

---

*   Approximate wholesale prices; price to consumer will be higher. Prices are provided by generic name alphabetically; prices for both trade and generic name are provided for some products.

**   Indicates preparation for parenteral administration.

PREFERRED ANTIMICROBIAL AGENTS FOR SPECIFIC PATHOGENS
(Adapted in part from The Medical Letter on Drugs and Therapeutics 34:49, 1992)

Organism	Usual Disease	Preferred Agent	Alternatives
Achromobacter xylosoxidans	Meningitis, septicemia	Antipseudomonad penicillin (2) Imipenem	Cephalosporins - 3rd gen (5) Sulfa-trimethoprim Imipenem Ticarcillin + clavulanic acid
Acinetobacter calcoaceticus var antitratum (Herellea vaginicola); var lwoffi (Mima polymorpha)	Sepsis (esp line sepsis) Pneumonia	Imipenem Aminoglycoside (tobramycin or amikacin) + ceftazidime or antipseudomonad penicillin (2)	Fluoroquinolone (6) Cephalosporin - 3rd gen (5) Tetracycline (4) Antipseudomonad penicillin (2)
Actinobacillus actinomycetemcomitans	Actinomycosis	Penicillin	Clindamycin Tetracycline (4) Erythromycin Cephalosporins (5)
	Endocarditis	Penicillin + aminoglycoside (1)	Cephalosporin (5) + aminoglycoside (1)
Actinomyces israelii (also A. naeslundii, A. viscosus, A. odontolyticus and Arachnia propionica)	Actinomycosis	Penicillin G	Clindamycin Tetracycline (4) Erythromycin
Aeromonas hydrophila	Diarrhea	Fluoroquinolone (6) Sulfa-trimethoprim	Tetracycline (4)
	Bacteremia	Cephalosporin (3rd gen)	Sulfa-trimethoprim Aminoglycoside (1)

(continued)

15

Organism	Usual Disease	Preferred Agent	Alternatives
<u>Aeromonas hydrophila</u> (cont.)	Cellulitis/myositis/ osteomyelitis	Fluoroquinolone (6) Sulfa-trimethoprim	Aminoglycoside (1) Imipenem
<u>Afipia felix</u>	Cat scratch disease	Fluoroquinolone (6) (usually not treated)	Sulfa-trimethoprim Gentamicin Amoxicillin-clavulanate
<u>Bacillus anthracis</u>	Anthrax	Penicillin G Penicillin + streptomycin (meningitis or inhalation anthrax)	Erythromycin Tetracycline (4) Chloramphenicol
<u>Bacillus cereus</u>	Food poisoning Invasive disease	Not treated Clindamycin, erythromycin, vancomycin	
<u>Bacillus species</u>	Septicemia (comp host)	Vancomycin	Imipenem Aminoglycosides (1) Fluoroquinolones (6)
<u>Bacteroides bivius</u>	Female genital tract infections	Metronidazole Clindamycin Cefoxitin Cefotetan	Chloramphenicol Antipseudomonad penicillin (2) Imipenem Betalactam-betalactamase inhibitor (7)
"<u>B. fragilis</u> group"	Abscesses Bacteremia Intra-abdominal sepsis	Metronidazole Clindamycin Cefoxitin	Chloramphenicol Antipseudomonad penicillin (2) Imipenem Betalactam-betalactamase inhibitor (7) Cefmetazole
"<u>B. melaninogenicus</u> group"	Oral-dental & pulmonary infections Female genital tract infections	Metronidazole Clindamycin Cefoxitin	Chloramphenicol Betalactam-betalactamase inhibitor (7) Imipenem Cefotetan Cefmetazole

(continued)

Organism	Usual Disease	Preferred Agent	Alternatives
Bartonella bacilliformis	Bartonellosis	Chloramphenicol Penicillin	Tetracycline + streptomycin
Bordetella pertussis	Pertussis	Erythromycin	Sulfa-trimethoprim Ampicillin
Borrelia burgdorferi	Lyme disease	Tetracycline (4) (early disease) Ceftriaxone (late complications)	Penicillin G po or IV Amoxicillin Cefuroxime axetil Erythromycin/Azithromycin(?) Cefotaxime
Borrelia recurrentis	Relapsing fever	Tetracycline (4)	Penicillin G Erythromycin Chloramphenicol
Brucella	Brucellosis	Doxycycline + rifampin Doxycycline + gentamicin or streptomycin	Chloramphenicol ± streptomycin Sulfa-trimethoprim Rifampin + cephalosporin (3rd gen) (5) (CNS involvement)
Calymmatobacterium granulomatis	Granuloma inguinale	Tetracycline (4)	Sulfa-trimethoprim Erythromycin (pregnancy)
Campylobacter fetus	Septicemia, vascular infections, meningitis	Gentamicin Imipenem	Chloramphenicol Erythromycin Clindamycin Tetracycline (4)
Campylobacter jejuni	Diarrhea	Erythromycin Fluoroquinolone (6)	Tetracycline (4) Furazolidine Gentamicin
Capnocytophaga ochracea	Periodontal disease Bacteremia in neutropenic host Tonsillitis (?)	Clindamycin Erythromycin	Amoxicillin-clavulanic acid Imipenem Cefoxitin Cephalosporins (3rd gen) (5) Fluoroquinolone (6) Tetracycline (continued)

17

Organism	Usual Disease	Preferred Agent	Alternatives
Capnocytophaga canimorus (DF₂)	Dog and cat bites Bacteremia meningitis (asplenia)	Penicillin Clindamycin	Cephalosporins (3rd gen) (5) Imipenem Vancomycin Fluoroquinolones (6)
Cardiobacterium	Bacteremia Endocarditis	Penicillin + aminoglycoside	Cephalosporin (5) ± aminoglycoside (1)
Cat scratch disease, agent of	Cat scratch disease with lymphadenitis	Fluoroquinolone (6)	Gentamicin Amoxicillin-clavulanate Trimethoprim-sulfamethoxazole
<u>Chlamydia pneumoniae</u> (TWAR agent)	Pneumonia	Tetracycline (4) Erythromycin	Clarithromycin Azithromycin
<u>Chlamydia psittaci</u>	Psittacosis	Tetracycline (4)	Chloramphenicol
<u>Chlamydia trachomatis</u>	Urethritis Endocervicitis PID Epididymitis Urethral syndrome	Tetracycline (4) Azithromycin	Erythromycin Ofloxacin Sulfisoxazole
	Trachoma	Tetracycline (4) (topical + oral)	Sulfonamide (topical + oral)
	Lymphogranuloma venereum	Tetracycline (4)	Erythromycin
	Inclusion conjunctivitis	Erythromycin (topical or oral)	Sulfonamide
<u>Citrobacter diversus</u>	Urinary tract infections, pneumonia	Aminoglycoside (1) Cephalosporin (2nd & 3rd gen) (5) Sulfa-trimethoprim	Tetracycline (4) Fluoroquinolone (6) Imipenem Piperacillin

(continued)

18

Organism	Usual Disease	Preferred Agent	Alternatives
Citrobacter freundii	Urinary tract infection, wound infection, septicemia, pneumonia	Imipenem Fluoroquinolone (6) Sulfa-trimethoprim Aminoglycoside (1)	Tetracycline (4) Cephalosporin (3rd gen) (5)
Clostridium difficile	Antibiotic-associated colitis	Vancomycin (oral) Metronidazole (oral)	Bacitracin (oral) Cholestyramine Lactobacilli Vancomycin + rifampin
Clostridium sp.	Gas gangrene Sepsis Tetanus Botulism Crepitant cellulitis	Penicillin G Tetanus immune globulin or IGIV Trivalent equine antitoxin (CDC)*	Chloramphenicol Metronidazole Antipseudomonad penicillin (2) Clindamycin Imipenem
Corynebacterium diphtheriae	Diphtheria	Penicillin or erythromycin + antitoxin (CDC)*	
Corynebacterium JK strain	Septicemia	Vancomycin	Penicillin G + gentamicin Fluoroquinolone (6)
Corynebacterium minutissimum	Erythrasma	Erythromycin	
Corynebacterium ulcerans	Pharyngitis	Erythromycin	
Coxiella burnetii	Q fever	Tetracycline (4)	Chloramphenicol Ciprofloxacin (6) Rifampin (7)
Dysgonic fermenter type 2 (DF₂)	See Capnocytophaga canimoris		

(continued)

19

Organism	Usual Disease	Preferred Agent	Alternatives
Edwardsiella tarda	Gastroenteritis (usually not treated) Wound infection Bacteremia, liver abscesses	Ampicillin	Cephalosporin (5) Aminoglycoside (1) Chloramphenicol Tetracycline (4)
Ehrlichia canis	Ehrlichiosis	Tetracycline (4)	Chloramphenicol (7)
Eikenella corrodens	Oral infections, bite wounds	Ampicillin/amoxicillin Penicillin G	Tetracycline (4) Amoxicillin-clavulanic acid Cephalosporin (5) Imipenem
Enterobacter aerogenes, E. cloacae	Sepsis, pneumonia, wound infections	Aminoglycoside (1) Sulfa-trimethoprim Fluoroquinolone (6)	Aztreonam Imipenem Antipseudomonad penicillin (2) Cephalosporin-3rd gen (5)
	Urinary tract infection	Sulfa-trimethoprim Cephalosporin-3rd gen (5)	Antipseudomonad penicillin (2) Aminoglycoside Fluoroquinolone (6) Imipenem
Enterococcus (E. faecalis and E. faecium)	Urinary tract infections	Ampicillin/amoxicillin	Penicillin + aminoglycoside (1) Vancomycin Nitrofurantoin Fluoroquinolone (6)
	Wound infections, intra-abdominal sepsis	Ampicillin	Vancomycin Penicillin + aminoglycoside (1) Imipenem (E. faecalis)
	Endocarditis	Penicillin G/ampicillin + gentamicin, streptomycin or amikacin	Vancomycin + gentamicin or streptomycin

(continued)

20

Organism	Usual Disease	Preferred Agent	Alternatives
Enterococcus (Vancomycin-resistant)		Moderate resistance: high dose penicillin + vancomycin ± aminoglycoside(MIC ≤ 32 μg/ml) High resistance + deep infection: ciprofloxacin ± rifampin and gentamicin	Teicoplanin (many strains resistant)
Erwinia agglomerans	Urinary tract infections Bacteremia Pneumonia	Aminoglycosides (1)	Fluoroquinolone (6) Chloramphenicol Cephalosporins (5)
Erysipelothrix rhusiopathiae	Localized cutaneous	Penicillin	Erythromycin
	Endocarditis/ disseminated	Penicillin	Cephalosporins (5)
E. coli	Septicemia Intra-abdominal sepsis Wound infection	Cephalosporin (3rd gen) (5) Ampicillin (if sensitive)	Aminoglycoside (1) Sulfa-trimethoprim Imipenem Fluoroquinolone (6) Cephalosporin (1st or 2nd gen) (5) Aztreonam Antipseudomonad penicillin (2)
	Urinary tract infection	Ampicillin (if sensitive) Tetracycline (4) Sulfa-trimethoprim Aminoglycoside (1) Cephalosporin (5) Antipseudomonad penicillin (2)	Imipenem Aztreonam Fluoroquinolone (6) Sulfonamide
Flavobacterium meningosepticum	Sepsis	Vancomycin	Sulfa-trimethoprim Erythromycin Clindamycin Imipenem Fluoroquinolone (6)

(continued)

21

Organism	Usual Disease	Preferred Agent	Alternatives
Francisella tularensis	Tularemia	Streptomycin or gentamicin	Tetracycline (4) Chloramphenicol (7)
Fusobacterium	Oral/dental/pulmonary infection; liver abscess	Penicillin G Metronidazole	Cefoxitin/cefotetan Chloramphenicol Imipenem Clindamycin
Gardnerella vaginalis	Vaginitis	Metronidazole	Clindamycin (po or topical)
Haemophilus aphrophilus	Sepsis, endocarditis	Penicillin G + aminoglycoside (1)	Cephalosporin-3rd gen (5) + aminoglycoside (1)
H. ducreyi	Chancroid	Ceftriaxone Erythromycin	Sulfa-trimethoprim Amoxicillin + clavulanic acid Fluoroquinolone (6)
H. influenzae	Meningitis	Cefotaxime, ceftriaxone Chloramphenicol	
	Epiglottitis Pneumonia Arthritis Cellulitis	Cephalosporin - 3rd gen (5) Sulfa-trimethoprim Cefamandole/cefuroxime Ampicillin (if sensitive)	Chloramphenicol ± ampicillin Betalactam-betalactamase inhibitor (7)
	Otitis Sinusitis Bronchitis	Sulfa-trimethoprim Ampicillin/amoxicillin (if sens)	Erythromycin - sulfonamide Cephalosporin - 2nd or 3rd gen (5) Tetracycline (4) Betalactam-betalactamase inhibitor (7) Fluoroquinolone (6)
Hafnia alvei	Pneumonia, wound infection, urinary tract infection	Aminoglycosides (1)	Ciprofloxacin (6) Chloramphenicol Antipseudomonad penicillin (2)

(continued)

22

Organism	Usual Disease	Preferred Agent	Alternatives
Helicobacter pylori (Campylobacter pylori)	Gastritis Recurrent duodenal ulcer disease	Bismuth subcitrate plus metronidazole plus tetracycline	Bismuth plus metronidazole plus amoxicillin Omeprazole plus amoxicillin
Kingella sp.	Endocarditis Septic arthritis	Penicillin + aminoglycoside	Cephalosporin (5) + aminoglycoside (1)
Klebsiella pneumoniae, K. oxytoca	Septicemia Pneumonia Intra-abdominal sepsis	Cephalosporin (3rd gen) (5)	Aminoglycoside (1) Sulfa-trimethoprim Piperacillin/mezlocillin Imipenem Betalactam-betalactamase inhibitor (7) Aztreonam Fluoroquinolone (6)
Klebsiella sp.	Urinary tract infection	Sulfa-trimethoprim Cephalosporin (5) Tetracycline (4)	Aminoglycoside (1) Betalactam-betalactamase inhibitor (7) Fluoroquinolone (6) Piperacillin/mezlocillin Imipenem
Legionella sp.	Legionnaires' disease	Erythromycin ± rifampin	Sulfa-trimethoprim + rifampin Fluoroquinolone (6) + rifampin Clarithromycin (7) Azithromycin (7)
Leptospira	Leptospirosis	Penicillin G or ampicillin	Tetracycline (4)
Leptotrichia buccalis	Orodental infections "Vincent's infection"	Penicillin G	Tetracycline (4) Clindamycin Erythromycin Metronidazole

(continued)

23

Organism	Usual Disease	Preferred Agent	Alternatives
Listeria monocytogenes	Meningitis Septicemia	Ampicillin or penicillin ± gentamicin	Sulfa-trimethoprim
Moraxella	Ocular infections Bacteremia	Aminoglycoside (1) Penicillins	Cephalosporin - 3rd gen (5) Imipenem Fluoroquinolone (6) Antipseudomonad penicillin (2)
Moraxella catarrhalis (Branhamella catarrhalis)	Otitis, sinusitis, pneumonitis	Sulfa-trimethoprim	Amoxicillin-clavulanic acid Erythromycin Clarithromycin/azithromycin Tetracycline (4) Cephalosporin (5) Fluoroquinolone (6)
Morganella morganii	Bacteremia Urinary tract infection Pneumonia Wound infection	Aminoglycoside Fluoroquinolone (6) Imipenem Cephalosporin (3rd gen) (5)	Sulfa-trimethoprim Aztreonam Antipseudomonad penicillin (2) Betalactam-betalactamase inhibitor (7) Tetracycline (4)
Mycobacterium tuberculosis (See page 126)	Tuberculosis	INH + rifampin pyrazinamide, ± ethambutol	Streptomycin, Capreomycin or Kanamycin Ciprofloxacin or Ofloxacin Ethionamide PAS Cycloserine
M. kansasii (See page 133)	Pulmonary infection	INH + rifampin + ethambutol ± streptomycin	Ethionamide Cycloserine

(continued)

24

Organism	Usual Disease	Preferred Agent	Alternatives
M. avium-intracellulare (See page 133)	Pulmonary infection	INH + rifampin + ethambutol + streptomycin	Clofazimine (extrapul dis) Clarithromycin Ethionamide Amikacin Cycloserine Ciprofloxacin/Ofloxacin
	Disseminated infection (AIDS)	Clarithromycin + ethambutol or clofazimine ± ciprofloxacin (6) 3-5 of the following: rifampin, ethambutol, amikacin, kanamycin, clofazimine, clarithromycin, ciprofloxacin	Rifampin or rifabutin Ethionamide Cycloserine Pyrazinamide Imipenem Amikacin
M. chelonae (See page 134)	Skin and soft tissue	Amikacin and/or cefoxitin, clofazimine or clarithromycin, then sulfonamide, rifampin, doxycycline or erythromycin	Clofazimine Clarithromycin Cefoxitin Doxycycline Imipenem
M. fortuitum (See page 133)	Soft tissue and wound infections	Amikacin, ciprofloxacin + sulfonamide	Ciprofloxacin (6)
M. marinum (See page 133)	Soft tissue infections	Rifampin + ethambutol or Sulfa-trimethoprim or Minocycline (doxycycline)	
M. ulcerans	Pulmonary	INH, rifampin + ethambutol	
M. leprae	Leprosy	Sulfone sensitive strains: Dapsone + rifampin Sulfone resistant strains: Clofazimine ± rifampin	Ethionamide (Protionamide) Minocycline Ofloxacin

(continued)

25

Organism	Usual Disease	Preferred Agent	Alternatives
<u>Mycoplasma fermentans</u>	Genital tract infections	Doxycycline	
<u>Mycoplasma pneumoniae</u>	Pneumonia	Erythromycin Tetracycline (4)	Clarithromycin (?) Azithromycin (?) Fluoroquinolone (?)
<u>Neisseria gonorrhoeae</u>	Urethritis Salpingitis Cervicitis Arthritis-dermatitis	Ceftriaxone Cefixime Fluoroquinolone (6)	Spectinomycin Sulfa-trimethoprim Cefotaxime, Cefoxitin Ceftizoxime Cefuroxime axetil
<u>N. meningitidis</u>	Meningitis Bacteremia Pericarditis Pneumonia	Penicillin G	Ampicillin Chloramphenicol Sulfa-trimethoprim Cephalosporin-cefotaxime, ceftizoxime, ceftriaxone
	Prophylaxis	Rifampin Fluoroquinolone (6)	
<u>Nocardia asteroides</u>	Nocardiosis: pulmonary infection, abscesses - skin, lung, brain	Sulfonamide (usually sulfadiazine) Sulfa-trimethoprim (sulfa level maintained at 10-20 mg/dl)	Sulfisoxazole Imipenem ± amikacin Minocycline ± sulfa Amikacin ± sulfa Cycloserine
<u>Pasteurella multocida</u>	Animal bite wound	Penicillin G	Tetracycline (4) Ciprofloxacin (6) Amoxicillin-clavulanic acid
	Septicemia Septic arthritis/ osteomyelitis	Penicillin G	Cephalosporins (5) Betalactam-betalactamase inhibitor (7) Chloramphenicol

(continued)

Organism	Usual Disease	Preferred Agent	Alternatives
Peptostreptococcus	Oral/dental/pulmonary infection; intra-abdominal sepsis; gynecologic infection	Penicillin G Ampicillin/amoxicillin	Clindamycin Metronidazole Cephalosporin (5) Chloramphenicol Erythromycin Vancomycin Imipenem
Plesiomonas shigelloides	Diarrhea (usually not treated)	Sulfa-trimethoprim Tetracycline (4) Fluoroquinolone (6)	Chloramphenicol Aminoglycosides (1)
	Extra-intestinal infection	Cephalosporin-3rd gen (3) Aminoglycoside (1)	Aztreonam Sulfa-trimethoprim Imipenem Fluoroquinolone (6)
Propionibacterium acnes	Acne	Tetracycline (4)	Clindamycin (topical)
	Systemic infection	Penicillin	Clindamycin
Proteus mirabilis	Septicemia Urinary tract infection Intra-abdominal sepsis Wound infection	Ampicillin	Aminoglycosides (1) Cephalosporins (5) Sulfa-trimethoprim Antipseudomonad penicillin Aztreonam Imipenem Fluoroquinolone (6)
Proteus indole positive	Septicemia Urinary tract infection	Cephalosporin-3rd gen (5)	Aminoglycoside (1) Sulfa-trimethoprim Antipseudomonad penicillin (2) Aztreonam Imipenem Betalactam-betalactamase inhibitor (7) Fluoroquinolone (6)

(continued)

27

Organism	Usual Disease	Preferred Agent	Alternatives
Providencia rettgeri	Septicemia Urinary tract infection	Cephalosporin-3rd gen (5)	Aminoglycoside (1) Antipseudomonad penicillin (2) Imipenem Aztreonam Sulfa-trimethoprim Fluoroquinolone (6)
Providencia stuartii	Septicemia Urinary tract infection	Cephalosporin-3rd gen (5)	Aminoglycoside (1) Antipseudomonad penicillin (2) Sulfa-trimethoprim Imipenem Aztreonam Fluoroquinolone (6) Betalactam-betalactamase inhibitor (7)
Pseudomonas aeruginosa	Septicemia, pneumonia Intra-abdominal sepsis	Aminoglycoside (tobramycin) ± antipseudomonad penicillin (2)	Aminoglycoside (1) ± cefoperazone, imipenem or ceftazidime Aztreonam Ciprofloxacin (6)
	Urinary tract infections	Aminoglycoside (1) Antipseudomonad penicillin (2) Fluoroquinolone (6)	Imipenem Ceftazidime Cefoperazone Aztreonam
Ps. cepacia	Septicemia Pneumonia	Sulfa-trimethoprim	Betalactam-betalactamase inhibitor (7) Ceftazidime Fluoroquinolone (6)
Ps. mallei	Glanders	Streptomycin + tetracycline	Chloramphenicol + streptomycin
Ps. maltophilia (Xanthomonas maltophilia)	Septicemia	Sulfa-trimethoprim	Ticarcillin-clavulanic acid

Organism	Usual Disease	Preferred Agent	Alternatives
Ps. pseudomallei	Melioidosis	Ceftazidime ± sulfa-trimethoprim	Sulfa-trimethoprim Tetracycline (4) + chloramphenicol Imipenem Cefotaxime Amoxicillin + clavulanate
Ps. putida	Septicemia, pneumonia, urinary tract infections	Aminoglycosides (1) Fluoroquinolone (6)	
Rhodococcus equi	Pneumonia, pulmonary abscess, bacteremia	Vancomycin ± ciprofloxacin, imipenem or amikacin	Imipenem Erythromycin Ciprofloxacin (6) Amikacin
Rickettsia	Rocky Mountain spotted fever, Q fever, tick bite fever, murine typhus, scrub typhus, typhus, trench fever	Tetracycline (4)	Chloramphenicol Fluoroquinolone (6)
Rochalimaea henselae	(See Afipia felix)		
Rochalimaea quintana	Bacillary angiomatosis	Erythromycin	Aminoglucosides Aztreonam Sulfa-trimethoprim Tetracycline (4)
Salmonella typhi	Typhoid fever	Ceftriaxone	Chloramphenicol Sulfa-trimethoprim Ampicillin/amoxicillin Fluoroquinolones (6) Cefotaxime/cefoperazone/ceftriaxone

(continued)

29

Organism	Usual Disease	Preferred Agent	Alternatives
Salmonella sp. (other)	Enteric fever Mycotic aneurysm	Cefotaxime/cefoperazone/ ceftriaxone	Ampicillin/amoxicillin Sulfa-trimethoprim Chloramphenicol Fluoroquinolone (6)
Serratia marcescens	Septicemia Urinary tract infection Pneumonia	Cephalosporin-3rd gen (5)	Gentamicin or amikacin ± antipseudomonad penicillin or cephalosporin-3rd gen (5) Cephalosporins-3rd gen (5) Sulfa-trimethoprim Antipseudomonad penicillin (2) Imipenem Fluoroquinolone (6) Aztreonam
Shigella	Colitis	Sulfa-trimethoprim	Ampicillin Tetracycline (4) Ciprofloxacin/nalidixic acid (6)
Spirillum minus	Rat bite fever	Penicillin G	Tetracycline (4) Streptomycin
Staphylococcus aureus Methicillin-sensitive	Septicemia Pneumonia Wound infection	Penicillinase resistant penicillin (3) ± rifampin or gentamicin Cephalosporins-1st gen (5) Cefuroxime/cefamandole	Erythromycin/clindamycin Vancomycin Betalactam-betalactamase inhibitor (7) Imipenem Fluoroquinolone (6) Clindamycin
Methicillin-resistant		Vancomycin ± rifampin or gentamicin	Sulfa-trimethoprim Fluoroquinolones (6) Minocycline Teicoplanin (investigational)

(continued)

Organism	Usual Disease	Preferred Agent	Alternatives
Staph. saprophyticus	Urinary tract infections	Sulfa-trimethoprim Ampicillin/amoxicillin Fluoroquinolone (6)	Cephalosporins (5) Tetracycline (4)
Staph. epidermidis	Septicemia Infected prosthetic devices	Vancomycin	Sulfa-trimethoprim Penicillinase resistant penicillin (3) Cephalosporin (5) Fluoroquinolone (6) Imipenem
Streptococcus, Group A,B, C,G; bovis, milleri, pneumoniae, viridans, anaerobic	Pharyngitis Soft tissue infection Pneumonia Abscesses	Penicillin G or V	Cephalosporin (5) Clindamycin Vancomycin Erythromycin Clarithromycin
	Endocarditis	Penicillin G ± streptomycin or gentamicin	Cephalosporin (5) Vancomycin
	Meningitis	Penicillin G	Chloramphenicol Cephalosporin-3rd gen (5)
S. pneumoniae (resistant strains)		Vancomycin ± rifampin (for meningitis) Erythromycin	Chloramphenicol Sulfa-trimethoprim Tetracycline
Streptobacillus moniliformis	Rat bite fever Haverhill fever	Penicillin G	Tetracycline (4) Streptomycin
Treponema carateum	Pinta	Penicillin G	Tetracycline
Treponema pallidum	Syphilis	Penicillin G	Tetracycline (4) Erythromycin Ceftriaxone
Treponema pallidum ss endemicum	Bejel	Penicillin G	

(continued)

Organism	Usual Disease	Preferred Agent	Alternatives
Treponema pallidum ss pertenue	Yaws	Penicillin G	Tetracycline (4)
Ureaplasma urealyticum	Urethritis Endocervicitis PID (?)	Erythromycin	Tetracycline (4)
Vibrio cholerae	Cholera	Tetracycline (4)	Erythromycin Sulfa-trimethoprim Furazolidone Fluoroquinolone (6)
Vibrio vulnificus	Septicemia Wound infection	Tetracycline (4)	Cefotaxime
Xanthomonas maltophilia	Septicemia UTI Pneumonia	Sulfa-trimethoprim	Ceftazidine Fluoroquinolone (6)
Yersinia enterocolitica	Enterocolitis (usually not treated) Mesenteric adenitis (usually not treated)	Sulfa-trimethoprim	Cephalosporin-3rd gen (5) Ciprofloxacin (6) Tetracycline (4)
	Septicemia	Aminoglycoside (gentamicin)	Chloramphenicol Cephalosporins-3rd gen (5)
Yersinia pestis	Plague	Streptomycin	Chloramphenicol Tetracycline (4) Gentamicin
Yersinia pseudotuberculosis	Mesenteric adenitis (usually not treated) Septicemia	Aminoglycoside (1) Ampicillin	Sulfa-trimethoprim Tetracycline (4)

(continued)

* Available from CDC 404-639-3670

1. Aminoglycosides = Gentamicin, tobramycin, amikacin, netilmicin
2. Antipseudomonad penicillin = Ticarcillin, piperacillin, mezlocillin; carbenicillin and azlocillin are no longer available
3. Penicillinase resistant penicillins: Nafcillin, oxacillin, methicillin, cloxacillin, dicloxacillin
4. Tetracycline = Tetracycline, doxycycline, minocycline
5. Cephalosporins
   1st generation: Cefadroxil, cefprozil, cefazolin, cephalexin, cephalothin, cephapirin, cephradine
   2nd generation: Cefaclor, cefamandole, cefonicid, cefuranide, cefotetan, cefoxitin, cefuroxime, cefmetazole
   3rd generation: Cefotaxime, ceftizoxime, ceftazidime, cefoperazone, ceftriaxone, moxalactam, cefixime, cefpodoxime, ceftibutin,
   Carbacefems: Loracarbef, cefprozil
6. Fluoroquinolones: Norfloxacin, ciprofloxacin, ofloxacin and lomefloxacin. Systemic infections are usually treated with ciprofloxacin,
   exoxacin, lomefloxacin or ofloxacin; all may be used for urinary tract infections. With regard to spectrum: Ps. aeruginosa
   -- ciprofloxacin; S. pneumoniae -- ofloxacin; Mycobacteria -- ciprofloxacin or ofloxacin; C. trachomatis -- ofloxacin
7. Betalactam-betalactamase inhibitor: Amoxicillin + clavulanate, ticarcillin + clavulanate and ampicillin + subactam

ANTIMICROBIAL DOSING REGIMENS IN RENAL FAILURE

A. **General Principles**

1. The initial dose is not modified.
2. Adjustments in subsequent doses for renally excreted drugs may be accomplished by a) giving the usual maintenance dose at extended intervals, usually 3 half lives (extended interval method); b) giving reduced doses at the usual intervals (dose reduction method); or c) a combination of each.
3. Adjustments in dose are usually based on creatinine clearance that may be estimated as follows:

    a. Formula: Males: $$\frac{\text{weight (kg) x (140-age in yrs)}}{\text{72 x serum creatinine (mg/dl)}}$$

    Females: above value x 0.85

    b. Nomogram (Kampmann J et al. Acta Med Scand 196:617,1974).

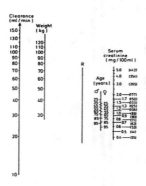

Use a straight edge to connect the patient's weight (2nd line on the left) and the patient's age (4th line). Mark intercept on R (3rd line) and swing straight edge to serum creatinine (5th line). Intercept on first line provides creatinine clearance

c. Pitfalls and notations with calculations

(1) Elderly patient: Serum creatinine may be deceptively low with danger of overdosing) due to reduced muscle mass.

(2) Pregnancy and volume expansion: GFR may be increased (with danger of underdosing) in third trimester of pregnancy and patients with normal renal function who receive massive parenteral fluids.

(3) Obese patients: Use lean body weight.

(4) Renal failure: Formulas assume stable renal function; for patients with anuria or oliguria assume CCr of 5-8 ml/min.

B. Aminoglycoside Dosing

1. Guidelines of Johns Hopkins Hospital Clinical Pharmacology Department

Agent	Loading dose (regardless of renal function)	Susequent doses (prior to level measurements) CCr>70 ml/mm	CCr<70 ml/mm	Therapeutic levels (1 hr after infusion over 20-30 min)
Gentamicin	2 mg/kg	1.7-2 mg/kg/8h	0.3 x CCr=mg/kg/8h	5-10 mcg/ml
Tobramycin	2 mg/kg	1.7-2 mg/kg/8h	0.3 x CCr=mg/kg/8h	5-10 mg/ml
Netilmicin	2.2 mg/kg	2-2.2 mg/kg/8h	0.3 x CCr=mg/kg/8h	5-10 mg/ml
Amikacin	8 mg/kg	7.5-8 mg/kg/8h	.12 x CCr=mg/kg/8h	20-40 mg/ml
Kanamycin	8 mg/kg	7.5-8 mg/kg/8h	.12 x CCr=mg/kg/8h	20-40 mg/ml

Note:
1. CCr = creatinine clearance.
2. Doses for gentamicin, tobramycin and netilmicin should be written in multiples of 5 mg; doses of amikacin and kanamycin should be written in multiples of 25 mg.
3. For obese patients use calculated lean body weight plus 40% of excess adipose tissue.
4. For patients who are oliguric or anuric use CCr of 5-8 ml/min.

Mayo Clinic guidelines (Van Scoy RE and Wilson WR, Mayo Clin Proc 62:1142, 1987)
a. Initial dose: Gentamicin, tobramycin, netilmicin: 1.5-2 mg/kg
Amikacin, kanamycin, streptomycin: 5.0-7.5 mg/kg
b. Maintenance dose: Usual daily dose x CCr/100

Reduced dose nomogram developed for tobramycin

Weight lbs	kg	Usual dose (q8h) 1 mg/kg	1.7 mg/kg
264	120	120	200
242	110	110	185
220	100	100	165
198	90	90	150
176	80	80	135
154	70	70	115
132	60	60	100
110	50	50	85
88	40	40	65

Source: Package insert of Tobramycin.

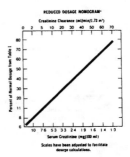

REDUCED DOSAGE NOMOGRAM*

Creatinine Clearance (ml/min/1.73 m²)

Percent of Normal Dosage from Table I

Serum Creatinine (mg/100 ml)

Scales have been adjusted to facilitate dosage calculations.

4. Guidelines for AMA Drug Evaluations, American Medical Assoc., Chicago, Vol. II 6:3, 1990 and Drug Information 92, American Hospital Formulary Service, pg 57, 1992

a. Loading dose based on estimated ideal body weight

Agent	Dose (mg/kg ideal wt)	Peak conc. (mcg/ml)
Tobramycin	1.5-2 mg/kg	4-10
Gentamicin	1.5-2 mg/kg	4-10
Netilmicin	1.3-3.25 mg/kg	4-12
Amikacin	5-7.5 mg/kg	15-30
Kanamycin	5-7.5 mg/kg	15-30

b. Maintenance dose as % of loading dose according to desired dosing interval and the corrected creatinine clearance CCr*

$$CCr\ (male) = \frac{(140 - age)}{serum\ creatinine}$$

$$CCr\ (female) = 0.85 \times CCr\ male$$

CCr (ml/min)	Half life (hrs)**	Dosing 8	Interval 12	(hr) 24
90	3.1	84%	-	-
80	3.4	80%	91%	-
70	3.9	76%	88%	-
60	4.5	71%	84%	-
50	5.3	65%	79%	-
40	6.5	57%	72%	92%
30	8.4	48%	63%	86%
25	9.9	43%	57%	81%
20	11.9	37%	50%	75%
17	13.6	33%	46%	70%
15	15.1	31%	42%	67%
12	17.9	27%	37%	61%
10***	20.4	24%	34%	56%
7	25.9	19%	28%	47%
5	31.5	16%	23%	41%
2	46.8	11%	16%	30%
0	69.3	8%	11%	21%

* From: Sarubbi FA Jr, Hull JH. Ann Intern Med, 89:612, 1978.
** Maintenance dose may be one half the loading dose at an interval approximately the estimated half life.
*** Serum concentrations should be measured to assist dose selection when the CCr is < 10 ml/min.

C. DRUG THERAPY DOSING GUIDELINES

(Adapted from Bennett WM, et al Ann Intern Med 93:62,1980, AMA Drug Evaluations, 1990, section 13, pp 1:1-8:35 and Drug Information 92, American Formulary Service, 1990, pp 33-481, 1992)

Drug	Major excretory route	Half life (hr) Normal	Half life (hr) Anuria	Usual regimen Oral	Usual regimen Parenteral	Maintenance regimen renal failure* GFR 50-80	10-50	<10
Acyclovir	Renal	2-2.5	20	200 mg 2-5x/day; 800 mg 5x/day; --	--; --; 5-12 mg/kg q8h	Usual; Usual; Usual	Usual; 800 mg q8h; 5-12 mg/kg q12-24h	200 mg q12h; 800 mg q12h; 2.5-6 mg/kg q24h
Amantidine	Renal	15-20	170	100 mg bid	--	100-150 mg q day	100-200 mg 2-3 x/wk	100-200 mg q wk
Amdinocillin	Renal	1	3.3	--	10 mg/kg q4-6h	Usual	10 mg/kg q6h	10 mg/kg q8h
Amikacin	Renal	2	30	--	7.5 mg/kg	↑ ↑ ↑ ↑	See pages 35, 36	↓ ↓ ↓ ↓ ↓
Amoxicillin	Renal	1	15-20	250-500 mg q8h	--	.25-.5 gm q12h	.25-.5 gm q12-24h	.25-.5 gm q12-24h
Amoxicillin-clavulanic acid	Renal	1	8-16	250-500 mg q8h	--	Usual	0.25-0.5 gm q12h	0.25-0.5 gm q20-36h
Amphotericin B	Nonrenal	15 days	15 days	--	0.3-1.4 mg/kg/day	Usual	Usual	Usual
Ampicillin	Renal	1	8-12	.25-0.5 gm q6h	1-3 gm q4-6h	Usual	Usual	Usual
					1-2 gm IV q6h	Usual	1-2 gm IV q8h	1-2 gm IV q12h

(continued)

37

Drug	Major excretory route	Half life (hr) Normal	Half life (hr) Anuria	Usual regimen Oral	Usual regimen Parenteral	Maintenance regimen renal failure* Glomerular filtration rate in mL/min 50-80	10-50	<10
Ampicillin-sulbactam	Renal	1	8-12	--	1-2 gm q6h	1-2 gm IV q8h	1-2 gm IV q8h	1-2 gm IV q12h
Atovaquone	Gut	69.6	69.6	750 mg tid w/food	--	Usual	Usual	Unknown
Azlocillin	Renal	1	5	--	2-4 gm q4-6h	Usual	1.5-2 gm q8h	1.5-3 gm q12h
Azithromycin	Hepatic	68	68	250 mg/d	--	Usual	No data -- "use caution"	Usual
Aztreonam	Renal	1.7-2	6-9	--	1-2 gm q6h	1-2 gm q8-12h	1-2 gm q12-18h	1-2 gm q24h
Bacampicillin	Renal	1	8-12	0.4-0.8 gm q12h	--	Usual	Usual	Usual
Capreomycin	Renal	4-6	50-100	1 gm q day-2x/wk	--	Usual	7.5 mg/kg q 1-2 days	7.5 mg/kg 2x/wk
Carbenicillin	Renal	1	13-16	.5-1 gm q6h --	5-6 gm IV q4h	Usual Usual	Usual 2-3 gm q6h	Avoid 2 gm q12h
Cefaclor	Renal	0.75	2.8	.25-0.5 gm q8h	--	Usual	Usual	Usual
Cefadroxil	Renal	1.4	20-25	.5-1 gm q12-24h	--	Usual	.5 gm q12-24h	.5 gm q36h
Cefamandole	Renal	0.5-2.1	10	--	0.5-2 gm q4-8h	.5-2 gm q6h	1-2 gm q8h	0.5-1 gm q12h
Cefazolin	Renal	1.8	18-36	--	0.5-2 gm	0.5-1.5 q8h	.5-1 gm q8-12h	0.25-0.75 gm q18-24h

(continued)

Drug	Major excretory route	Half life (hr)		Usual regimen		Maintenance regimen renal failure* Glomerular filtration rate in mL/min		
		Normal	Anuria	Oral	Parenteral	50-80	10-50	<10
Cefixime	Renal	3-4	12	200 mg q12h	--	Usual	300 mg/d	200 mg/d
Cefmetazole	Renal	1.2		--	2 gm q6-12h	1-2 gm q12h	1-2 gm q16-24h	1-2 gm q 48h
Cefonicid	Renal	4-5	50-60	--	.5-2 gm q24h	8-25 mg/kg q24h	4-15 mg/kg q24-48h	3-15 mg/kg q3-5d
Cefoperazone	Gut	1.9-2.5	2-2.5	--	1-2 gm q 6-12h	Usual	Usual	Usual
Ceforanide	Renal	3	20-40	--	0.5-1 gm q12h	Usual	0.5-1 gm q24h	0.5-1 gm q48-72h
Cefotaxime	Renal	1.1	3	--	1-2 gm q8-12h	Usual	1-2 gm q12-24h	1-2 gm q24h
Cefotetan	Renal	3-4	12-30	--	1-2 gm q12h	Usual	1-2 gm q24h	1-2 gm q48h
Cefoxitin	Renal	0.7	13-22	--	1-2 gm q6-8h	1-2 gm q8-12h	1-2 gm q12-24h	0.5-1 gm q12-48h
Cefprozil	Renal	1.3	5-6	0.25-0.5 gm q12h	--	Usual	0.25-0.5 gm q24h	0.25 gm q12-24h
Ceftazidime	Renal	0.9-1.7	15-25	--	1-2 gm q8-12h	Usual	1 gm q12-24h	0.5 gm q24-48h
Ceftizoxime	Renal	1.4-1.8	25-35	--	1-3 gm q6-8h	0.5-1.5 gm q8h	.25-1 gm q12h	.25 gm q12h

(continued)

(continued)

Drug	Major excretory route	Half life (hr) Normal	Half life (hr) Anuria	Usual regimen Oral	Usual regimen Parenteral	Maintenance regimen renal failure* Glomerular filtration rate in mL/min 50-80	10-50	<10
Ceftriaxone	Renal & gut	6-9	12-15	--	0.5-1 gm q12-24h	Usual	Usual	Usual
Cefuroxime	Renal	1.3-1.7	20	--	.75-1.5 gm q8h	Usual	0.75-1.5 gm q8-12h	0.75 gm q24h
Cefuroxime axetil	Renal	1.2	20	250 mg q12h	--	Usual	Usual	250 mg q24h
Cephalexin	Renal	0.9	5-30	0.25-1.0 gm q6h	--	Usual	0.25-1.0 gm q8-12h	0.25-1 gm q24-48h
Cephalothin	Renal	0.5-0.9	3-8	--	.5-2 gm q4-6h	Usual	1.0-1.5 gm q6h	.5 gm q8h
Cephapirin	Renal	0.6-0.9	2.4	--	0.5-2 gm q4-6h	0.5-2 gm q6h	0.5-2 gm q8h	0.5-2 gm q12h
Cephradine	Renal	.7-1	8-15	0.25-1.0 gm q6h / --	0.5-2 gm q4-6h	Usual	0.5 gm q6h / 0.5-1 gm q6-24h	0.25 gm q12h / 0.5-1 gm q24-72h
Chloramphenicol	Hepatic	2.5	3-7	.25-1.0 gm q6h	.25-1 gm q6h	Usual	Usual	Usual
Chloroquine	Renal & metabolized	48-120	?	300-600 mg po qd	--	Usual	Usual	150-300 mg po qd

40

Drug	Major excretory route	Half life (hr) Normal	Anuria	Usual regimen Oral	Parenteral	Maintenance regimen renal failure* Glomerular filtration rate in mL/min 50-80	10-50	<10
Cinoxacin	Renal	1.5	8.5	.25-.5 gm q12h	--	.25 gm q8h	.25 gm q12h	.25 gm q24h
Ciprofloxacin	Renal & hepatic metabolism	4	5-10	.25-.75 gm q12h	400 mg q12h	Usual / Usual	.25-.5 gm q12h / .4 gm q18h	.25-.5 gm q18h / .4 gm q24h
Clarithromycin	Hepatic metabolism & renal	4	slight†	250-500 mg q12h	--	Usual	Usual	250-500 mg q24h
Clindamycin	Hepatic	2-2.5	2-3.5	150-300 mg q6h	300-900 mg q6-8h	Usual	Usual	Usual
Clofazimine	Hepatic	8 days	8 days	50 mg qd 100 mg tid	--	Usual	Usual	Usual
Cloxacillin	Renal	0.5	0.8	0.5-1.0 gm q6h	--	Usual	Usual	Usual
Colistin	Renal	3-8	10-20	--	1.5 mg/kg q6-12h day	2.5-3.8 mg/kg q24-36h	1.5-2.5 mg/kg	.6 mg/kg q24h
Cyclacillin	Renal	0.6		0.5-1.0 gm q6h	--	Usual	Usual	0.5-1.0 q12h
Cycloserine	Renal	8-12	?	250-500 mg bid	--	Usual	250-500 mg qd	250 mg qd
Dapsone	Hepatic metabolism	30	slight†	50-100 mg/day	--	Usual	Usual	(No data)
Dicloxacillin	Renal	0.5-0.9	1-1.6	0.25-0.5 gm 96h	--	Usual	Usual	Usual

41

(continued)

Drug	Major excretory route	Half life (hr) Normal	Half life (hr) Anuria	Usual regimen Oral	Usual regimen Parenteral	Maintenance regimen renal failure* Glomerular filtration rate in mL/min 50-80	10-50	<10
Dideoxyinosine (ddI)	Renal & nonrenal	1.3-1.6	?	200 mg bid	--	Usual	Consider dose reduction; note Mg load -- 60 mEq/tab	0.75 mg po qd
Dideoxycytidine (ddC, zalcitabine)	Renal	2	8	0.75 mg tid	--	Usual	0.75 mg bid	0.75 mg bid
Doxycycline	Renal & gut	14-25	15-36	100 mg bid	100 mg bid	Usual	Usual	Usual
Enoxacin	Renal & hepatic metabolism	3-6		200-400 mg mg bid	--	Usual	½ usual dose	½ usual dose
Erythromycin	Hepatic	1.2-2.6	4-6	.25-.5 gm q6h	1 gm q6h	Usual	Usual	Usual
Ethambutol	Renal	3-4	8	15-25 mg/kg q24h	--	15 mg/kg q24h	15 mg/kg q24-36h	15 mg/kg q48h
Ethionamide	Metabolized	4	9	.5-1 gm/day 1-3 doses	--	Usual	Usual	5 mg/kg q24h
Fluconazole	Renal	20-50	100	100-200 mg/day	100-200 mg/day	Usual	50-100 mg/day	25-50 mg/day
Flucytosine	Renal	3-6	70	37 mg/kg q6h	--	Usual	37 mg/kg q12-24h	Not recommended
Foscarnet induction maintenance	Renal	3	†	--	60 mg/kg q8h; 90 mg/kg qd; 120 mg/kg qd	40-50 mg/kg q8h; 60-70 mg/kg qd; 80-90 mg/kg qd	20-30 mg/kg q8h; 50-70 mg/kg qd; 60-80 mg/kg qd	Contraindicated (CrCl<20/ml); Contraindicated (CrCl<20/ml); Contraindicated (CrCl<20/ml)

42

(continued)

(continued)

Drug	Major excretory route	Half life (hr) Normal	Half life (hr) Anuria	Usual regimen Oral	Usual regimen Parenteral	Maintenance regimen renal failure* Glomerular filtration rate in ml/min 50-80	10-50	<10
Ganciclovir - induction doses (maintenance - 1/2 dose)	Renal	1.5-3	10	--	5.0 mg/kg bid 50 mg/kg/d	2.5 mg/kg bid 2.5 mg/kg/d ↑	2.5 mg/kg qd 1.2 mg/kg/d	1.25 mg/kg qd ↓ ↓ ↓ ↓ 0.6 mg/kg/d
Gentamicin	Renal	2	48	--	1.7 mg/kg q8h	↑ ↑ ↑ ↑ ↑ See pages 35, 36	See pages 35, 36	See pages 35, 36 ↓ ↓ ↓ ↓
Griseofulvin microsize	Hepatic metabolism	24	24	.5-1 gm qd	--	Usual	Usual	Usual
ultramicrosize	(Same)	(Same)	(Same)	.33-.66 gm qd	--	Usual	Usual	Usual
Imipenem	Renal	.8-1	3.5	--	0.5-1 gm q6h	0.5 gm q6-8h	0.5 gm q8-12h	0.25-0.5 mg q12h
Isoniazid	Hepatic	0.5-4	2-10	300 mg q24h	300 mg q24h	Usual	Usual	Slow acetylators 1/2 dose
Itraconazole	Hepatic	20-60	20-60	100-200 mg/day	--	Usual	Usual	Usual
Kanamycin	Renal	2-3	27-30	--	7.5 mg/kg	↑ ↑ ↑ ↑ See pages 35, 36	See pages 35, 36	↓ ↓ ↓ ↓
Ketoconazole	Hepatic metabolism	1-4	1-4	200-400 mg q12-24h	--	Usual	Usual	Usual
Lomefloxacin	Renal	8	45	400 mg q24h	--	Usual	400 mg; then 200 mg qd	Usual
Loracarbef	Renal	1	32	200-400 mg q12h	--	Usual	200-400 mg q24h	200-400 mg q 3-5 days
Mefloquine	Hepatic	2-4 wks	2-4 wks	1250 mg x 1 250 mg q wk	--	Usual	Usual	Usual

43

Drug	Major excretory route	Half life (hr) Normal	Half life (hr) Anuria	Usual regimen Oral	Usual regimen Parenteral	Maintenance regimen renal failure* Glomerular filtration rate in mL/min 50-80	10-50	<10
Methenamine hippurate	Renal	3-6	?	1 gm q12h	--	Usual	Avoid	Avoid
mandelate	Renal	3-6	?	1 gm q12h	--	Usual	Avoid	Avoid
Methicillin	Renal (hepatic)	0.5	4	--	1-2 gm q4-6h	1-2 gm q6h	1-2 gm q8h	1-2 gm q12h
Metronidazole	Hepatic	6-14	8-15	.25-7.5 gm tid	.5 gm q6h	Usual	Usual	Usual
Mezlocillin	Renal	1	1.5	--	3-4 gm q4-6h	Usual	3 gm q8h	2 gm q8h
Miconazole	Hepatic	0.5-1	0.5-1	--	0.4-1.2 gm q8h	Usual	Usual	Usual
Minocycline	Hepatic & metabolized	11-26	17-30	100 mg q12h	100 mg q12h	Usual	Usual	Usual or slight decrease
Moxalactam	Renal	2	20	--	1-4 gm q8-12h	3 gm q8h	2-3 gm q12h	1 gm 12-24h
Nafcillin	Hepatic metabolism	0.5	1.2	0.5-1 gm 96h	0.5-2 gm q4-6h	Usual	Usual	Usual
Nalidixic acid	Renal & hepatic metabolism	1.5	21	1 gm q6h	--	Usual	Usual	Avoid
Netilmicin	Renal	2.5	35	--	2.0 mg/kg q8h	↑ ↑ ↑ ↑	See pages 35, 36	↓ ↓ ↓ ↓
Nitrofurantoin	Renal	0.3	1	50-100 mg q6-8h	--	Usual	Avoid	Avoid

(continued)

44

Drug	Major excretory route	Half life (hr) Normal	Anuria	Usual regimen Oral	Parenteral	Maintenance regimen renal failure* Glomerular filtration rate in mL/min 50-80	10-50	<10
Norfloxacin	Renal & hepatic metabolism	3.5	8	400 mg bid	--	Usual	400 mg qd	400 mg qd
Nystatin	Not absorbed	--	--	.4-1 mil units 3-5 x daily	--	Usual	Usual	Usual
Ofloxacin	Renal	6	40	200-400 mg bid	--	Usual	200-400 mg qd	100-200 mg qd
				--	200-400 mg q12h	Usual	200-400 mg q24h	100-200mg q24h
Oxacillin	Renal	0.5	1	0.5-1 gm	0.5-2 gm	Usual	Usual	Usual
Penicillin G crystalline	Renal	0.5	7-10	0.4-0.8 mil units q6h	1.4 mil units q4-6h	Usual	Usual	1/2 usual dose
procaine	Renal	24		--	0.6-1.2 mil units IM q12h	Usual	Usual	Usual
benzathine	Renal	days		--	0.6-1.2 mil units IM	Usual	Usual	Usual
V	Renal	0.5-1.0	7-10	0.4-0.8 mil units q6h	--	Usual	Usual	Usual
Pentamidine	Non-renal	6	6-8	--	4 mg/kg q24h	Usual	4 mg/kg q24-36h	4 mg/kg q48h
Piperacillin	Renal	1	3	--	3-4 gm	Usual q4-6h	3 gm q8h	3 gm q12h
Polymyxin B	Renal	6	48	--	.8-1.2 gm IV q12h	1-1.5 mg/kg qd	1-1.5 mg/kg q2-3d	1 mg/kg q5-7d

(continued)

Drug	Major excretory route	Half life (hr) Normal	Anuria	Usual regimen Oral	Parenteral	Maintenance regimen renal failure* Glomerular filtration rate in mL/min 50-80	10-50	<10
Praziquantel	Hepatic metabolism	0.8-1.5	?	10-25 mg/kg tid	--	Usual	Usual	Usual
Pyrazinamide	Metabolized	10-16	?	15-35 mg/kg daily	--	Usual	Usual	12-20 mg/kg/day
Pyrimethamine	Non-renal	1.5-5 days	?	25-75 mg/day	--	Usual	Usual	Usual
Quinine	Hepatic metabolism	4-5	4-5	650 mg tid	7.5-10 mg/kg q8h	Usual	Usual	Usual
Quinacrine	Renal	5 days		100-200 mg q6-8h	--	Usual	?	?
Rifampin	Hepatic	Early 2-5 Late 2	2-5	600 mg/kg/day	600 mg/day	Usual	Usual	Usual
Spectinomycin	Renal	1-3	?	--	2 gm IM/day	Usual	Usual	Usual
Streptomycin	Renal	2.5	100-110	--	500 mg q12h	7.5 mg/kg q24h	7.5 mg/kg q24-72h	7.5 mg/kg q72-96h
Sulfadiazine	Renal	8-17	22-34	0.5-1.5 gm q4-6h	--	Usual	0.5-1.5 gm q8-12h	0.5-1.5 gm q12-24h
				--	30-50 mg/kg q6-8h	Usual	30-50 mg/kg q12-18h	30-50 mg/kg q18-24h
Sulfisoxazole	Renal	3-7	6-12	1-2 gm q6h	--	Usual	1 gm q8-12h	1 gm q12-24h
Teicoplanin	Renal	6	41	--	6-12 mg/kg/d	Usual	1/2 usual dose	1/3 usual dose

(continued)

46

Drug	Major excretory route	Half life (hr) Normal	Half life (hr) Anuria	Usual regimen Oral	Usual regimen Parenteral	Maintenance regimen renal failure* Glomerular filtration rate in mL/min 50-80	10-50	<10
Tetracycline	Renal	8	50-100	.25-.5 gm q6h	.5-1 gm q12h	Usual	Use doxycycline	
Ticarcillin	Renal	1-1.5	16	--	3 gm q4h	Usual	2-3 gm q6-8h	2 gm q12h
Ticarcillin + clavulanic acid	Renal	1-1.5	16	--	3 gm q4h	Usual	2-3 gm q6-8h	2 gm q12h
Tobramycin	Renal	2.5	56	--	1.7 mg/kg q8h	↑ ↑ ↑ ↑	See pages 35, 36	↓ ↓ ↓ ↓
Trimethoprim	Renal	8-15	24	100 mg q12h q18-24h	--	Usual	100 mg	Avoid
Trimethoprim-sulfamethoxazole	Renal	T:8-15 S:7-12	T:24 S:22-50	2-4 tabs/d or 1-2 DS/day	--	Usual	Half dose	Avoid
Vancomycin	Renal	6-8	200-250	.125-.5 gm q6h	15 mg/kg q12h	Usual dose 1 gm q24h	Usual dose 1 gm q3-10d	0.125 mg po 1 gm q5-10d
Vidarabine	Renal	3.5	--	--	15 mg/kg/day	Usual	Usual	10 mg/kg/day
Zidovudine AZT	Hepatic metabolism to G-AZT → renal	1	3	100 mg q4h x 5/d	--	Usual	Usual	100 mg q8h

D. **ANTIMICROBIAL DOSING REGIMENS DURING DIALYSIS**
(Adapted from: Norris S, Nightengale CH and Mandell GL: In: Principles and Practice of Infectious Diseases, 3rd Ed., Churchill Livingstone, NY 1990, pp 440-457; American Hospital Formulary Service Drug Information 92, pp 33-481, 1992, and Berns JS et al, J Amer Soc Neph 1:1061, 1991.)

	Hemodialysis	Peritoneal dialysis
Acyclovir	2.5-5.0 mg/kg/day + dose post-dialysis	2.5 mg/kg/day
Amdinocillin	No extra dose	--
Amikacin	2.5-3.75 mg/kg post-dialysis	Loading dose predialysis 9-20 mg/L dialysate*
Amoxicillin	0.25 gm post-dialysis	Usual regimen
Amoxicillin + clavulanic acid	0.50 gm (amoxicillin) + .125 (CA) halfway through dialysis and another dose at end	Usual regimen
Amphotericin B	Usual regimen	Usual regimen
Ampicillin	Usual dose post-dialysis	Usual regimen
Ampicillin + sulbactam	2 gm ampicillin post-dialysis	Usual regimen
Atovaquone	Unknown	Unknown
Azithromycin	Usual regimen	Usual regimen
Aztreonam	One-eighth initial dose (60-250 mg) post-dialysis	Usual loading dose, then one-fourth usual dose at usual intervals
Carbenicillin	.75-2.0 gm post-dialysis	2 gm 6-12h
Cefaclor	Repeat dose post-dialysis	Usual regimen
Cefadroxil	0.5-1 gm post-dialysis	0.5 gm/day
Cefamandole	Repeat dose post-dialysis	0.5-1 gm q12h
Cefazolin	0.25-0.5 gm post-dialysis	0.5 gm q12h
Cefixime	300 mg/day	200 mg/day
Cefonicid	No extra dose	Usual regimen
Cefoperazone	Schedule dose post-dialysis	Usual regimen

(continued)

48

	Hemodialysis	Peritoneal dialysis
Cefotaxime	0.5-2 gm daily plus supplemental dose post-dialysis	1-2 gm/day
Cefotetan	One-fourth usual dose q24h on non-dialysis days and one-half dose on dialysis days	1 gm/day
Cefoxitin	1-2 gm post-dialysis	1 gm/day
Cefprozil	250-500 mg post-dialysis	0.25 gm q12-24h
Ceftazidime	1 gm loading 1 gm post-dialysis	0.5-1 gm loading then 0.5 gm/day or 250 mg in each 2 L dialysate
Ceftizoxime	Scheduled dose post-dialysis	1 gm/day
Ceftriaxone	No extra dose	Usual regimen
Cefuroxime	Repeat dose post-dialysis	15 mg/kg post-dialysis or 750 mg/day
Cephalexin	0.25-1 gm post-dialysis	250 mg po tid
Cephalothin	Supplemental dose post-dialysis	Option to add $\leq$ 6 mg/dL to dialysate
Cephapirin	7.5-15 mg/kg before dialysis and q12h after	1-2 gm q12h
Cephradine	250 mg pre-dialysis, then at 12 and 36-48 hr later	1 gm/day (IV) 250 mg bid (po)
Chloramphenicol	Schedule dose post-dialysis	Usual regimen
Ciprofloxacin	250-500 mg q24h post-dialysis	250-500 mg/day
Clindamycin	Usual regimen	Usual regimen
Cloxacillin	Usual regimen	Usual regimen

(continued)

	Hemodialysis	Peritoneal dialysis
Clofazamine	Usual regimen	Usual regimen
Dicloxacillin	Usual regimen	Usual regimen
Doxycycline	Usual regimen	Usual regimen
Erythromycin	Usual regimen	Usual regimen
Ethambutol	15 mg/kg/day post-dialysis	15 mg/kg/day
Fluconazole	Usual dose post-dialysis	½ usual dose
Flucytosine	20-37.5 mg/kg post-dialysis	0.5-1 gm/day
Ganciclovir	1.25 mg/kg q24h given post-dialysis on dialysis days	?
Gentamicin	1.0-1.7 mg/kg post-dialysis	Loading dose predialysis 2-4 mg/L dialysate*
Isoniazid	5 mg/kg post-dialysis	Daily dose post-dialysis or ½ usual dose
Imipenem	Supplemental dose post-dialysis and q12h thereafter	500 mg/day
Itraconazole	Usual regimen	Usual regimen
Kanamycin	4-5 mg/kg post-dialysis	3.75 mg/kg/day
Ketoconazole	Usual regimen	Usual regimen
Metronidazole	Usual regimen	Usual regimen
Mezlocillin	2-3 gm post-dialysis then 3-4 gm q12h	3 gm q12h
Minocycline	Usual dose	Usual dose
Moxalactam	1-2 gm post-dialysis	1-2 gm/day
Nafcillin	Usual regimen	Usual regimen
Netilmicin	2 mg/kg post-dialysis	Loading dose predialysis 3-5 mg/L dialysate*

(continued)

	Hemodialysis	Peritoneal dialysis
Ofloxacin	Usual regimen	200-400 mg/day
Oxacillin	Usual regimen	Usual regimen
Penicillin G	500,000 units post-dialysis	
Penicillin V	0.25 gm post-dialysis	
Pentamidine	Usual regimen	Usual regimen
Piperacillin	1 gm post-dialysis, then 2 gm q8h	3-6 gm/day
Pyrazinamide	Usual dose post-dialysis	(Avoid)
Rifampin	Usual regimen	Usual regimen
Streptomycin	0.5 gm post-dialysis	
Tetracycline	500 mg post-dialysis	(Use Doxycycline)
Ticarcillin	3 gm post-dialysis, then 2 gm q12h	2-3 gm q12h
Ticarcillin + clavulanic acid	3 gm (ticarcillin) post-dialysis, then 2 gm q12h	2-3 gm (ticarcillin) q12h
Tobramycin	1 mg/kg post-dialysis	Loading dose predialysis 2-4 mg/L dialysate*
Trimethoprim-sulfa	4-5 mg/kg (as trimethoprim) post-dialysis	0.16/0.8 q48h
Vancomycin	1 gm/wk	0.5-1 gm/wk
Vidarabine	Scheduled dose post-dialysis	
Zidovudine (AZT)	300 mg/day	300 mg/day

* Aminoglycosides given for prolonged periods to patients receiving continuous peritoneal dialysis have been associated with high rates of ototoxicity. Monitor level after loading dose and follow for symptoms of ototoxicity.

USE OF ANTIMICROBIAL AGENTS IN HEPATIC DISEASE

Many antimicrobial agents are metabolized by the liver and/or excreted via the biliary tract. Nevertheless, relatively few require dose modifications in hepatic disease; with few exceptions, doses are usually modified only if there is concurrent renal failure and/or the liver disease is either acute or is associated with severe hepatic failure as indicated by ascites or jaundice. The following recommendations are adopted from Drug Information 92, American Hospital Formulary Service, Amer Soc Hosp Pharmacists, Bethesda, MD, pp 33-481, 1992.

Agent: Recommended dose modification

Aztreonam: Some recommend a dose reduction of 20-25%.

Carbenicillin: Maximum of 2 gm/day for patients with severe renal and hepatic insufficiency.

Cefoperazone: Maximum dose is 4 gm/day; if higher monitor levels; with coexisting renal impairment maximum dose is 1-2 gm/day.

Ceftriaxone: Maximum daily dose of 2 gm with severe hepatic and renal impairment.

Chloramphenicol: Use with caution with renal and/or hepatic failure; monitor serum levels to achieve levels of 5-20 ug/mL.

Clindamycin: Dose reduction recommended only for severe hepatic failure.

Isoniazid: Use with caution and monitor hepatic function for mild-moderate hepatic disease; acute liver disease or history of INH-associated hepatic injury is contraindication to INH.

Metronidazole: Modify dose for severe hepatic failure although specific guidelines are not provided; peak serum levels with 500 mg doses are 10-20 ug/ml.

Mezlocillin: Reduce dose by 50% or double the dosing interval.

Nafcillin: Metabolized by liver and largely eliminated in bile; nevertheless, dose modifications are suggested only for combined hepatic and renal failure.

Penicillin G: Dose reduction for hepatic failure only when accompanied by renal failure.

Rifampin: Induces hepatic enzymes responsible for inactivating methadone, corticosteroids, oral antidiabetic agents, digitalis, quinidine, cyclosporine, oral anticoagulants, estrogens, oral contraceptives and chloramphenicol. Concurrent use of these drugs with rifampin and use of rifampin in patients with prior liver disease requires careful review.

Ticarcillin: For patients with hepatic dysfunction and creatinine clearance < 10 mL/min, give 2 gm IV/day in one or two doses.

Ticarcillin/Clavulanate K: For patients with hepatic dysfunction and creatinine clearance < 10 mL/min give usual loading dose (3.1 gm) followed by 2 gm once daily.

ADVERSE REACTIONS TO ANTIMICROBIAL AGENTS

A. ADVERSE REACTIONS BY CLASS

	Frequent	Occasional	Rare
Acyclovir	Irritation at infusion site	Rash; nausea and vomiting; diarrhea; renal toxicity (esp with rapid IV infusion, prior renal disease and nephrotoxic drugs); dizziness; abnormal liver function tests; itching; headache	CNS-agitation, encephalopathy; lethargy, disorientation, seizures; hallucinations; anemia; hypotension; neutropenia; thrombocytopenia
Amantadine	Insomnia, lethargy, dizziness, inability to concentrate (5-10% of healthy young adults receiving 200 mg/day)	GI intolerance especially nausea (5-10%); rash	CNS--lethargy, tremor, confusion, obtundation, delirium, psychosis, seizures (primarily IV admin.); heart failure; eczematoid dermatitis; photosensitivity; oculogyric episodes; orthostatic hypotension; peripheral edema; bone marrow suppression
Aminoglycosides Tobramycin Gentamicin Amikacin Netilmicin Kanamycin	Renal failure: related to dose duration and hydration status (monitor creatinine 3-7x/wk and output; monitor peak levels when dose is high, treatment long or toxicity noted)	Vestibular and auditory damage: related to dose and duration (most common with prior high frequency loss, tinnitis, vertigo, renal failure and other ototoxic drugs -- note dizziness, vertigo, roaring, tinnitis, hearing loss)	Fever; rash; blurred vision; neuromuscular blockage esp with myesthenia; or Parkinson's; eosinophilia Allergic reactions -- usually due to sulfites in some preparations
Aminosalicylic acid (PAS)	GI intolerance	Liver damage; allergic reactions; thyroid enlargement	Acidosis; vasculitis; hypoglycemia (diabetes); hypokalemia; encephalopathy; decreased prothrombin activity; myalgias; renal damage; gastric hemorrhage
Amoxicillin + clavulanic acid	(Similar to amoxicillin - See penicillins)		

(continued)

53

	Frequent	Occasional	Rare
Amphotericin B	Fever (maximal at 1 hr) and chills (at 2 hrs) (Prevent/ reduce with hydrocortisone, ibuprophen, ASA, aceto-minophen, meperidine); renal damage -- dose dependent and reversible in absence of prior renal damage and dose <3 gm; reduce with hydration and sodium supplementation; hypokalemia; anemia, phlebitis and pain at injection site	Hypomagnesemia; nausea, vomiting, metallic taste; headache	Hypotension; rash; pruritus; blurred vision; peripheral neuropathy; convulsions; hemorrhagic gastroenteritis; arrhythmias; diabetes insipidus; hearing loss; pulmonary edema; anaphylaxis; acute hepatic failure; eosinophilia; leukopenia; thrombocytopenia
Ampicillin + subactam	(Similar to those for ampicillin alone - See penicillins)		
Atovaquone		Rash (usually macro-papular and rarely treatment-limiting; nausea, vomiting, mild diarrhea; headache	Fever, elevated aminotransferases (generally mild), abdominal pain
Aztreonam	Eosinophilia	Phlebitis at infusion site; rash; diarrhea; nausea; eosinophilia; abnormal liver function tests	Thrombocytopenia; colitis; hypotension; unusual taste; seizures; chills
Bacitracin			Rash; blood dyscrasias
Capreomycin	Nephrotoxicity (proteinuria, oliguria, azotemia); pain with IM use	Ototoxicity (vestibular > auditory should: assess vestibular and auditory function before and during treatment); electrolyte abnormalities; pain, induration and sterile abscesses at injection sites	Allergic reactions; leukopenia; leuko-cytosis; neuromuscular blockage (large IV doses - reversed with neostigmine); hypersensitivity reactions; hepatitis?

54

(continued)

	Frequent	Occasional	Rare
Cephalosporins	Phlebitis at infusion sites; diarrhea (esp cefoperazone); pain at IM injection sites (less with cefazolin)	Allergic reactions (anaphylaxis rare); diarrhea and colitis; hypoprothrombinemia (cefamandole, cefoperazone, moxalactam, cefmetazole and cefotetan); platelet dysfunction (moxalactam); eosinophilia; positive Coombs' test	Hemolytic anemia; interstitial nephritis (cephalothin); hepatic dysfunction); convulsions (high dose with renal failure); neutropenia; thrombocytopenia; serum sickness (esp cefaclor)
Chloramphenicol		GI intolerance (oral); marrow suppression (dose related)	Fatal aplastic anemia; fever; allergic reactions; peripheral neuropathy; optic neuritis
Chloroquine		Visual disturbances (related to dose and duration of treatment with dose used for rheumatoid arthritis); GI intolerance; pruritus	CNS-headache, confusion, dizziness, psychosis; peripheral neuropathy; cardiac toxicity; hemolysis (G-6-PD deficiency); marrow suppression; exacerbate psoriasis
Ciprofloxacin	(See quinolones)		
Clindamycin	Diarrhea (frequency of C. difficile toxin is 5% for all clindamycin recipients and 15-25% for those with antibiotic associated diarrhea)	Rash; colitis and PMC, usually due to C. difficile; GI intolerance (oral)	Blood dyscrasias; hepatic damage; neutropenia; neuromuscular blockage; eosinophilia; fever; metallic taste; phlebitis at IV infusion sites
Clofazimine	Ichthyosis; and dry skin; pink to brownish-black discoloration of skin, cornea, retina and urine (up to 75-100% with prolonged use, first noted in 1-4 wks, resolves 6-12 months after drug is stopped but traces may persist); GI intolerance	Persistent abdominal pain, diarrhea and weight loss (high dose over 3 months); dry, burning, irritated eyes; pruritis, rash	Bowel obstruction with docs >300 mg/day (may be fatal, cause is unknown); GI bleeding; splenic infarction; eosinophilic enteritis; vision loss

(continued)

55

	Frequent	Occasional	Rare
Colistimethate	(See Polymyxins)		
Cycloserine	CNS-anxiety, confusion, depression, somnolence, disorientation, headache, hallucinations, tremor, hyper-reflexia, increased CSF protein and pressure (dose related and reversible) (Contraindicated in active alcoholics; twitching and seizures prevented with large doses pyroxidine -- 100 mg tid)	Liver damage; malabsorption; peripheral neuropathy; folate deficiency; anemia	Coma; seizures (contraindicated in epileptics); hypersensitivity reactions; heart failure, arrhythmias
Dapsone	Hemolytic anemia (dose dependent)	Blood dyscrasias (methemoglobulinemia and sulfahemoglobinemia ± G6PD deficiency); nephrotic syndrome; allergic reactions; insomnia; irritability; headache (transient); GI intolerance	Hypoalbuminemia; epidermal necrolysis; optic atrophy; agranulocytosis; peripheral neuropathy; aplastic anemia; "Sulfone syndrome" -- fever, exfoliative dermatitis, jaundice, adenopathy, methemoglobinemia and anemia -- treat with steroids
Didecoxyinosine (ddI; didanosine)	Diarrhea (15-30%) Pancreatitis (5-9%, fatal in 6% of cases) Peripheral neuropathy (painful feet, 5-12%) All are dose related	Nausea; vomiting; rash; marrow suppression; hyperuricemia; hepatitis with transaminase levels >5x normal in up to 10%	Cardiomyopathy; hepatic failure
Didecoxycytidine (ddC; zalcitabine)	Peripheral neuropathy (17-31%, frequency is related to cumulative dose)	Aphthous oral and esophageal ulcers; pancreatitis (1%); flu-like complaints; hepatitis with transaminase levels > 5x normal in up to 10%	Thrombocytopenia; leukopenia
Diloxanide		Flatulence, diarrhea, nausea	Dizziness, diplopia, headache

(continued)

56

	Frequent	Occasional	Rare
Emetine	Arrhythmias; precordial pain; muscle weakness; phlebitis	Diarrhea; vomiting; neuropathy; heart failure	
Erythromycins	GI intolerance (oral-dose related); phlebitis (IV)	Diarrhea; stomatitis; cholestatic hepatitis (esp estolate-reversible); phlebitis (IV administration); generalized rash	Allergic reactions; colitis; hemolytic anemia; reversible ototoxicity (esp high dose and renal failure)
Ethambutol		Optic neuritis (decreased acuity, reduced color discrimination, constricted fields, scotomata – dose related and infrequent with with 15 mg/kg); GI intolerance; confusion; precipitation of acute gout	Hypersensitivity Peripheral neuropathy; thrombocytopenia; toxic epidermal necrolysis; lichenoid skin rash
Ethionamide	GI intolerance (CNS effect)	Allergic reactions; peripheral neuropathy (prevented with pyroxidine); reversible liver damage (9%) with jaundice (1-3%) – monitor transaminase q2-4 wks; gynecomastia; menstrual irregularity	Optic neuritis; gouty arthritis; hypothyroidism; impotence; hypothyroidism; purpura; poor diabetic control; rash
Fluconazole		Nausea; vomiting; bloating, abdominal pain; transaminase elevating to ≥ 8x normal (1%); headache; rash; diarrhea; prolonged protime with coumadin	Hepatitis; Stevens-Johnson syndrome; thrombocytopenia; anaphylaxis
Flucytosine	GI intolerance (including nausea, vomiting, diarrhea and ulcerative colitis)	Marrow suppression with leukopenia or thrombocytopenia (dose related, esp with renal failure, >100 mg/ml, or concurrent amphotericin); confusion; rash; hepatitis (dose related)	Hallucinations; eosinophilia; granulocytosis; fatal hepatitis

(continued)

	Frequent	Occasional	Rare
Foscarnet	Renal failure (usually reversible; 30% get creatinine > 2 mg/dl; discontinue if creatinine > 2.9 mg/dl	Mineral and electrolyte changes -- (calcium, magnesium, phosphorus, ionized calcium, potassium); seizures (10%), fever, GI intolerance, anemia	Marrow suppression, arrhythmias
Furazolidone	GI intolerance	Allergic reactions; pulmonary infiltrates; headache	Hemolytic anemia (G-6-PD deficiency); hypotension; polyneuropathy; hypoglycemia; agranulocytosis
Ganciclovir (DHPG) (Cytovene)	Neutropenia (ANC < 500/mm³ in 15-20%, usually early in treatment and responds within 3-7 days to drug holiday or to G-CSF/ GM-CSF; thrombocytopenia (platelet count < 20,000/mm³ in 10%, reversible)	Anemia; fever; rash; CNS-headache, seizures, confusion; changes in mental status; abnormal liver function tests (2-3%)	Psychosis; neuropathy; impaired reproductive function (?); hematuria; renal failure; nausea; vomiting; GI bleeding or perforation myocardiopathy; hypotension; ataxia; coma; somnolence
Griseofulvin	Headache (often resolves with continued treatment)	Photosensitivity	GI disturbances; allergic reactions; liver paresthesias; exacerbation of lupus; liver damage; lymphadenopathy; blood dyscrasias; thrush; transient hearing loss; fatigue; dizziness; insomnia; psychosis
Imipenem		Phlebitis at infusion sites; allergic reactions; nausea, vomiting and diarrhea; eosinophilia; hepatotoxicity (transient)	Seizures; myoclonus; colitis; bone marrow suppression; renal toxicity
Interferon alpha	Flu-like illness (80% with > 5 mil units/d; fever, fatigue, anorexia, headache, myalgias, depression, abdominal pain, diarrhea	Marrow suppression -- Leukopenia, anemia ± thromboctytopenia (3-70%, dose related, usually transient and well tolerated); Neuro-psychiatric effects -- psychosis,	Edema; arrhythmias; cardiomyopathy; renal failure; hearing loss

(continued)

58

	Frequent	Occasional	Rare
Interferon alpha (continued)	Starts within 6 hrs and lasts 2-12 hrs; pretreat with NSAIA	Confusion, somnolence, anxiety); hepatitis -- dose related and up to 40% receiving high doses; alopecia (8%); rash	CNS-optic neuritis; psychosis; convulsions; toxic encephalopathy; twitching; coma; blood dyscrasias; hyperglycemia; lupus-like syndrome; keratitis; pellagra-like rash
Isoniazid	Hepatitis - age related < 20 yrs-nil; 35-6%; 45-11%; 55-18%. Patient should be warned of symptoms and drug should be discontinued if transaminase levels are 3x normal limit	Allergic reactions; fever; peripheral neuropathy (reduce with pyridoxine), esp with alcoholism, diabetes, pregnancy, malnutrition	Hepatitis (1/1000)
Itraconazole		Headache; nausea (10%); vomiting; rash (8%)	
Ketoconazole	GI intolerance (dose related) Temporary increase in transaminase levels (2-5%)	Endocrine-decreased steroid and testosterone synthesis with impotence; gynecomastia, oligospermia, reduced libido; menstrual abnormalities (prolonged use and dose related, usually ≥ 600 mg/day); headache; dizziness; asthenia; pruritus; rash	Abrupt hepatitis (1:15,000), rare cases of fatal hepatic necrosis; anaphylaxis; lethargy; arthralgias; fever; marrow suppression; hypothyroidism (genetically determined)
Mefloquine	Vertigo; light-headedness; nausea; nightmares; headache; visual disturbances (dose related)	Psychosis and seizures (dose related -- rare at doses used for prophylaxis); GI intolerance; dizziness	Prolonged cardiac conduction
Methenamine	GI intolerance; metallic taste; headache	GI intolerance; dysuria (reduced dose or acidification)	Allergic reactions; edema; tinnitus; muscle cramps
Metronidazole		Peripheral neuropathy (prolonged use-reversible); phlebitis at injection sites; Antabuse-like reaction	Seizures; ataxic encephalitis; colitis; leukopenia; dysuria; pancreatitis; allergic reactions; mutagenic in Ames test

(continued)

59

	Frequent	Occasional	Rare
Miconazole		Phlebitis at injection sites; chills; pruritus; rash; dizziness; blurred vision; hyperlipidemia; nausea; vomiting; hyponatremia	Marrow suppression - anemia and thrombocytopenia; renal damage; anaphylaxis; psychosis; cardiac arrest
Nalidixic acid	(See Quinolones)		
Nitrofurantoin	GI intolerance	Hypersensitivity reactions; pulmonary infiltrates (acute, subacute or chronic; ± fever, eosinophilia, rash or lupus-like reaction)	Peripheral neuropathy; hepatitis; hemolytic anemia (G-6-PD deficiency); lactic acidosis; parotitis; pancreatitis
Nystatin		GI intolerance	Allergic reactions
Ofloxacin	(See Quinolones)		
Penicillins	Hypersensitivity reactions; rash (esp ampicillin and amoxicillin); diarrhea (esp ampicillin)	GI intolerance (oral agents); fever; Coombs' test positive; phlebitis at infusion sites and sterile abscesses at IM sites; Jarisch-Herxheimer reaction (syphilis or other spirochetal infections)	Anaphylaxis; leukopenia; thrombocytopenia; colitis (esp ampicillin); hepatic damage; renal damage; CNS-seizures, twitching (high doses in patients with renal failure); hyperkalemia (penicillin G infusion); abnormal platelet aggregation with bleeding diathesis (carbenicillin and ticarcillin)
Pentamidine	Nephrotoxicity - in 25%, usually reversible with discontinuation; Aerosol administration - cough (30%)	Hypotension (administer IV over 60 min); hypoglycemia (5-10%, usually occurs after day 5 of treatment including past treatment, may last days or weeks, treat with IV glucose), rash (including Stevens-Johnson syndrome; marrow suppression (common in AIDS patients); GI intolerance; Aerosol administration - asthma reaction (5%)	Hepatotoxicity; leukopenia; thrombocytopenia; pancreatitis; hyperglycemia, insulin-dependent diabetes

(continued)

60

	Frequent	Occasional	Rare
Polymyxins	Pain and phlebitis at injection sites; neurotoxicity (ataxia, paresthesias); nephrotoxicity		Allergic reactions; neuromuscular blockade
Primaquine		Hemolytic anemia (G-6-PD deficiency); GI intolerance	Headache; pruritus
Pyrazinamide	Non-gouty polyarthralgia; asymptomatic; hyperuricemia	Hepatitis (dose related, frequency not increased when given with INH or rifampin, rarely serious); GI intolerance; gout (treat with allopurinol and probenecid)	Rash; fever; porphyria; photosensitivity
Pyrimethamine		Folic acid deficiency with megaloblastic anemia and pancytopenia (dose related and reversed with leucovorin); allergic reactions	CNS-ataxia, tremors, seizures (dose related), fatigue
Quinine		GI intolerance; cinchonism (tinnitus, headache, visual disturbances); hemolytic anemia (G-6-PD deficiency)	Arrhythmias; hypotension with rapid IV infusion; hypoglycemia; hepatitis; thrombocytopenia
Quinolones	(Animal studies show arthropathies in weight bearing joints of immature animals; significance in humans is not known, but this class is considered contraindicated in children and pregnancy)	GI intolerance; CNS-headache; malaise; insomnia; dizziness; allergic reactions	Papilledema; nystagmus; visual disturbances; diarrhea; pseudomembranous colitis; abnormal liver function tests including hepatic necrosis; marrow suppression; photosensitivity anaphylaxis; seizures; toxic psychosis; CNS stimulation -- tremors, restlessness; confusion

(continued)

	Frequent	Occasional	Rare
Rifampin	Orange discoloration of urine, tears (contact lens), sweat (See drug interactions)	Hepatitis (frequency not increased when given with INH); jaundice (usually reversible with dose reduction and/or continued use); GI intolerance; hypersensitivity reactions; increases hepatic metabolism of steroids to increase steroid requirement in adrenal insufficiency and require alternative to birth control meds (See drug interactions); flu-like syndrome with intermittent use characterized by dyspnea, wheezing	Thrombocytopenia; leukopenia; hemolytic anemia, eosinophilia; renal damage; proximal myopathy; hyperuricemia; anaphylaxis
Spectinomycin		Pain at injection site; urticaria; fever; insomnia; dizziness; nausea; headache	Anaphylaxis; fever; anemia; renal failure and abnormal liver function tests (multiple doses)
Sulfonamides	Allergic reactions - rash, pruritis (appears to be dose related), fever (usually 7-10 days of initial dose). Cross reactions noted between sulfonamides including thiazide diuretics and antidiabetic agents	Periarteritis nodosum, lupus, Stevens-Johnson syndrome, serum sickness; crystalluria with renal damage, urolithiasis and oliguria (prevent with increasing urine pH hydration and use of sulfonamide -- sulfonamide combinations); GI intolerance; photosensitivity	Myocarditis; psychosis; neuropathy; dizziness, depression; hemolytic anemia (G-6-PD deficiency); marrow suppression; agranulocytosis
Tetracyclines	GI intolerance (dose related); stains and deforms teeth in children up to 8 yrs; vertigo (minocycline); negative nitrogen balance and increased azotemia with renal failure (except doxycycline); vaginitis	Hepatotoxicity (dose related, esp pregnant women); esophageal ulcerations; diarrhea; candidiasis (thrush and vaginitis); photosensitivity (esp demeclocycline); phlebitis with IV treatment and pain with IM injection	Malabsorptions; allergic reactions; visual disturbances; aggravation of myasthenia; hemolytic anemia; colitis

(continued)

	Frequent	Occasional	Rare
Ticarcillin + clavulanic acid	Similar to those for ticarcillin alone (See Penicillins)		
Trimethoprim	GI intolerance (dose related); rash (up to 24% receiving ≥ 400 mg/d x 14 days)	Marrow suppression -- megaloblastic anemia, neutropenia, thrombo-cytopenia (hematologic toxicity increased with folate depletion and high doses -- treat with leucovorin, 3-15 mg/day x 3 days)	Pancytopenia; erythema multiforme, Stevens-Johnson syndrome, TEN
Trimethoprim-sulfamethoxazole	Fever, leukopenia, rash (AIDS patients); reactions noted above for sulfonamides and trimethoprim		
Vancomycin	Phlebitis at injection sites	"Red-man syndrome" (flushing over chest and face) or hypotension (infusion too rapid); rash; fever; neutro-penia; eosinophilia; allergic reactions with rash	Anaphylaxis; ototoxicity and nephrotoxicity (dose related); peripheral neuropathy; marrow suppression
Vidarabine	GI intolerance; phlebitis at infusion site; fluid overload		Blood dyscrasias; CNS-confusion and neurologic deterioration (esp with renal failure)
Zidovudine (AZT, Retrovir)	Marrow suppression: anemia and/or leukopenia (dose and stage related: marrow toxicity with Hgb < 7.5 g/dL or ANC < 750/ml is 3%/yr for asymptomatic patients and 40% for AIDS patients)	Subjective complaints: headaches (50%); malaise; insomnia; myalgias; nausea (often resolves with dose reduction and/or continued use); myopathy with myalgias or weakness plus elevated CPK -- responds to drug withdrawal within 2 wks	Seizures (reversible); allergy (rash, anaphylaxis); twitching; mania; hepatitis; esophageal ulceration

B.   **Penicillin Allergy**

1.   Classification of penicillin hypersensitivity reactions

Type	Mechanism	Clinical expression
I	IgE	Urticaria, angioedema, anaphylaxis, laryngeal edema, asthma frequency - 0.02%, mortality - 10%
II	Cytotoxic Ab of IgG class	Hemolytic anemia
III	Immune complexes IgG & IgM Ab	Serum sickness
IV	Cell-mediated	Contact dermititis
Idiopathic	Unknown	Maculopapular rash (common), interstitial nephritis, drug fever, eosinophilia, exfoliative dermititis, Stevens- Johnson syndrome

2.   Cross reactions among betalactam agents
      Allergy to one penicillin indicates allergy to all.
      Allergy to penicillins may indicate allergy to cephalosporins and imipenem;
       it is generally considered safe to give cephalosporins to patients with
       non-IgE- medicated reactions to penicillins such as maculopapular rashes.
      There is no apparent cross reaction with aztreonam.

3.   Skin testing: This is considered a safe, rapid and effective method to
      exclude an IgE mediated response with ≥ 98% assurance (MMWR 38:S13,1989)

      a.   Patients with a history of severe reactions during the past year
            should be tested in the hospital setting with antigens diluted 100-
            fold; others may be tested in a physician staffed clinic.

      b.   Patients with a history of penicillin allergy and a negative skin
            test should receive penicillin, 250 mg po and be observed for one
            hour prior to treatment with therapeutic doses. Those with a positive
            skin test should be desensitized.

      c.   Penicillin allergy skin testing (adapted from Beall*)
            Note: If there has been a severe, generalized reaction to penicillin
            in the previous year, the antigens should be diluted 100-fold, and
            patients should be tested in a controlled environment. Both major and
            minor determinants should be available for the tests to be interpre-
            table. The patient should not have taken antihistamines in the previous
            48 hours.

Reagents

Major determinants:
   Benzylpenicilloyl-polylysine (major, Pre-Pen [Taylor Pharmacal
      Co., Decatur, Illinois], 6×10^{-5}M)
   Benzylpenicillin (10^{-2} or 6000 U/mL)
Minor determinants:
   Benzylpenicilloic acid (10^{-2}M)
   Benzylpenilloic acid (10^{-2}M)
Positive control (histamine, 1 mg/mL)
Negative control (buffered saline solution)

   Dilute the antigens 100-fold for preliminary testing if there
has been an immediate generalized reaction within the past year.

Procedure

   Epicutaneous (scratch or prick) test: apply one drop of material to
volar forearm and pierce epidermis without drawing blood; observe for
20 minutes. If there is no wheal $\geq$ 4mm, proceed to intradermal test.

   Intradermal test: Inject 0.02 ml intradermally with a 27- gauge
short-bevelled needle; observe for 20 minutes.

   Interpretation: For the test to be interpretable, the negative (saline)
control must elicit no reaction and the positive (histamine) control must
elicit a positive reaction.

   Positive test: A wheal > 4mm in mean diameter to any penicillin
reagent; erythema must be present.

   Negative test: The wheals at the site of the penicillin reagents
are equivalent to the negative control.

   Indeterminate: All other results

---

*Reprinted with permission from Beall GN, Penicillins, pp 205-9.
In: Saxon A, moderator. Immediate hypersensitivity reactions to
beta-lactam antibiotics. Ann Intern Med 1987;107:204-15.

4.   Penicillin desensitization (Adapted from the Medical Letter on Drugs and
     Therapeutics 30:77,1988 and MMWR 38:S13,1989).

   a.   Penicillin densensitization should be done in a hospital because IgE
        mediated reactions can occur, although they are rare. Desensitization
        may be done orally or intravenously, although oral administration is
        often considered safer, simpler and easier.

   b.   Parenteral desensitization: Give 1 unit penicillin IV and then double
        the dose at 15 minute intervals or increase the dose 10-fold at 20-30
        minute intervals.

c.   Oral-desensitization protocol (from Wendel)

Dose*	Penicillin V Suspension (units/ml)	Amount[T] ml	Amount[T] units	Cumulative dose (units)
1	1,000	0.1	100	100
2	1,000	0.2	200	300
3	1,000	0.4	400	700
4	1,000	0.8	800	1,500
5	1,000	1.6	1,600	3,100
6	1,000	3.2	3,200	6,300
7	1,000	6.4	6,400	12,700
8	10,000	1.2	12,000	24,700
9	10,000	2.4	24,000	48,700
10	10,000	4.8	48,000	96,700
11	80,000	1.0	80,000	176,700
12	80,000	2.0	160,000	336,700
13	80,000	4.0	320,000	656,700
14	80,000	8.0	640,000	1,296,700

Observation period: 30 minutes before parenteral administration of penicillin.
*Interval between doses, 15 minutes; elapsed time, 3 hours and 45 minutes; cumulative dose, 1.3 million units
[T]The specific amount of drug was diluted in approximately 30 ml of water and then given orally.

Adapted with permission from the New England Journal of Medicine 312:1229-32, 1985.

5.   Management of allergic reactions
    Epinephrine: IgE mediated reactions
    Antihistamines: Accelerated and late urticaria, maculopapular rashes
    Glucocorticoids: Severe urticaria, prolonged systemic anaphylaxis, serum
        sickness, contact dermatitis, exfoliative and bullous skin reactions,
        interstitial nephritis, pulmonary and hepatic reactions

6.   Anaphylactic shock

	Epinephrine dose
Initial treatment	
Subcutaneous (preferred) or intramuscular	0.3-0.5 ml (1:1000)
Repeat every 20-30 min prn up to 3x	
Severe shock or inadequate response to IM or SC; administration intravenous	3-5 ml at 5-10 min intervals (1:1000)

C. Adverse Reactions during Pregnancy (Adapted from Drug Evaluations, 6th Edition, AMA, Chicago, 1986, pp 44-46)

Agent	1st trimester (Embryonic development)	2nd & 3rd trimesters (Fetal development)	Labor-delivery
Antibacterial agents			
Aminoglycosides	8th nerve damage**	8th nerve damage**	-
Chloramphenicol	-	Gray-baby syndrome*	Gray-baby syndrome*
Dapsone	-	-	Carcinogenic*** Hemolytic reactions*
Metronidazole	Tumors***	-	-
Nitrofurantoin	-	Hyperbilirubinemia* Hemolytic anemia*	Hyperbilirubinemia* Hemolytic anemia*
Streptomycin	8th nerve damage multiple defects, micromelia*	8th nerve damage*	-
Sulfamethoxazole-trimethoprim	Malformations****	-	-
Sulfonamides	-	Hyperbilirubinemia*	Hyperbilirubinemia*
Tetracycline	Inhibit bone growth* Micromelia** Syndactyly**	Stain deciduous teeth* Inhibit bone growth* Enamel hypoplasia**	-
Antimalarial agents			
Chloroquine	8th nerve damage**	8th nerve damage**	-
Quinine	Malformations, abortions, 8th nerve damage*	Deafness Thrombocytopenia	-
Antituberculous agents			
Isoniazid	CNS effects***	-	-
Rifampin	CNS effects***	-	-
Streptomycin (see above)			

* Generally well documented in humans   *** Documented in animals only
Suspected in humans   ** Questionable effects in humans

D. Relative Safety of Antimicrobial Agents During Pregnancy (classification according to the Medical Letter 29:61,1987 and data from Drug Information - 1992, American Hospital Formulary Service, Amer Soc Hosp Pharmac, Bethesda, pp 33-481, 1992)

Note: Drugs are listed by category of microbes. Medical Letter classifies drug in 3 categories: Probably safe, Use with caution, or Contraindicated. PDR and FDA recommendations usually state that any drug used in pregnant women is justified only when the medical need justifies the risk to the fetus or that safety in pregnancy is not established.

ANTIBACTERIAL AGENTS	Experimental animal studies (often 5-20x human dose)	Experience in Pregnant Women	Recommendation (including Medical Letter recommendations)
Aminoglycosides	---	Several reports of congenital deafness with streptomycin	Use only with life-threatening infections where no alternatives are available. Warn patient of risk. <u>Med Letter</u>: Caution
Aztreonam	Harmless except slightly reduced survival in off-spring with very high doses	No studies	Use with caution. <u>Med Letter</u>: Probably safe
Cephalosporins	Harmless	No adverse effects reported	Use with caution. <u>Med Letter</u>: Probably safe
Chloramphenicol	---	Gray baby syndrome with administration in late pregnancy or labor	Use with great caution at term or labor. <u>Med Letter</u>: Caution
Clindamycin	---	No studies	<u>Med Letter</u>: Caution
Dapsone	---	No adverse effects reported	Use with caution. <u>Med Letter</u>: Caution
Erythromycin	Harmless	No studies	Use only when clearly needed, although CDC recommends erythromycin for treatment of chlamydia and syphilis in pregnancy. Avoid estolate. <u>Med Letter</u>: Probably safe
Imipenem	Harmless	No studies	Use with caution. <u>Med Letter</u>: Caution
Methenamine	Harmless	No adverse effects reported	Safety not definitely established. <u>Med Letter</u>: Probably safe
Metronidazole	Fetotoxicity (with parenteral administration only)		Contraindicated during first trimester. <u>Med Letter</u>: Caution

(continued)

68

ANTIBACTERIAL AGENTS	Experimental animal studies (often 5-20x human dose)	Experience in Pregnant Women	Recommendation (including Medical Letter recommendations)
Nitrofurantoin	---	Hemolytic anemia in neonate due to immature enzyme systems. Drug appears safe in early pregnancy	Contraindicated at term. <u>Med Letter:</u> Caution
Penicillins	Harmless	No adverse effects reported	Use only when necessary, although CDC recommends penicillin G for syphilis and gonorrhea during pregnancy. <u>Med Letter:</u> Probably safe
Quinolones	Arthropathy in immature animals with erosions in joint cartilage	No studies	Contraindicated. <u>Med Letter:</u> Contraindicated
Spectinomycin		No studies	CDC recommends for pregnant women with gonorrhea. <u>Med Letter:</u> Probably safe
Sulfonamides	Cleft palate and bone abnormalities with high doses	Extensive use -- no complication except one case of agranulocytosis (possibly associated) Risk of sulfa-induced kernicterus when used in last term -- risk is low	Use with caution and avoid in last trimester when feasible. Contraindicated at term. <u>Med Letter:</u> Caution
Tetracyclines		Retardation of skeletal development and bone growth. Enamel hypoplasia and discoloration of teeth of fetus	Contraindicated. <u>Med Letter:</u> Contraindicated
Trimethoprim	Teratogenic	No studies	Use with caution due to effect on folic acid metabolism. <u>Med Letter:</u> Caution
Trimethoprim-sulfamethoxazole	Teratogenic	No congenital abnormalities in 35 children born to women who received TMP-SMX in first trimester	Use with caution due to effect on folic acid metabolism. Contraindicated at term due to kernicterus from sulfonamides. <u>Med Letter:</u> Caution
Vancomycin		No studies	Use with caution. <u>Med Letter:</u> Caution

(continued)

ANTIFUNGAL AGENTS	Experimental animal studies (often 5-20x human dose)	Experience in Pregnant Women	Recommendation (including Medical Letter recommendations)
Amphotericin B	---	No studies	Use with caution. Med Letter: Caution
Fluconazole	---	No studies	Use with caution. Med Letter: Caution
Flucytosine	Teratogenic	No studies	Use with caution. Med Letter: Caution
Griseofulvin	Embryotoxic and teratogenic	Congenital malformations and conjoined twins reported; relationship to drug debated	Contraindicated. Med Letter: Contraindicated
Itraconazole	Embryotoxic and teratogenic	No studies	Use with caution.
Ketoconazole	Embryotoxic and teratogenic	No studies	Use with caution. Med Letter: Caution
Miconazole	Harmless	No studies	Med Letter: Caution
Nystatin	---	No complications reported	Safe. Med Letter: Probably safe

ANTIMYCO-BACTERIAL AGENTS	Experimental animal studies (often 5-20x human dose)	Experience in Pregnant Women	Recommendation (including Medical Letter recommendations)
Aminosalicylic acid (PAS)	---	No studies	Use with caution. Med Letter: Caution
Capreomycin	Teratogenic -- "wavy rib"	No studies	Use with caution. Med Letter: Caution
Ethambutol	Teratogenic	No adverse effects reported	Use with caution. Med Letter: Caution
Ethionamide	Teratogenic	No studies	Use with caution. Med Letter: Caution
Isoniazide	Embryocidal. No teratogenic effects	No adverse effects reported	AAP recommendation: Pregnant women with positive PPD should receive INH if HIV pos., recent contact or x-ray showing old TB; begin after 1st trimester if possible; otherwise delay prophylaxis until postdelivery. Give with pyridoxine. Med Letter: Caution

(continued)

ANTIMYCO-BACTERIAL AGENTS	Experimental animal studies (often 5-20x human dose)	Experience in Pregnant Women	Recommendation (including Medical Letter recommendations)
Pyrazinamide	---	No studies	Use with caution. <u>Med Letter</u>: Caution
Rifampin	Congenital malformations -- cleft palate, spina bifida Embryotoxicity	Isolated cases of fetal abnormalities Administration in last weeks of pregnancy may cause postnatal hemorrhage	Use with caution. <u>Med Letter</u>: Caution

ANTIPARASITIC AGENTS	Experimental animal studies (often 5-20x human dose)	Experience in Pregnant Women	Recommendation (including Medical Letter recommendations)
Chloroquine	Accumulates in melanin of fetal eyes	Use with lupus: 8th nerve deficits, postcolumn defects, mental retardation. Use for malaria: No adverse effects	CDC and WHO conclude benefits with malaria exposure outweigh risk. <u>Med Letter</u>: Probably safe
Iodoquinol	---	No studies	<u>Med Letter</u>: Caution
Mebendazole	Embryotoxic, teratogenic	170 patients -- no adverse effects	Use with caution esp in 1st trimester and warn patient of risk. <u>Med Letter</u>: Caution
Mefloquine			Contraindicated: CDC advises contraception during prophylaxis and for 2 months after.
Niclosamide	Harmless	No studies	Usually can delay therapy. <u>Med Letter</u>: Probably safe
Oxamniquine	Embryocidal	No studies	Use with caution.
Paromomycin	---	No studies	<u>Med Letter</u>: Probably safe
Pentamidine	---	Spontaneous abortion reported during aerosol administration (causal relationship not established)	Avoid use of aerosolized pentamidine including those planning to become pregnant

(continued)

71

ANTIPARASITIC AGENTS	Experimental animal studies (often 5-20x human dose)	Experience in Pregnant Women	Recommendation (including Medical Letter recommendations)
Piperazine	---	Limited experience	Safety not clearly established <u>Med Letter</u>: Caution
Praziquantel	Harmless except increased rates of abortion	No studies	Use with caution <u>Med Letter</u>: Probably safe
Primaquine	---	No studies; theoretical concern is hemolytic anemia in G-6-PD deficient fetus	CDC: Chloroquine for relapsing malaria until postdelivery, then use primaquine for radical care
Pyrantel pamoate	Harmless	No studies	Self-medicate under direction of physician
Pyrimethamine	Teratogenic; stunted fetus; malformations	No reported adverse effects	Use with caution: indicated for toxoplasmosis in pregnancy. Fansidar indicated when risk of chloroquine resistant malaria cannot be avoided <u>Med Letter</u>: Caution
Quinacrine	Teratogenic	No studies	Usually can delay treatment of cestodiasis <u>Med Letter</u>: Caution
Quinine	Teratogenic	Stillbirths reported. Congenital malformations with large doses used for attempted abortions. Preferred.	Contraindicated. CDC previously recommended use for life-threatening malaria, but quinidine gluconate is now recommended <u>Med Letter</u>: Caution
Thiabendazole	Harmless except when suspended in olive oil	No experience	Use with caution. <u>Med Letter</u>: Caution

ANTIVIRAL AGENTS	Experimental animal studies (often 5-20x human dose)	Experience in Pregnant Women	Recommendation (including Medical Letter recommendations)
Acyclovir	Not teratogenic but potential to cause chromosomal damage at high doses	Limited data from BW registry -- no adverse effects; report to 1-800-722-9292	CDC: Use for life-threatening disease; do not use for treatment or prophylaxis of genital herpes. <u>Med Letter</u>: Caution

(continued)

ANTIVIRAL AGENTS	Experimental animal studies (often 5-20x human dose)	Experience in Pregnant Women	Recommendation (including Medical Letter recommendations)
Amantadine	Embryotoxic and teratogenic	Single case of 1st trimester exposure with single ventricle	Use with great caution. Med Letter: Contraindicated
Foscarnet	Skeletal abnormalities (<5%)	No studies	Use only if clearly needed.
Ganciclovir	Teratogenic and embryogenic, growth retardation, aplastic organs	No studies	Use only when necessary and warn patient of teratogenic and embryogenic effects Med Letter: Caution
Vidarabine	Teratogenic, maternal toxicity, fetal abnormalities	No studies	Use only when necessary. Med Letter: Caution
Zidovudine	Fetal resorptions; teratogenic and fetal hematologic toxicity with extremely high doses	No adverse effects with 160 patients reported to BW registry	Use only when necessary and report to registry 800-722-9292 Med Letter: Caution

DRUG INTERACTIONS

(Adapted from The Medical Letter Handbook of Adverse Drug Interactions, Medical Letter, pp 6-282, 1991; AMA Drug Evaluations and Drug Information 92; American Hospital Formulary Service; Amer Soc Hosp Pharmacists, Bethesda, MD, pp 33-481, 1992)

Drug	Effect of Interaction
Acyclovir	
Narcotics	Increased meperidine effect
Probenecid	Possible increased acyclovir toxicity
Amantadine	
Anticholinergics	Hallucination, confusion, nightmares
Thiazide diuretics	Increased amantadine toxicity with hydroclorothiazide-triameterene combination
Aminoglycosides	
Amphotericin	Increased nephrotoxicity
Bumetanide	Ototoxicity
Cephalosporins	Increased nephrotoxicity
Cisplatin*	Increased nephrotoxicity
Cyclosporine*	Increased nephrotoxicity
Enflurane*	Increased nephrotoxicity
Ethacrynic acid*	Increased ototoxicity
Furosemide*	Increased oto- and nephrotoxicity
MgSO₄	Increased neuromuscular blockage
Methotrexate	Possible decreased methotrexate activity with oral aminoglycosides
Vancomycin	Increased nephrotoxicity and possible increased ototoxicity
Aminosalicylic acid (PAS)	
Anticoagulants, oral	Increased hypoprothrombenia
Digitalis	Decreased digoxin effect
Probenecid	Increased PAS toxicity
Rifampin	Decreased rifampin effectiveness (give as separate doses by 8-12 hr)
Amphotericin B	
Aminoglycosides	Increased nephrotoxicity
Capreomycin	Increased nephrotoxicity
Corticosteroids	Increased hypokalemia
Cisplatin	Increased nephrotoxicity
Cyclosporine*	Increased nephrotoxicity
Digitalis	Increased cardiotoxicity (?)
Diuretics	Increased hypokalemia
Methoxyflurane	Increased nephrotoxicity
Skeletal muscle relaxants	Increased effect of relaxants
Vancomycin	Increased nephrotoxicity
AZT (Retrovir, Zidovudine)	
Amphotericin B	Increased anemia

(continued)

Drug	Effect of Interaction
Cancer chemotherapy (adriamycin, vinblastin, vincristine)	Increased marrow toxicity
Dapsone	Increased marrow toxicity
Flucytosine	Increased leukopenia
Ganciclovir*	Increased leukopenia, concurrent use contraindicated except with G-CSF
Interferon	Increased leukopenia
Phenytoin	Decreased phenytoin levels
Probenecid	Increased AZT levels (and rash)

Capreomycin

Aminoglycosides*	Increased oto- and nephrotoxicity
Theophylline	Increased theophylline effect and toxicity

Cephalosporins

Alcohol	Disulfiram-like reaction for those with tetrazolethiomethyl side chain: Cefamandole, cefoperazone, cefotetan, cefmetazole, moxalactam
Aminoglycosides	Possibly increased nephrotoxicity
Ethacrynic acid	Increased nephrotoxicity
Furosemide	Increased nephrotoxicity
Probenecid	Increased concentrations of most cephalosporins

Chloramphenicol

Anticoagulants, oral	Increased hypoprothrombinemia
Chlorpropamide	Increased chlorpropamide activity
Dicumarol	Increased dicumarol activity
Phenobarbital	Decreased concentrations chloramphenicol
Phenytoin	Increased phenytoin activity
Rifampin*	Decreased concentrations chloramphenicol
Tolbutamide	Increased tolbutamide activity

Ciprofloxacin (See Fluoroquinolones)

Clindamycin

Antiperistaltic agents (Lomotil, loparamide)	Increased risk and severity of C. difficile colitis

Cycloserine

Alcohol*	Increased alcohol effect or convulsions; warn patients
Ethionamide	Increased CNS toxicity
Isoniazid	CNS toxicity, dizziness, drowsiness
Phenytoin	Increased phenytoin effect (toxicity)

Dapsone

Coumadin	Increased prothrombin time
ddI	Decreased levels of dapsone
Primaquine	Increased hemolysis with G-6-PD deficiency
Probenecid	Increased dapsone levels
Pyrimethamine	Increased marrow toxicity (Monitor CBC)
Rifampin	Decreased levels of dapsone
Trimethoprim	Increased levels of both drugs

(continued)

Drug	Effect of Interaction

ddC (HIVID, zalcitabine, dideoxycytidine)

Agents associated with peripheral neuropathy:	Cisplatin, dapsome, ddI, disulfiram, ethionamide, glutethimide, gold, hydralazine, Iodoquinol, INH, metronidazole, nitrofurantoin, phenytoin, ribivirin, vincristine
Agents associated with pancreatitis:	Pentamidine, ddI, rifampin

ddI (videx, didanosine)

Dapsone	Decreased dapsone absorption, give ≥ 2hrs before ddI
Ketoconazole	Decreased ketoconazole absorption, give ≥ 2hrs before ddI
Tetracycline	Decreased tetracycline absorption, give ≥ 2hrs before ddI
Quinolones	Decreased quinolone absorption, give ≥ 2hrs before ddI

Note: All drugs that require gastric acidity for absorption should be given ≥ 2hrs before ddI

Alcohol	Increased frequency of pancreatitis
Pentamidine	Increased frequency of pancreatitis

Erythromycins

Anticoagulants (oral)	Increased hypoprothrombinemia
Carbamazepine	Increased carbamazepine toxicity
Corticosteroids	Increased effect of methylprednisolone
Cyclosporine	Increased cyclosporine toxicity (nephrotoxicity)
Digoxin	Increased digitalis toxicity
Disopyramide	Increased disopramide toxicity
Ergot alkaloids	Increased ergot toxicity
Phenytoin	Increased or decreased phenytoin effect
Seldane	Ventricular arrhythmias
Theophylline	Increased theophylline effect
Triazolam	Increased triazolam toxicity

Ethionamide

Cycloserine	Increased CNS toxicity
Isoniazid	Increased CNS toxicity

Fluconazole

Coumadin	Increased prothrombin time
Cyclosporine	Increased cyclosporine in renal transplant recipients
Phenytoin	Increased phenytoin effect
Sulfonylureas	Increased levels with hypoglycemia

Fluoroquinolones (ciprofloxacin, norfloxacin, ofloxacin, lomefloxacin)

Antacids	Decreased fluoroquinolone absorption with Mg, Ca or Al containing antacids or sucralfate: Give antacid > 2hrs after fluoroquinolone
Anticoagulants (oral)	Increased hypoprothrombinemia
Caffeine	Increased caffeine effect; significance?; not noted with ofloxacin
Cyclosporine	Possible increased nephrotoxicity
Iron*	Decreased ciprofloxacin absorption

(continued)

Drug	Effect of Interaction
Nonsteroidal anti-inflammatory agents	Possible seizures and increased epileptogenic potential of theophylline, opiates, tricyclics and neuroleptics
Probenecid	Increased fluoroquinolone levels
Theophylline	Increased theophylline toxicity -- esp ciprofloxacin and enoxacin (seizures, cardiac arrest, respiratory failure)
Zinc	Decreased ciprofloxacin absorption

Foscarnet

Aminoglycosides	Increased renal toxicity
Amphotericin B	Increased renal toxicity
Pentamidine	Increased hypocalcemia

Ganciclovir

Azathriaprim	Increased marrow suppression.
AZT (Retrovir)*	Increased leukopenia or give G-CSF
Imipenem	Increased frequency of seizures (?)

Griseofulvin

Alcohol	Possibly potentiates effect of alcohol
Anticoagulant (oral)	Decreased anticoagulant effect
Contraceptive	Decreased contraceptive effect
Phenobarbital	Decreased griseofulvin levels

Isoniazid

Alcohol	Increased hepatitis; Decreased INH effect in some
Antacids	Decreased INH with Al containing antacids
Anticoagulants (oral)	Possible increased hypoprothrombinemia
Benzodiazepines	Increased effects of benzodiazepines
Carbamazepine*	Increased toxicity of both drugs
Cycloserine	Increased CNS toxicity, dizziness, drowsiness
Disulfiram*	Psychotic episodes, ataxia
Ethionamide	Increased CNS toxicity
Enflurane*	Possible nephrotoxicity
Ketoconazole*	Decreased ketoconazole effect
Phenytoin	Increased phenytoin toxicity
Rifampin	Possible increased hepatic toxicity
Theophylline	Increased theophylline levels
Tyramine (rich foods & fluids)	Palpitations, sweating, urticaria, headache, vomiting, with consumption of cheese, wine, some fish

Itraconazole

Coumadin	Increased hypoprothrombinemia
Cyclosporine	Increased cyclosporine levels
Digoxin	Increased digoxin levels
H_2 antagonists	Decreased itraconazole levels
Hypoglycemics (oral)	Severe hypoglycemia
INH	Decreased itraconazole levels
Phenytoin	Decreased itraconazole levels
Rifampin	Decreased itraconazole levels
Terfenadine	Cardiac dysrhythmias

(continued)

Drug	Effect of Interaction
Ketoconazole	
Alcohol	Possible disulfiram-like reaction
Antacids	Decreased ketoconazole effect
Anticoagulants, oral	Increased hypoprothrombinemia
Corticosteroids	Increased methylprednisolone effect
Cyclosporine	Increased cyclosporine toxicity
H2 antagonists*	Decreased ketoconazole effect; use sucralfate or antacids given 2 hrs before
Isoniazid*	Decreased ketoconazole effect
Phenytoin	Altered metabolism of both drugs
Rifampin*	Decreased activity of both drugs
Seldane*	Ventricular arrhythmias
Theophylline	Increased theophylline activity
Mebendazole	
Phenytoin and Carbamazepine	Decreased mebendazole concentrations: clinically significant only for extraintestinal helminthic infections
Metronidazole	
Alcohol	Disulfiram-like reaction
Anticoagulants, oral	Increased hypoprothrombinemia
Barbiturates	Decreased metronidazole effect with phenobarbital
Corticosteroids	Decreased metronidazole effect
Cimetidine*	Possible increased metronidazole toxicity
Disulfiram*	Organic brain syndrome
Fluorouracil	Transient neutropenia
Lithium	Lithium toxicity
Miconazole	
Aminoglycosides	Possible decreased tobramycin levels
Anticoagulant, oral	Increased hypoprothrombinemia
Hypoglycemics	Severe hypoglycemia with sulfonylurea
Phenytoin	Increased phenytoin toxicity
Nalidixic acid	
Anticoagulants, oral	Increased hypoprothrombinemia
Nitrofurantoin	
Antacids	Possible decreased nitrofurantoin effect; give 6 hrs apart
Probenecid	Decreased nitrofurantoin effect (for UTIs)
Penicillins	
Allopurinol	Increased frequency of rash with ampicillin
Anticoagulants, oral	Decreased anticoagulant effect with nafcillin and dicloxacillin
Cephalosporins	Increased cefotaxime toxicity with mezlocillin + renal failure
Contraceptives	Possible decreased contraceptive effect with ampicillin or oxacillin
Cyclosporine	Decreased cyclosporine effect with nafcillin and increased cyclosporin toxicity with ticarcillin
Lithium	Hypernatremia with ticarcillin

(continued)

Drug	Effect of Interaction
Methotrexate	Possible increased methotrexate toxicity
Probenecid	Increased concentrations of penicillins
Pentamidine	
Aminoglycosides	Increased nephrotoxicity
Amphotericin B	Increased nephrotoxicity
Capreomycin	Increased nephrotoxicity
Foscarnet	Increased nephrotoxicity
Piperazine	
Chlorpromazine	Possibly induces seizures
Polymyxin B and colistimethate	
Aminoglycoside	Increased nephrotoxicity; increased neuromuscular blockade
Neuromuscular blocking agents	Increased neuromuscular blockade
Vancomycin	Increased nephrotoxicity
Pyrazinamide	
Allopurinal*	Failure to decrease hyperuricemia
Pyrimethamine	
Antacids	Possible decreased pyrimethamine absorption
Dapsone*	Agranulocytosis reported
Kaolin	Possible decreased pyrimethamine absorption
Phenothiazines	Possible chlorpromazine toxicity
Rifampin	
Aminosalicylic acid (PAS)	Decreased effectiveness of rifampin; give in separate doses by 8-12 h
Anticoagulants	Increased hypoprothrombinemia
Barbiturates	Decreased barbiturate effect
Benzodiazepines	Possible decreased benzodiazepine effect
ß-adrenergic blockers	Decreased B blocker effect
Chloramphenicol*	Decreased chloramphenicol effect
Clofazimine	Reduced rifampin effect
Clofibrate	Decreased clofibrate effect
Contraceptives	Decreased contraceptive effect
Corticosteroids*	Decreased corticosteroid effect
Cyclosporine*	Decreased cyclosporine effect
Dapsone	Decreased dapsone effect (not significant with treatment of leprosy)
Digitalis	Decreased digitalis effect
Disopyramide*	Decreased disopyramide effect
Doxycycline	Decreased doxycycline effect
Estrogens	Decreased estrogen effect
Haloperidol	Decreased haloperidol effect
Hypoglycemics	Decreased hypoglycemic effect of sulfonurea
Isoniazid	Increased hepatotoxicity
Ketoconazole*	Decreased effect of ketoconazole and rifampin (concurrent use contraindicated)

(continued)

Drug	Effect of Interaction
Methadone	Methadone withdrawal symptoms
Mexiletin	Decreased antiarrhythmic effect
Phenytoin	Decreased phenytoin effect
Progestins	Decreased norethindrome effect
Quinidine	Decreased quinidine effect
Theophyllines	Decreased theophylline effect
Trimethoprim	Decreased trimethoprim levels
Verapamil	Decreased verapamil effect

Spectinomycin

Lithium	Increased lithium toxicity

Sulfonamides

Anticoagulants, oral	Increased hypoprothrombinemia
Barbiturates	Increased thiopental effect
Cyclosporine	Decreased cyclosporine effect with sulfamethazine
Digoxin	Decreased digoxin effect with sulfasalazine
Hypoglycemics	Increased hypoglycemic effect of sulfonylurea
Methotrexate	Possible increased methotrexate toxicity
Monoamine oxidase inhibitors	Possible increased phenelzine toxicity with sulfisoxazole
Phenytoin	Increased phenytoin effect except with sulfisoxazole

Tetracycline

Alcohol	Decreased doxycycline effect in alcoholics
Antacids*	Decreased tetracycline effect with antacids containing Ca^{++}, Al^{++}, Mg^{++} and $NaHCO_3$ (give 3 hrs apart)
Anticoagulants, oral	Increased hypoprothrombinemia
Antidepressants, tricyclic*	Localized hemosiderosis with amitriptyline and minocycline
Antidiarrhea agents	Agents containing kaolin and pectin or bismuth subsalicylate decrease tetracycline effect
Barbiturates*	Decreased doxycycline effect
Bismuth subsalicylate (Pepto-Bismol)	Decreased tetracycline effect
Carbamazepine (Tegretol)*	Decreased doxycycline effect
Contraceptives, oral*	Decreased contraceptive effect
Digoxin	Increased digoxin effect (10% of population)
Iron, oral	Decreased tetracycline effect (except with doxycycline) and decreased iron effect; give 3 hrs before
Laxatives	Agents containing Mg^{++} decrease tetracycline effect
Lithium	Possible increased lithium toxicity (single case)
Methotrexate	Possible increased methotrexate toxicity
Methoxyflurane anesthesia (Penthrane)	Possibly lethal nephrotoxicity
Milk	Decreased absorption of tetracycline. Does not apply to doxycycline or minocycline
Molindone	Decreased tetracycline effect
Phenformin*	Decreased doxycycline effect
Phenytoin	Decreased doxycycline effect
Rifampin	Possible decreased doxycycline effect
Theophylline	Possible increased theophylline toxicity
Zinc*	Decreased tetracycline effect (continued)

Drug	Effect of Interaction
Thiabendazole	
Theophyllines	Increased theophylline toxicity
Trimethoprim	
Azathioprine	Leukopenia
Cyclosporine*	Increased nephrotoxicity
Dapsone	Increased levels of both drugs; increased methemoglobinemia
Digoxin	Possible increased digitalis effect
Phenytoin	Increased phenytoin effect
Thiazide diuretics	Possible increased hyponatremia with concomitant use of amiloride with thiazide diuretics
Trimethoprim-sulfamethoxazole	
Anticoagulants, oral	Increased hypothrombinemia
Mercaptopurine*	Decreased mercaptopurine activity
Methotrexate*	Megaloblastic anemia
Paromycin	Increased nephrotoxicity
Phenytoin	Increased phenytoin toxicity
Procainamide	Increased procainamide
Vancomycin	
Aminoglycosides	Increased nephrotoxicity and possible increased ototoxicity
Amphotericin B	Increased nephrotoxicity
Cisplatin	Increased nephrotoxicity
Digoxin	Possible decreased digoxin effect
Paromomycin	Increased nephrotoxicity
Polymyxin	Increased nephrotoxicity
Vidarabine	
Allopurinol	Increased neurotoxicity, nausea, pain and pruritus
Theophyllines	Increased theophylline effect

* Concurrent use to be avoided if possible

A. Vaccines available in the United States, by type and recommended routes of administration (MMWR 38:207,1989)

Vaccine	Type	Route
BCG (Bacillus of Calmette and Guérin)	Live bacteria	Intradermal or subcutaneous
Cholera	Inactivated bacteria	Subcutaneous or intradermal*
DTP (D=Diphtheria) (T=Tetanus) (P=Pertussis)	Toxoids and inactivated bacteria	Intramuscular
HB (Hepatitis B)	Inactive viral antigen	Intramuscular
Haemophilus influenzae b -Polysaccharide (HbPV) -or Conjugate (HbCV)	Bacterial polysaccharide or Polysaccharide conjugated to protein	Subcutaneous or intramuscular[T] Intramuscular
Influenza	Inactivated virus or viral components	Intramuscular
IPV (Inactivated Poliovirus Vaccine)	Inactivated viruses of all 3 serotypes	Subcutaneous
Measles	Live virus	Subcutaneous
Meningococcal	Bacterial polysaccharides of serotypes A/C/Y/W-135	Subcutaneous
MMR (M=Measles) (M=Mumps) (R=Rubella)	Live viruses	Subcutaneous
Mumps	Live virus	Subcutaneous
OPV (Oral Poliovirus Vaccine)	Live viruses of all 3 serotypes	Oral
Plague	Inactivated bacteria	Intramuscular
Pneumococcal	Bacterial polysaccharides of 23 pneumococcal types	Intramuscular or subcutaneous
Rabies	Inactivated virus	Subcutaneous or intradermal[‡]
Rubella	Live virus	Subcutaneous
Tetanus	Inactivated toxin (toxoid)	Intramuscular'
Td or DT** (T=Tetanus) (D or d=Diphtheria)	Inactivated toxins	Intramuscular'
Typhoid	Inactivated bacteria	Subcutaneous[TT]
Yellow fever	Live virus	Subcutaneous

*The intradermal dose is lower.
[T]Route depends on the manufacturer; consult package insert for recommendation for specific product use.
[‡]Intradermal dose is lower and used only for preexposure vaccination.
'Preparations with adjuvants should be given intramuscularly.
** DT=tetanus and diphtheria toxoids for use in children aged <7 years. Td= tetanus and diphtheria toxoids for use in persons aged ≥7 years. Td contains the same amount of tetanus toxoid as DTP or DT but a reduced dose of diphtheria toxoid.
[TT]Boosters may be given intradermally unless acetone-killed and dried vaccine is used.

B. GUIDE FOR ADULT IMMUNIZATION

(Adapted from: Guide for Adult Immunization, American College of Physicians, 2nd Ed., Philadelphia, PA 1-178,1990; MMWR 40(RR12):1-94,1991)

Category	Vaccine	Comments
AGE		
18-24 yrs	Td* (0.5 ml IM)	Booster every 10 yrs at mid-decades (age 25, 35, 45, etc) for those who completed primary series
	Measles** (MMR, 0.5 ml SC x 1 or 2)	Post-high school institutions should require two doses of live measles vaccine (separated by 1 month), the first dose preferably given before entry
	Mumps*** (MMR, 0.5 ml SC x 1)	Especially susceptible males
	Rubella*** (MMR, 0.5 ml SC x 1)	Especially susceptible females; pregnancy now or within 3 months post-vaccination is contraindication to vaccination
	Influenza	Advocated for young adults at increased risk of exposure (military recruits, students in dorms, etc)
25-64 yrs	Td*	As above
	Mumps***	As above
	Measles** (MMR, 0.5 ml SC x 1)	Persons vaccinated between 1963 and 1967 may have received inactivated vaccine and should be revaccinated
	Rubella*** (MMR, 0.5 ml SC x 1)	Principally females $\leq$ 45 yrs with child-bearing potential; pregnancy now or within 3 months post-vaccination is contraindication to vaccination
$\geq$ 65 yrs	Td*	As above
	Influenza (0.5 ml IM)	Annually, usually in November
	Pneumococcal (23 valent, 0.5 ml IM)	Single dose; efficacy for elderly not established, but case control and epidemiology studies suggest 60-70% effectiveness in preventing pneumococcal bacteremia (NEJM 325:1453, 1991)
SPECIAL GROUPS		
Pregnancy		All pregnant women should be screened for hepatitis B surface antigen (HBsAg) and rubella antibody
		Live virus vaccines**** should be avoided unless specifically indicated
		It is preferable to delay vaccines and toxoids until 2nd or 3rd trimester
		Immune globulins are safe; most vaccines are a theoretical risk only

(continued)

Category	Vaccine	Comments
	Td* (0.5 ml IM)	If not previously vaccinated - dose at 0, 4 wks (preferably 2nd and 3rd trimesters) and 6-12 mo.; boost at 10 yr intervals; protection to infant is conferred by placental transfer of maternal antibody
	Measles	Risk for premature labor and spontaneous abortion; exposed pregnant women who are susceptible** should receive immune globulin within 6 days and then MMR post delivery at least 3 months after immune globulin (MMR is contraindicated during pregnancy)
	Mumps	No sequelae noted, immune globulin is of no value and MMR is contraindicated
	Rubella	Rubella during 1st 16 wks carries great risk, e.g., 15-20% rate of neonatal death and 20-50% incidence of congenital rubella syndrome; history of rubella is unreliable indicator of immunity. Women exposed during 1st 20 weeks should have rubella serology and if not immune should be offered abortion.
	Hepatitis A	Immune globulin within 2 weeks of exposure
	Hepatitis B	All pregnant women should have prenatal screening for HBsAg; newborn infants of HBsAg carriers should receive HBIG and HBV vaccine; pregnant women who are HBsAg negative and at high risk should receive HBV vaccine
	Inactivated oral polio vaccine (0.5 ml SC)	Advised if exposure is imminent in women who completed the primary series over 10 yrs ago. Unimmunized women should receive 2 doses separated by 1-2 mo.; unimmunized women at high risk who need immediate protection should receive oral live polio vaccine
	Influenza Pneumococcal vaccine	Not routinely recommended, but can be given if there are other indications
	Varicella (VZIG, 12.5 U/kg IM)	Varicella-zoster immune globulin (VZIG) may prevent or modify maternal infection
<u>Family member exposure</u>		**Recommendations generally apply to household contacts**
	H. influenzae type B	H. influenzae meningitis: Rifampin prophylaxis for all household contacts in households with another child <4 yrs; contraindicated in pregnant women
	Hepatitis A	Immune globulin within 2 weeks of exposure

(continued)

84

Category	Vaccine	Comments
	Hepatitis B	HBV vaccine (3 doses) for those with intimate contact and no serologic evidence of prior infection
	Influenza	Influenza case should be treated with amantadine to prevent spread; unimmunized high risk family members should receive amantadine (x 14 days) and vaccine
	Meningococcal infection	Rifampin or sulfonamide for family contacts of meningococcal meningitis
	Varicella-zoster	No treatment unless immunocompromised: consider VZIG

ENVIRONMENTAL SETTINGS
Residents of nursing homes

	Influenza (0.5 ml IM)	Annually; vaccination rates of 80% required to prevent outbreaks
	Pneumococcal vaccine (23 valent, 0.5 ml IM)	Single dose, efficacy not clearly established
	Td* (0.5 ml IM)	Booster dose at mid-decades

Residents of institutions for mentally retarded

	Hepatitis B	Screen all new admissions and long term residents: HBV vaccine for susceptibles (Seroprevalence rates are 30-80%)

Prison inmates	Hepatitis B	As above

Homeless	Td*	
	Measles, rubella, mumps	MMR 0.5 ml SC (young adults)
	Influenza	
	Pneumococcal vaccine	

OCCUPATIONAL GROUPS
Health care workers

	Hepatitis B (3 doses)	Personnel in contact with blood or blood products; serologic screening with vaccination only of seronegatives is optional; serologic studies show 5% are nonresponders (neg for anti-HBs) even with repeat vaccinations
	Influenza	Annual
	Rubella (MMR, 0.5 ml SC)	Personnel who might transmit rubella to pregnant patients or other health care workers should have documented immunity or vaccination

(continued)

85

Category	Vaccine	Comments
	Mumps (MMR, 0.5 ml SC)	Personnel with no documented history of mumps or mumps vaccine should be vaccinated
	Measles (MMR, 0.5 ml SC)	Personnel who do not have immunity** should be vaccinated; those vaccinated in or after 1957 should receive an additional dose and those who are unvaccinated should receive 2 doses separated by at least 1 month; during outbreak in medical setting vaccinate (or revaccinate) all health care workers with direct patient contact
	Polio	Persons with incomplete primary series should receive inactivated polio vaccine
Immigrants and refugees		
	Td*	Immunize if not previously done
	Rubella, Measles, Mumps	Most have been vaccinated or had these conditions, although MMR is advocated except for pregnant women
	Polio	Adults will usually be immune
	Hepatitis B	Screen for HBsAg and vaccinate family members and sexual partners of carriers; screening is especially important for pregnant women
LIFESTYLES		
Homosexual men		
	Hepatitis B	Prevaccination serologic screening advocated since 30-80% have serologic evidence of HBV markers
IV drug abusers		
	Hepatitis B	As above; seroprevalence rates of HBV marker are 50-80%
IMMUNODEFICIENCY		
HIV infection	Measles	Postexposure prophylaxis with immune globulin (0.25 ml/kg IM)
	Pneumococcal vaccine	Recommended
	H. influenzae b conjugate vaccine	Consider
	Influenza (0.5 ml IM)	Annual; consider amantadine during epidemics
Asplenia	Pneumococcal vaccine (23 valent, 0.5 ml IM)	Recommended, preferably given 2 weeks before elective splenectomy; revaccinate those who received the 14 valent vaccine and those vaccinated > 6 yrs previously
	Meningococcal vaccine	Indicated
	H. influenzae b conjugate	Consider

(continued)

Category	Vaccine	Comments
Renal failure	Hepatitis B	For patients whose renal disease is likely to result in dialysis or transplantation; double dose and periodic boosters advocated
	Pneumococcal vaccine	Pneumococcal vaccine
	Influenza	Annual
Alcoholics	Pneumococcal vaccine	
Diabetes & other high risk diseases	Influenza	
	Pneumococcal vaccine	
TRAVEL* (Recommendations of Med Lett 34:41,1992; and CDC Information for International Travel 1992, HHS Publication #92-8280)		For travelers to developed countries (Canada, Europe, Japan, Australia, New Zealand) the risk of developing vaccine-preventable disease is no greater than for traveling in the U.S.
		Each country has its own vaccine requirements
		Smallpox vaccination is no longer required and should not be given
	Yellow fever (see MMWR 39: RR6,1990)	Recommended for endemic area: Tropical S. America and most of Africa between 15° North & 15° South
		Available in U.S. only at sites designated by local or state health departments
		Contraindications: Immunocompromised host; pregnancy is a relative contraindication (live virus vaccine)
	Cholera	Not recommended since risk is low and vaccine has limited effectiveness (Lancet 1:270,1990)
	Typhoid fever	Recommended for travel to rural areas of countries where typhoid fever is endemic or any area of an outbreak. The live oral vaccine (one cap every other day x 4 starting 2 wks before travel) is preferred over the parenteral vaccine due to comparable efficacy and better tolerance (Lancet 336:891, 1990); available from Berna Products (800-533-5899)
	Hepatitis A	Immune globulin for susceptible travelers to areas with poor sanitation conditions; especially if contact with small children or work in health care areas; dose is 0.02 ml/kg (or 2 ml) IM for travel < 3 mo. and 0.06 ml/kg (or 5 ml) IM for travel > 3 mo. Repeat dose q 4-6 mo. while in endemic area. Susceptibility may be determined with tests for IgG antibody that are widely available (Lancet 1:1447,1988). (continued)

Category	Vaccine	Comments
	Hepatitis B	HBV vaccine if travel to endemic areas, and travel > 6 mo., sexual contact with local persons is likely or if contact with blood is likely. Major risk areas are Southeast Asia and sub-Saharan Asia.
	Rabies	Consider human diploid cell rabies vaccine (HDCV) or rabies vaccine absorbed (RVA) for extended travel to endemic area
	Japanese encephalitis (1 ml SC x 3 1-2 wks apart)	Vaccine recommended for > 1 mo. in rural rice-growing areas with extensive exposure to mosquitoes. Potential problem countries include Bangladesh, Cambodia, Indonesia, Laos, Malasia, Burma, Pakistan, China, Korea, Taiwan, Thailand, Vietnam, India, Nepal, Sri Lanka and the Philippines (NEJM 319: 641,1988). Available through U.S. embassies in Asia
	Measles	Susceptible persons** should receive a single dose before travel
	Meningococcal vaccine	Recommended for travel to areas of epidemics, most frequently sub-Saharan Africa (Dec-Jan), Middle East, India and Napal
	Polio	Travelers to developing countries should receive a primary series of inactivated polio vaccine if not previously immunized If protection is needed within 4 wks: single dose eIPV or trivalent (live) OPV recommended. Previously immunized travelers should receive one booster of OPV or eIPV

* Td - Diphtheria and tetanus toxoids absorbed (for adult use). Primary series is 0.5 ml IM at 0, 4 wks and 6-12 months; booster doses at 10-year intervals are single doses of 0.5 ml IM. Adults who have not received at least 3 doses of Td should complete the primary series. Persons with unknown histories should receive the series.

** Persons are considered immune to measles if there is documentation of receipt of two doses of live measles vaccine after the first birthday, prior physician diagnosis of measles, laboratory evidence of measles immunity or birth before 1957.

*** Persons are considered immune to mumps if they have a record of adequate vaccination, documented physician diagnosed disease, or laboratory evidence of immunity. Persons are considered immune to rubella if they have a record of vaccination after their first birthday or laboratory evidence of immunity. (A physician diagnosis of rubella is considered non-specific).

** ***The preferred vaccine for persons susceptible to measles, mumps or rubella is MMR given as 0.5 ml SC for measles (one or two doses), mumps (one dose) or rubella (one dose). Pregnant women should not be vaccinated until after delivery.

**** Live virus vaccines = measles, rubella, yellow fever, oral polio vaccine

C. SPECIFIC VACCINES

1. Influenza Vaccine (Recommendations of the Advisory Committee on Immunization Practice: MMWR 41:315, 1992; 41 RR-9, 1992)

<u>Preparations</u>: Inactivated egg grown viruses that may be split (chemically treated to reduce febrile reactions in children) or whole. For the 1992-93 season the FDA Vaccine Advisory Panel has recommended a trivalent vaccine with A/Texas/36/91-like (H1N1), A/Beijing/353/89-like (H3N2) and B/Panama/45/90-like viruses. Product information available from Connaught (800) 822-2463, Parke Davis (800) 223-0432 and Wyeth (800) 321-2304. A history of prior vaccination in any prior year does not preclude the need for revaccination. Remaining 1991-92 season vaccine should not be used.

<u>Administration (over 12 years)</u>: Whole or split virus vaccine, 0.5 ml x 1 IM in the deltoid muscle, preferrably in November and as early as September.

Target groups

<u>Groups at increased risk for influenza-related complications</u>
1. Persons ≥ 65 years
2. Residents of nursing homes and other chronic care facilities housing persons of any age with chronic medical conditions
3. Persons with chronic disorders of the pulmonary or cardiovascular system, including those with asthma
4. Adults and children who require regular medical follow-up or hospitalization during the prior year due to chronic metabolic diseases (diabetes), renal dysfunction, hemoglobulinopathies or immunosuppression
5. Children and teenagers who are receiving long-term aspirin therapy (risk of Reye's syndrome)

<u>Groups that can transmit influenza to high risk patients</u>
1. Physicians, nurses and other personnel who have contact with high risk patients
2. Employees of nursing homes and chronic care facilities who have contact with patients or residents
3. Providers of home care to high risk persons
4. Household members of high risk persons

<u>Other groups</u>
1. Persons who desire it
2. Persons who provide essential community services
3. Persons in institutional settings
4. Persons with HIV infection
5. Elderly and other high risk persons embarking on international travel: Tropics -- all year; Southern hemisphere -- April thru September

Contraindications
1. Severe allergy to eggs
2. Persons with acute febrile illness (delay until symptoms abate); persons with minor illnesses such as URIs may be vaccinated

89

3. Pregnancy: There has been no excess in the influenza-associated mortality among
    pregnant women since the 1957-1958 pandemic. Influenza vaccine is not routinely
    recommended, but pregnancy is not viewed as a contraindication in women with
    other high risk conditions; it is preferred to vaccinate after the first trimester
    unless the first trimester corresponds to the influenza season.

Adverse reactions:
1. Soreness at the vaccination site for up to 2 days in about one-third.
2. Fever, malaise, etc. - infrequent and most common in those not previously exposed
    in influenza antigens, e.g. young children. Reactions begin 6-12 hrs post-
    vaccination and persist 1-2 days.
3. Allergic reactions - rare and include hives, angioedema, asthma, anaphylaxis;
    usually allergy to egg protein.

2. **Measles Prevention: Revised recommendations of the Advisory Committee on
    Immunization Practices (MMWR 40 RR 12:20-21, 1991)**

Category	Recommendations
Routine childhood schedule	Two doses*, 1st at 12 months (high risk area) or 15 months (most areas); 2nd dose at 4-6 yrs.
Adults	Single dose unless documentation of at least one dose of live measles vaccine ≥ 1 yr** or other evidence of immunity***
Colleges and other educational institutions	Two doses* unless documentation of receipt of two doses** live measles vaccine at ≥ 1 yr or other evidence of immunity***, ****
Medical personnel beginning employment	Two doses* for all persons who do not have proof of two** doses live measles vaccine at ≥ 1 yr or other evidence of immunity***, ****
Outbreaks in institutions or medical facilities	Two doses* for all persons born after 1956 who do not have proof of two** doses of live measles vaccine ≥ 1 yr or other evidence of immunity***, ****
Exposures	Vaccine preferred if given < 72 h after exposure. Alternative is immune globulin (0.25 ml/kg IM, maximum 15 ml), acceptable if given within 6 days. Live measle vaccine should be given 3 mo. after IG

*   Usually MMR (0.5 ml SC). Two doses in adults should include 2nd dose ≥ 1 month
     after first.
** Single dose of live measles vaccine given at ≥ 1 yr of age should provide long-lasting
     immunity in 95%. In some settings a 5% rate of susceptibility provides enough non-
     immune persons to sustain an epidemic. Persons vaccinated with killed measles vaccine
     (1963-67) are considered unvaccinated.
*** Born before 1957, physician diagnosed measles or laboratory evidence of immunity
     (measles-specific antibody). Serologic studies in health care workers showed 9% of
     persons born before 1957 were not immune, and 29% of health care workers who
     acquired measles (1985-89) were born before 1957. Therefore, vaccine should be offered
     to those born before 1957 if there is reason to consider them susceptible.

3. **Rabies Vaccine (Recommendation of Advisory Committee on Immunization Practice) MMWR 40RR-3:1-16,1991)**

There are two types of immunizing products
1. Rabies vaccine to induce active immune response; this response requires 7-10 days and persists ≥ 2 years.
    a. Rabies Vaccine, Human Diploid Cell: HDCV for intramuscular or intradermal injection (Connaught Labs, 800-VACCINE).
    b. Rabies Vaccine Absorbed: RVA (distributed by Biologics Products Program, Michigan Department of Public Health (517) 335-8050.
2. Rabies immune globulins (RIG) to give rapid passive protection with half life of 21 days available from Cutter Biological and Connaught Laboratories.

Table 1. Rabies postexposure prophylaxis. United States, 1991

Animal type	Evaluation and disposition of animal	Postexposure prophylaxis recommendations
Dogs and cats	Healthy and available for 10 days observation	Should not begin prophylaxis unless animal develops symptoms of rabies*
	Rabid or suspected rabid	Immediate vaccination
	Unknown (escaped)	Consult public health officials
Skunks, raccoons, bats, foxes, and most other carnivores; woodchucks	Regarded as rabid unless geographic area is known to be free of rabies or until animal proven negative by laboratory test[r]	Immediate vaccination
Livestock, rodents, and lagomorphs (rabbits and hares)	Consider individually	Consult public health officials. Bites of squirrels, hamsters, guinea pigs, gerbils, chipmunks, rats, mice, other rodents, rabbits, and hares almost never require antirabies treatment.

* During the 10-day holding period, begin treatment with HRIG and HDCV or RVA at first sign of rabies in a dog or cat that has bitten someone. The symptomatic animal should be killed immediately and tested.
[r] The animal should be killed and tested as soon as possible. Holding for observation is not recommended. Discontinue vaccine if immunofluorescence test results of the animal are negative.

Table 2. Rabies postexposure prophylaxis schedule. United States, 1991

Vaccination status	Treatment	Regimen*
Not previously vaccinated	Local wound cleaning	All postexposure treatment should begin with immediate thorough cleansing of all wounds with soap and water.
	HRIG	20 IU/kg body weight. If anatomically feasible, up to one-half the dose should be infiltrated around the wound(s) and the rest should not be administered in the same syringe or into the same anatomical site as vaccine. Because HRIG may partially suppress active production of antibody, no more than the recommended dose should be given.
	Vaccine	HDCV or RVA. 1.0 ml. IM (deltoid area[T]), one each on days 0, 3, 7, 14 and 28.
Previously vaccinated[TT]	Local wound	All postexposure treatment should begin with immediate thorough cleansing of all wounds with soap and water.
	HRIG	HRIG should not be administered.
	Vaccine	HDCV or RVA. 1.0 ml. IM (deltoid area[T]), one each on days 0 and 3.

* These regimens are applicable for all age groups, including children.
[T] The deltoid area is the only acceptable site of vaccination for adults and older children. For younger children, the outer aspect of the thigh may be use. Vaccine should never be administered in the gluteal area.
[TT] Any person with a history of pre-exposure vaccination with HDCV or RVA, prior postexposure prophylaxis with HDCV or RVA, or previous vaccination with any other type of rabies vaccine and a documented history of antibody response to the prior vaccination.

4.   **Tetanus Prophylaxis** (MMWR 40:RR10,1991)

History of Tetanus toxoid	Clean, minor wounds		Other wounds**	
	Td*	TIG*	Td*	TIG*
Unknown or < 3 doses	Yes	No	Yes	Yes
≥ 3 doses***	No, unless > 10 yrs since last dose	No	No, unless > 5 yrs since last dose	No

*   Td = Tetanus toxoid; TIG = Tetanus immune globulin
**   Wounds contaminated with dirt, stool, soil, saliva, etc; puncture wounds; avulsions; wounds from missiles, crushing, burns and frostbite.
*** If only three doses of toxoid, a fourth should be given.

5.   **Pneumococcal Vaccine** - Advisory Committee on Immunization Practices, Centers For Disease Control, American Thoracic Society, The Infectious Diseases Society of America, American College of Physicians: MMWR 40 RR-12:1-94, 1991 and Guide for Adult Immunization ACP (2nd Edition) - 91-96, 1990.

<u>Vaccine</u>: 23 valent polysaccharide vaccine for the <u>S</u>. pneumoniae contains antigens for serotypes responsible for 87% of bacteremic pneumococcal disease in the U.S. Most adults show a 2x rise in type specific antibody at 2-3 weeks after vaccination. Efficacy estimated at 45-65%; it is not established in immunosuppressed populations (NEJM 325:1453, 1991).

<u>Recommendations for adults</u>

1.   Immunocompetent adults at increased risk of pneumococcal disease or its complications due to chronic illness (e.g. cardiovascular disease, pulmonary disease, diabetes, alcoholism, cirrhosis, or cerebrospinal fluid leaks) or who are ≥ 65 years old.

2.   Immunocompromised adults at increased risk of pneumococcal disease or its complications (e.g. splenic dysfunction or anatomic asplenia, lymphoma, Hodgkin's disease, multiple myeloma, chronic renal failure, nephrosis organ transplant recipients, HIV infection and other conditions associated with immunosuppression).

3.   Persons in special environments or social settings with identified risk of pneumococcal disease (Native Americans, homeless, etc.).

   Notations: 1) Vaccine should be given at least 2 weeks before elective splenectomy; 2) Vaccine should be given as long as possible before planned immunosuppressive treatment; 3) Hospital discharge is a convenient time for vaccination since 2/3's of patients with serious pneumococcal infections have been hospitalized within the prior 5 years; 4) May be given simultaneously with influenza vaccine (separate injection sites).

4.   Patients with HIV infection should be given vaccine early in the course of disease for adequate antibody response. (continued)

<u>Adverse reactions</u>
1. Pain and erythema at injection site: 50%
2. Fever, myalgia, severe local reaction: < 1%
3. Anaphylactoid reactions: 5/million
4. Frequency of severe reactions is increased with revaccination
   < 13 months after primary vaccination; severe reactions are
   no more frequent when revaccination occurs > 4 yrs after
   primary vaccination.

<u>Revaccination</u>: Should be strongly considered for high risk patients vaccinated 6 or more years previously; revaccination after 3-5 years is recommended for transplant recipients, patients with renal failure and patients with nephrotic syndrome.

6. **Hepatitis Vaccine (Recommendations of the Advisory Council on Immunization Practices) (MMWR 39:RR-2, 1-26, 1990)**

a.   <u>HAV</u>: Immune globulin (IG)

	Dose ml/kg IM	Frequency
(1) Pre-exposure		
Workers with non-human primates	0.06	q 4-6 mo.
Travelers to developing countries		
Visit less than 3 mo.	0.02	Once
Visit over 3 mo.	0.02	q 4-6 mo.

(2) Post-exposure (must be given within two weeks of exposure)

Close personal contacts and sexual partners

Day care centers: Staff and attendees when one case or at least two cases in families of attendees

Institutions for custodial care: Residents with staff with close contact with cases

Common source exposure: food and waterborne outbreaks if recognized within the 2 week post-exposure period of effectiveness

Food handlers: Other food handlers, but not patrons unless uncooked food was handled without gloves and patrons can be located within 2 weeks of exposure

Hospitals: Not recommended for hospital personnel

[The above post-exposure items share: Dose 0.02 ml/kg IM, Frequency Once]

b.   <u>Hepatitis B</u> (MMWR 36:353-366,1987; MMWR 37:342-351,1987; MMWR 39:1-26,1990):

<u>Vaccine preparations</u>
(1)   Heptavax B: Plasma-derived vaccine available since 6/82; 20 ug HBsAg/ml; use is now restricted to hemodialysis patients, other immunocompromised hosts and persons with yeast allergy.

(2)   Recombivax HB: Recombinant vaccine produced by <u>Saccharomyces cerevisiae</u> (baker's yeast) and available since 7/86; 10 or 40 μg HBsAg/ml; usual adult dose is 3 1 ml doses (10 μg) at 0,1 and 6 mo.

(3)   Engerix-B: Recombinant vaccine available since 1989; 20 μg HBsAg/ml; usual adult dose regimen is 3 1 ml doses (20 μg) at 0, 1 and 6 months; alternative schedule is 4 1 ml doses (20 μg) at 0, 1, 2 and 12 mo. (for more rapid induction of immunity)

<u>Pre-exposure vaccination</u>:

(1)   <u>Regimen</u>: Three IM doses (deltoid) at 0 time, 1 month and 6 months. The usual adult dose is 1 ml (20 μg Engerix B or 10 μg of Recombivax HB); hemodialysis patients and possibly other immunocompromised patients should receive 2-4x the usual adult dose (usually 40 μg doses of either recombinant vaccine preparation)

(2)   <u>Response rates</u>: > 90% of healthy adults develop adequate antibody response (> 10 million Internat. Units/ml) and field trials show 80-95% efficacy.

(3)   <u>Postvaccination serologic testing</u>: Recommended only when clinical management depends on knowledge of immune status, i.e., infants born to HBsAg positive mother, dialysis staff and patients, persons with HIV infection and exposed health care workers. When done, test at 1-6 mo. after last dose.

(4)   <u>Revaccination</u>: Revaccination of non-responders will produce response in 15-25% with one additional dose and in 30-50% with 3 doses. 13-60% of responders lose detectable antibody within 9 years, although implications for revaccination are unclear since protective efficacy persists at least 9 years. At present, booster doses are not recommended (MMWR 40:RR-13, 1991).

(5)   <u>Prevaccination serologic testing</u>: Testing groups at highest risk is usually cost effective if the prevalence of HBV markers is > 20% (see table). Routine testing usually consists of one antibody test: either anti-HBc or anti-HBs. Anti-HBc detects both carriers (HBsAg) and non-carriers (anti-HBsAg), but does not distinguish between them. Average wholesale price of 3 dose vaccine regimen is $160; usual cost of serologic testing for anti-HBs or anti-HBc is $12-$20.

Prevalence of hepatitis B serologic markers

Population group	Prevalence of serologic markers of HBV infection	
	HBsAg (%)	Any marker(%)
Immigrants/refugees from areas of high HBV endemicity	13	70-85
Alaskan Natives/Pacific Islanders	5-15	40-70
Clients in institutions for the developmentally disabled	10-20	35-80
Users of illicit parenteral drugs	7	60-80
Sexually active homosexual men	6	35-80
Household contacts of HBV carriers	3-6	30-60
Patients of hemodialysis units	3-10	20-80
Health-care workers - frequent blood contact	1-2	15-30
Prisoners (male)	1-8	10-80
Staff of institutions for the developmentally disabled	1	10-25

(continued)

| | Prevalence of serologic markers of HBV infection | |
Population group	HBsAg (%)	Any marker(%)
Heterosexuals with multiple partners	0.5	5-20
Health-care workers - no or infrequent blood contact	0.3	3-10
General population (NHANES II)		
Blacks	0.9	14
Whites	0.2	3

(6)   <u>Side-effects</u>: Pain at injection site (3-29%) and fever > 37.7°C (1-6%). Note: These side effects are no more frequent than in placebo recipients in controlled studies. Experience in over 4 million adults shows rare cases of Guillain-Barré syndrome with plasma-derived vaccine and no serious side effects with recombinant vaccines. Adverse reactions should be reported to 1-800-822-7967.

(7)   <u>Vaccine efficacy</u>: 80-95% for preventing HBV infection and virtually 100% if protective antibody response (≥ 10 mIU/mL is achieved

(8)   <u>Candidates for vaccination</u>

     a.   Health care workers who perform tasks involving contact with blood or bloody fluids. This should be done during training before contact with blood.

     b.   Public safety personnel who perform tasks involving contact with blood or bloody fluids. If exposure is infrequent, consider timely post-exposure prophylaxis.

     c.   Clients* and staff of institutions for developmentally disabled. For nonresidential day care of developmentally disabled, the staff should be vaccinated and clients "should have consideration of vaccination"

     d.   Hemodialysis patients*, preferably early in the course of renal disease since patients with uremia or receiving dialysis are less likely to respond.

     e.   Patients who receive clotting factor concentrates*

     f.   Adoptees, foster children or unaccompanied minors* from countries where HBV is endemic. If screening serology shows HBsAg, other family members should be vaccinated.

     g.   International travelers if 1) travel includes > 6 mo in HBV endemic area plus close contact with local population or 2) travel involves contact with blood or sexual contact with high risk residents. Vaccination should begin at least 6 mo. before travel; the alternative is the 4-dose schedule with 3 doses in 2 months

     h.   Parenteral drug abusers* who are susceptible; documentation of antiHBsAg response recommended for those with HIV infection

     i.   Sexually active gay men*; documentation of anti-HBsAg response recommended for those with HIV infection

     j.   Sexually active heterosexual men and women who 1) have recently acquired STDs, 2) prostitutes and 3) more then one partner in prior 6 months

     k.   Inmates of long-term correctional facilities*

     l.   Household and sexual contacts of HBsAg carriers*

*   *Indicates categories when prevaccination screening for susceptibility is clearly cost effective*

(continued)

(9)   Pregnant women (MMWR 40:RR-13, 1991). Risk of HBV transmission from HBsAg positive pregnant woman to infant is 10-85% depending on HBsAg status. Perinatal infection has a 90% risk of chronic HBV infection and 25% mortality due to liver disease -- cirrhosis or hepatocellular carcinoma. Children who do not acquire HBV perinatally are at increased risk for person-to-person spread during the first 5 years. Over 90% of these infections can be prevented using active and passive immunizations.

    Recommendations: All pregnant women should be tested for HBsAg during an early prenatal visit; infants born to HBsAg positive mothers should receive HBIG (0.5 ml) 1M x 1 (preferably within 12 hrs of delivery) and HB vaccine (0.5 ml) 1M x 3 (5 μg recombinant vaccine) at 0 time (concurrent with HBIG) at 1-2 mo. and at 6 mo. Test infants for HBsAg and anti-HBs at 12-15 mo.

(10)   Post-exposure vaccination (MMWR 40:RR-13,1991)
    a.   Acute exposure to blood
        Definition of exposure: percutaneous (needlestick, laceration or bite) or permucosal (ocular or mucous membrane) exposure to blood. Recommendations depend on HBsAg status of source and vaccination/vaccine response of exposed person. Note: HBIG, when indicated, should be given as soon as possible and value beyond 7 days post-exposure is unclear.

Recommendations for postexposure prophylaxis for percutaneous or permucosal exposure to hepatitis B, United States

	Treatment when source is:		
Exposed person	HBsAg* positive	HBsAg negative	Source not tested or unknown
Unvaccinated	HBIG^T x 1$_5$ and initiate HB^4 vaccine**	Initiate HB vaccine**	Initiate HB vaccine**
Previously vaccinated Known responder	Test exposed for anti-HBs^{TT} 1. If adequate,§§ no treatment 2. If inadequate, HB vaccine booster dose	No treatment	No treatment
Known nonresponder	HBIG x 2 or HBIG x 1 plus 1 HB vaccine	No treatment	If known high-risk source, may treat as if source were HBsAg positive
Response unknown	Test exposed for anti-HBs 1. If inadequate,§§ HBIG x 1 plus HB vaccine booster dose 2. If adequate, no treatment	No treatment	Test exposed for anti-HBs 1. If inadequate, HB vaccine booster dose 2. If adequate, no treatment

*HBsAg = Hepatitis B surface antigen.
^{T}HBIG = Hepatitis B immune globulin.
§HBIG dose 0.06 mL/kg IM.
^{4}HB = Hepatitis B.
**For HB vaccine dose, see page 93.
^{TT}Antibody to hepatitis B surface antigen.
§§Adequate anti-HBs is 10 SRU by radioimmunoassay or positive by enzyme immunoassay.

(continued)

b. Post-exposure immunoprophylaxis with other types of exposures (MMWR 40:RR13, pg 9, 1991)

Type of Exposure	Immunoprophylaxis	Comment
Perinatal (HBsAg positive mother)	HBIG + vaccination	HBIG plus vaccine within 12 hrs of birth
Sexual contact - Acute HBV	HBIG (0.06 ml/kg IM) ± vaccination	HBIG efficacy 75%; all susceptible partners should receive HBIG and start vaccination within 14 days of last exposure; testing susceptibility with anti-HBc recommended if it does not delay prophylaxis >14 days. Vaccination is optimal if exposed person is not in a high risk category and sex partner is HBsAg negative at 3 months
Sexual contact - Chronic carrier (HBsAg x 6 mo.)	Vaccination*	
Household contact - Acute HBV	None unless there is sexual contact or blood exposure (sharing tooth-brushes, razors, etc.)	With known exposure: HBIG ± vaccination
Household contact - Chronic carrier (HBsAg x 6 mo.)	Vaccination*	

* 1 ml IM x 3 at 0, 1, and 6 months

PROPHYLACTIC ANTIBIOTICS IN SURGERY

Antimicrobial Agents in Surgery (Adapted from the Medical Letter 31:105-108,1989 and Kaiser AB: N Engl J Med 315:1129-1138,1986; Rev Infect Dis Suppl 10, 13:S 779, 1991; Mayo Clin Proc 67:288, 1992)

Type of Surgery	Preferred regimen	Alternative	Comment
CARDIOTHORACIC Cardiovascular: Coronary by-pass; valve surgery	Cefazolin 2 gm IV pre-op (and 6qh x 48h)* Cefuroxime 1.5 gm IV ± q6-8h x 48h)*	Vancomycin** 15 mg/kg IV pre-op, after initiation of by-pass (10 mg/kg) (and q8h x 48h)	Single doses appear to be as effective as multiple doses providing high serum concentrations are maintained throughout the procedure (Antimicrob Ag Chemother 29-744, 1986). Some now use vancomycin routinely.
Pacemaker insertion	Cefazolin as above (see comments)	No alternative	Single doses appear to be as effective as multiple doses. Prophylaxis advocated only for centers with high infection rates.
Peripheral vascular surgery Abd. aorta and legs	Cefazolin 1-2 gm IV pre-op (± 1 gm q6h x 48h)*	Vancomycin** 15 mg/kg (and q8h x 48 h) Cefuroxime 1.5 gm IV q8h x 3	Recommended for procedures on abdominal aorta and procedures on leg that include groin incision. Some recommend prophylaxis for any implantation of prosthetic material or vascular access in hemodialysis (Ann Surg 188:283, 1978).
Carotid or brachial artery	None	Cefoxitin 1 gm IV	
Thoracic surgery: lobectomy, pneumonectomy	Cefazolin 1-2 gm IV pre-op (± 1 gm q6h x 48h)*		Optimal duration is unknown. Antibiotic prophylaxis is not recommended for thoracic trauma or chest tube insertion. Efficacy is not established (RID 13, Suppl 10:S869, 1991).
GASTROINTESTINAL Gastric surgery	Cefazolin 1-2 gm IV pre-op	Clindamycin 600 mg IV + gentamicin 1.7 mg/kg	Advocated only for high risk - bleeding ulcer, gastric cancer, gastric by-pass and percutaneous endoscopic gastrostomy. Prophylactic antibiotics are not indicated for uncomplicated duodenal ulcer surgery.

(continued)

Type of Surgery	Preferred regimen	Alternative	Comment
Biliary tract	Cefazolin 1-2 gm IV pre-op	Ampicillin 1 gm IV ± Gentamicin 1.7 mg/kg pre-op and q8h x 3	Advocated only for high risk - acute cholecystitis, obstructive jaundice, common duct stones, age over 70 yrs.
Colorectal and small bowel	Neomycin 1 gm po and erythromycin 1 gm po at 1 pm, 2 pm and 11 pm the day before surgery (19,18 and 11 hrs pre-op)	Cefoxitin 2 gm IV or Clindamycin 600-900 mg IV plus gentamicin 1.7 mg/kg IV or Metronidazole 1 gm IV plus gentamicin 1.7 mg/kg IV	Some advocate the combined use of an oral and parenteral prep, especially for low anterior resection. Some advocate 3 subsequent doses of parenteral agents at 8 hr intervals. Oral prep with metronidazole + neomycin or kanamycin are probably as effective as erythromycin + neomycin (RID 13, Suppl 10:S815, 1991).
Penetrating trauma abdomen	Cefoxitin 2 gm IV pre-op or Clindamycin 600 mg IV plus gentamicin 1.7 mg/kg pre-op	Antipseudomonad penicillin, ticarcillin-clavulanate or any combination of an aminoglycoside + metronidazole or clindamycin	Patients with intestinal perforation should receive these agents for 2-5 days. Most studies use suboptimal doses of aminoglycosides (RID 13, Suppl 10:S847, 1991).
Appendectomy	Cefoxitin 2 gm IV pre-op (and 1-5 days post-op - see comments)	Metronidazole 1 gm IV or clindamycin 600-900 mg IV plus gentamicin 1.7 mg/kg	For perforated or gangrenous appendix continue regimen for 3-5 days. For non-perforated appendix 1-4 doses are adequate (RID 13, Suppl 10:S813, 1991).
Laparotomy, lysis of adhesions, splenectomy, etc. without GI tract surgery	None		
GYNECOLOGY AND OBSTETRICS			
Vaginal and abdominal hysterectomy	Cefazolin 1-2 gm IV pre-op (and q6h x 2)*	Doxycycline 200 mg IV or doxycycline 100 mg po hs 3-4 hr pre-op	Single dose appears to be as effective as multiple doses. Recommendation for radical hysterectomy is cefazolin 1-2 gm pre-op (RID 13, Suppl 10:S821, 1991).
Cesarean section	Cefazolin 2 gm or ampicillin 2 gm IV after clamping cord (and q6h x2)*	Cefotetan 2 gm IV after clamping cord	Advocated primarily for high risk - active labor, premature rupture of membranes, but low risk patients may also benefit (RID 13, Suppl 10:S821, 1991). (continued)

Type of Surgery	Preferred regimen	Alternative	Comment
Abortion	Doxycycline 200 mg po before and 100 mg po 12 hrs later	Doxycycline 300-400 mg po Metronidazole 400 mg x 3 doses in perioperative period period	For patients with N. gonorrhoeae or C trachomatis, treat STD with minimum delay in abortion (Am J Ob Gyn 150:689, 1984 1984).
Hysterosalpingography	Doxycycline 200 mg po pre-procedure		(RID 13, Suppl 10:S845, 1991)
Placement of IUD	Doxycycline 200 mg po pre-procedure		(Brit J Ob Gyn 97:412, 1990)
Cervical cerclage	Cefazolin 2 gm IV pre-procedure		(Am J Ob Gyn 141:1065, 1981)
Cystocele or rectocele repair	None		
Tubal ligation	None		
HEAD AND NECK Tonsillectomy ± adenoidectomy	None		Controlled studies are limited.
Rhinoplasty	None		
Major surgery with entry via oral cavity or pharynx	Clindamycin 900 mg IV ± gentamicin 1.7 mg/kg IV pre-op and q6h x 1-2	Cefazolin 2 gm IV pre-op	Clindamycin study (J Otolaryng 19:197, 1990) Controlled study shows cefazolin dose of 2 gm superior to 0.5 gm (Ann Surg 207:108,1988).
ORTHOPEDIC SURGERY Joint replacement	Cefazolin 1-2 gm IV pre-op (± 1 gm q6h x 3 doses)*	Vancomycin** 1 gm IV Cefamandole is as effective as cefazolin	Cefazolin dose should be 2 gm for knee replacement with tourniquet (Orthop Rev 18:694, 1989). Antibiotic-impregnated cement appears to be effective (Int Orthop 11:241, 1987).

(continued)

Type of Surgery	Preferred regimen	Alternative	Comment
Open reduction of fracture/ internal fixation	Cefazolin 1 gm IV (± 1 gm q6h x 3 doses)*		Nafcillin or cephalothin x 48-72 hr appears effective for preventing post-op wound infections in closed hip fractures (J Bone Joint Surg 62A:457, 1980).
Compound fracture	Cefazolin 1-2 gm IV q8h x 5-10 days or Nafcillin 1-2 gm q4h	Vancomycin 1 gm IV q12h Clindamycin 900 mg IV q8h	Start treatment immediately and continue 5-10 days.
Amputation of leg	Cefoxitin 1-2 gm IV within 1 hr (± 2 gm q6h x 48h)*	Cefazolin 1-2 gm IV (± 1 gm q6h x 48h)*	(J Bone & Joint Surg 67:800, 1985)
NEUROSURGERY			
Cerebrospinal fluid shunt	Trimethoprim 160 mg plus sulfamethoxazole 800 mg IV pre-op and q12 h x 3 doses	Nafcillin or oxacillin ± rifampin x 1-2 days	Efficacy of antimicrobials not established (Ped Neurosci 15:111, 1989; RID 13, Suppl 10:S858, 1991)
Craniotomy	Vancomycin 1 gm IV ± gentamicin 1.5 mg/kg x 1	Clindamycin 300 mg IV and at 4 hr; cefazolin 1-2 gm plus gentamicin 1.5 mg/kg x 1; cefotaxime 2 gm x 2 repeated at 6 hr	Efficacy not clearly established, but advocated even for low risk procedures except where infection rates are <0.1% (Neurosurg 24:401, 1989)
Spinal surgery	None		
Ocular	Gentamicin or tobramycin topically for 2-24 hrs before surgery	Neomycin, gramicidin and polymyxin B topically 2-24 hrs pre-op	Some give subconjunctival injection (gentamicin, 10-20 mg ± cefazolin 100 mg) at end of surgery.
UROLOGY			
Prostatectomy Sterile urine	None (see Comment)		Cefazolin sometimes advocated for open prostatectomy (Urol Clin N Amer 17:595, 1990).
Infected urine	Continue agent active in vitro or give single pre-operative dose		Sterilization of urine before surgery is preferred.

(continued)

101

Type of Surgery	Preferred regimen	Alternative	Comment
Prostatic biopsy	None		
Dilation of urethra	None		
MISCELLANEOUS			
Inguinal hernia repair	Cefazolin 1gm IV pre-op (see Comment)		One study showed benefit of cefonicid, 1 gm IV 30 min. pre-op (R. Platt et al. NEJM 322:153,1990); sequel study showed diverse antibiotics (primarily cefazolin) in high risk patients was beneficial (R. Platt et al, JID 166:556, 1992).
Mastectomy	Cefazolin 1 gm IV pre-op (see Comment)		One study showed benefit of cefonicid for breast surgery (R. Platt et al. NEJM 322: 153,1990); sequel study (see above). Greatest risks were radical mastectomy and axillary node dissection.
Traumatic wound	Cefazolin 1 gm IV q8h		

* Single dose generally considered adequate; for dirty surgery, treatment should be continued 5-10 days.

** Vancomycin preferred for hospitals with a high rate of wound infections caused by methicillin-resistant S. aureus or S. epidermidis, and for patients with allergy to penicillins or cephalosporins.

PREVENTION OF BACTERIAL ENDOCARDITIS
Recommendations by the American Heart Association
(JAMA 264:2919,1990)

CARDIAC CONDITIONS

<u>Cardiac conditions considered at risk</u> (not all inclusive)
- Prosthetic cardiac valve, including bioprosthetic and homograph valves
- Prior endocarditis
- Most congenital malformations
- Rheumatic and other acquired valvular dysfunction
- Hypertrophic cardiomyopathy
- Mitral valve prolapse with valve regurgitation (Patients with mitral valve prolapse associated with thickening and/or redundancy of the valve may be at increased risk, esp. men $\geq$ 45 yrs.)

<u>Prophylaxis not recommended</u>
- Isolated secundum atrial septal defect
- Surgical repair without residual > 6 months of secundum atrial defect, ventricular septal defect or patent ductus
- Prior coronary by-pass surgery
- Mitral valve defect without regurgitation (see above)
- Physiologic or functional heart murmurs
- Prior rheumatic fever without valve disease
- Cardiac pacemakers and implanted defibrillators
- Prior Kawasaki disease without valve dysfunction

PROCEDURES

<u>Procedures that confer risk and require prophylaxis</u>
- Dental procedures that induce gingival or mucosal bleeding including professional cleansing
- Tonsillectomy and adenoidectomy
- Surgical procedures that involve the intestinal or respiratory mucosa
- Bronchoscopy with a rigid bronchoscope
- Sclerotherapy for esophageal varicies
- Esophageal dilatation
- Gallbladder surgery
- Cystoscopy
- Urethral dilatation
- Urethral catheterization with urinary tract infection (include treatment for likely urinary pathogen)
- Urinary tract surgery if urinary tract infection (include treatment for likely urinary pathogen)
- Prostatic surgery
- Incision and drainage of infected tissue (include treatment for likely pathogen)
- Vaginal hysterectomy
- Vaginal delivery in presence of infection (include treatment for likely pathogens)

Endocarditis prophylaxis not recommended*

    Dental procedures not likely to cause bleeding such as adjustment of
        orthodontic appliances or fillings above the gum line
    Injection of local intraoral anesthetic except intraligamentary injections
    Shedding primary teeth
    Tympanostomy tube insertion
    Bronchoscopy with flexible bronchoscopy with or without biopsy
    Endoscopy of GI tract with or without biopsy
    Cardiac catheterization
    Cesarean section
    Absence of infection for urethral catheterization, dilatation and curettage,
        uncomplicated vaginal delivery, therapeutic abortion, sterilization
        procedures or insertion or removal of intrauterine device

*   Patients at high risk may receive prophylactic antibiotics even for low risk
    procedures involving the lower respiratory, genitourinary or gastrointestinal
    tracts; these include patients with prosthetic valves, a history of endo-
    carditis or surgically constucted systemic - pulmonary shunts or conduits.

RECOMMENDED REGIMENS

Recommended regimens for dental, oral and upper respiratory procedures

Standard
    Amoxicillin: 3.0 gm orally 1 hr pre-procedure; then 1.5 gm 6 hr after first
    dose

Amoxicillin or penicillin allergy
    Erythromycin: Erythromycin ethylsuccinate, 800 mg or erythromycin
    stearate, 1 gm po 2 hr pre-procedure; then 1/2 initial dose 6 hr later
    Clindamycin: 300 mg orally 1 hr pre-procedure; 150 mg 6 hr later

Unable to take oral medications
    Ampicillin: 2.0 gm IM or IV 30 min pre-procedure; 1.0 gm ampicillin IM or
    IV or 1.5 gm amoxicillin orally 6 hr later

Amoxicillin or penicillin allergy and unable to take oral meds
    Clindamycin: 300 mg IV 30 min pre-procedure; then 150 mg IV or po 6 hr
    later

Patient considered high risk* and not a candidate for standard regimen
    Ampicillin: 2 gm IV plus gentamicin, 1.5 mg/kg 30 min pre-procedure; 1.5 gm
    amoxicillin po 6 hr later or repeat parenteral regimen 8 hr later

Amoxicillin or penicillin allergy in patient considered high risk*
    Vancomycin: 1 gm IV over 1 hr starting 1 hr pre-procedure; no repeat dose

<u>**Regimens for genitourinary and gastrointestinal procedures**</u>

> <u>Standard</u>
> Ampicillin, 2 gm IV or IM <u>plus</u> gentamicin, 1.5 mg/kg (not to exceed 80 mg)
> 30 min pre-procedure; amoxicillin, 1.5 gm po 6 hr later or repeat
> parenteral regimen 8 hr later
>
> <u>Ampicillin or penicillin allergy</u>
> Vancomycin, 1 gm IV over 1 hr plus gentamicin, 1.5 mg/kg IV or IM 1 hr
> pre-procedure; may be repeated once 8 hr later
>
> <u>Alternate low risk patient* regimen</u>
> Amoxicillin, 3.0 gm po 1 hr pre-procedure; 1.5 gm 6 hr later

* High risk: Prosthetic valve, history of endocarditis or surgically
  constructed systemic - pulmonary shunts or conduits

PROPHYLAXIS FOR DENTAL PATIENTS WITH PROSTHETIC JOINTS

1. Analysis by Gillespie showed no evidence of benefit (Infect Dis Clin N Amer 4:465,
    1990).

2. Position statement of the American Academy of Oral Medicine (Oral Surg, Oral Med,
    Oral Path 66:430, 1988):

    > It is the opinion of the American Academy of
    > Oral Medicine that there is insufficient scientific
    > evidence to support routine antibiotic prophylaxis
    > for patients with prosthetic joints who are
    > receiving dental care. Therefore it appears that a
    > blanket recommendation for antibiotic coverage
    > would be inappropriate at this time. This decision
    > should be determined by the dentist's clinical
    > judgment or in consultation with the patient's
    > surgeon.

3. Position of C.W. Norden (RID 13, S10, S845, 1991): Antibiotic prophylaxis is not
    recommended for routine dental work. Antibiotic prophylaxis is recommended for
    such individuals with periodontal or potential dental infections using an oral
    cephalosporin or clindamycin 1 hr before dental work and two subsequent doses.

PREVENTION OF DISEASES ASSOCIATED WITH TRAVEL

A. **INTERNATIONAL TRAVELER'S HOTLINE**

CDC 24 hr/day automated telephone system with advice for international travelers concerning malaria, food and water precautions, traveler's diarrhea, immunizations for children < 2 years, pregnant travelers disease outbreaks and vaccine requirements by geographic area. Call (404) 639-1610. Health Information for International Travel 1990 edition is available at $5.00/copy from Superintendent of Documents, U.S. Government Printing Office, Washington, D.C. 20402, (202) 783-3238, stock no. 017-023-00187-6.

B. **TRAVELER'S DIARRHEA (Adapted from NIH Consensus Development Panel, 1985. See JAMA 253:2700,1985; and Medical Letter 34:41-44,1992)**

<u>Risk</u>: <u>High risk areas</u> (incidence 20-50%): developing countries of Latin America, Africa, Middle East and Asia

<u>Intermediate risk</u>: Southern Europe and some Caribbean islands

<u>Low risk</u>: Canada, Northern Europe, Australia, New Zealand, United States

Agents

<u>Bacteria</u>	<u>Viruses</u>
<u>E. coli</u> (enterotoxigenic,* enteroinvasive, enteroadherent)	Norwalk agent
	Rotavirus (?)
<u>Salmonella</u>	
<u>Shigella</u>	<u>Parasites</u>
<u>Campylobacter jejuni</u>	<u>Giardia lamblia</u>
<u>Aeromonas hydrophila</u>	<u>Entamoeba histolytica</u>
<u>Plesiomonas shigelloides</u>	Cryptosporidia
<u>Vibrio cholerae</u> (non-01)	
<u>Vibrio fluvialis</u>	
<u>Vibrio parahaemolytica</u>	

* Most common

Prevention

Food and beverages: Risky foods - Raw vegetables, raw meat or raw seafood, tapwater, ice, unpasteurized milk and dairy products and unpeeled fruit; safe foods -- cooked foods that are still hot, fruits peeled by traveler, carbonated bottled water and other beverages.

Preventative agents with documented efficacy (efficacy of 50-85%)

Doxycycline: 100 mg po/day (photosensitivity reactions)

Sulfa-trimethoprim: 1 DS (double strength) tab po/day (serious skin reactions and hematological reactions reported).

Trimethoprim: 200 mg po/day

Ciprofloxacin: 500 mg po/day

Norfloxacin: 400 mg po/day

Bismuth subsalicylate (Pepto-Bismol): 2 300 mg tabs qid

<u>Treatment</u>

  <u>Oral intake</u> to maintain fluid and electrolyte balance:
    Potable fruit juice, caffeine-free soft drinks, salted crackers.
  For severe symptoms: WHO Oral Rehydration Salts may be formulated
    by - <u>Ingredients/L or qt. water</u>
    NaCl: 3.5 gm (3/4 tsp)
    $NaHCO_3$ (baking soda): 2.5 gm (1 tsp)
    KCl: 1.5 g (1 cup orange juice or 2 bananas)
    Sucrose (table sugar): 40 gm (4 level tbsp)
    May be ordered from: Jianas Bros, 2533 S.W. Blvd, Kansas City,
    MO; phone (816) 412-2880, fax (816) 421-2883
  <u>Antimotility drugs</u>
    Diphenoxylate (Lomotil) (2.5 mg tabs po 3-4 x daily)
    Loperamide (Imodium) (4 mg, then 2 mg after each loose stool to
      maximum of 16 mg/day)
    Bismuth subsalicylate (Pepto-Bismol) (30 ml or 2 tabs q 30 min x 8)
  <u>Antimicrobial agents</u> (empiric selection)
    Sulfa-trimethoprim: 1 DS tab bid x 5 days or 2 DS x 1
    Trimethoprim: 200 mg po bid x 5 days
    Doxycycline: 100 mg po bid x 5 days
    Ciprofloxacin: 500 mg po bid x 5 days
    Norfloxacin: 400 mg po bid x 5 days
    <u>Combination</u>: Sulfa-trimethoprim, 1 DS bid x 3 days <u>plus</u> Loperamide
      (above dose), appears more effective than either drug alone
      (JAMA 263:257,1990)

<u>Panel Recommendations</u>
1. Prophylactic drugs are not recommended (but prophylactic anti-
    microbial agents appear most cost-effective; see Reves RR et al:
    Arch Intern Med 148:2421,1988).

2. Travelers to risk areas should carry antimotility drugs (diphen-
    oxylate or loperamide) or bismuth subsalicylate <u>and</u> an antimicrobial
    agent (sulfa-trimethoprim, trimethoprim, doxycycline or flruoquinolone).
    a. Mild diarrhea (less than 3 stools/day, without blood, pus or
        fever): Loperamide, diphenoxylate or bismuth subsalicylate in
        doses noted above.
    b. Moderate or severe diarrhea: Antimicrobial agent (regimens
        noted above -- but some feel these are antiquated).
        Note: Medical Letter Consultants (34:41, 1992) recommends combined
        *   treatment for symptomatic adults using Imodium plus TMP-SMX 1*
        *   DS bid, ciprofloxacin 500 mg bid, norfloxacin 400 mg bid or*
        *   ofloxacin 300 mg bid for up to 3 days.*
        Many underdeveloped countries now have high rates of resistance among
        Enterotoxigenic <u>E</u>. <u>coli</u>, Shigella and other enteric bacterial pathogens. This
        accounts for the preference for fluoroquinolones for travel to many
        countries; TMP-SMX should still be appropriate for Mexico. Children
        <18 yrs should not take fluoroquinolones; furazolidine is a possible
        substitute.
    c. Persistent diarrhea with serious fluid loss, fever or stools
        showing blood or mucus: Seek medical attention.

3. Instruct patients regarding:
    Dietary precautions for prevention
    Oral rehydration
    Use of drugs including side effects

Cholera epidemic: South and Central America (see JAMA 267:1495, 1992)
        The cholera epidemic has involved primarily Peru (297,000 cases in 1991),
Ecuador (42,000), Columbia (11,000), Guatemala (2,900), Mexico (2,400), Panama (1,000),
El Salvador (900) and Brazil (600). Travelers should be warned to a) avoid raw or
partially cooked seafood, b) drink only boiled or bottled, carbonated water, c) avoid food
or drinks from street vendors and d) avoid uncooked vegetables. Cholera vaccine is
marginally effective and is not recommended. There are no cholera vaccine requirements
with entry or exit into Peru, Equador or the U.S. Call the traveler's hotline for updated
review: (404) 332-4559.

C. **IMMUNIZATIONS:**   See pages 87-88

D. **MALARIA PROPHYLAXIS AND TREATMENT (MMWR 39:1-10,1990, 40:727, 1991)
    and The Medical Letter on Drugs and Therapeutics 31:13,1990)**

    Centers for Disease Control Malaria Hotline: (404) 332-4555

    Risk areas: Most areas of Central and South America, Hispaniola, sub-
            Saharan Africa, the Indian Subcontinent, Southeast Asia, the Middle
            East and Oceania. During 1980-1990 there were 2,109 cases of
            P. falciparum in U.S. civilians: 1,721 (82%) acquired in sub-Saharan Africa;
            162 (8%) in Asia; 111 (5%) in the Caribbean and South America, and
            115 (5%) in other areas. All 43 cases of fatal infections were acquired in
            Africa south of the Sahara.

    Drug resistance of P. falciparum to chloroquine (CRFP) is probable or
            confirmed in all countries with P. falciparum except Central America -- west of
            the Panama Canal Zone, Mexico, Haiti, the Dominican Republic, and most
            of the Middle East. Resistance to both chloroquine and Fansidar is widespread
            in Thailand, Burma, Cambodia and the Amazon basin area of South America,
            and has been reported in sub-Saharan Africa.

    Advice to travelers
        1. Personal protection:
                Transmission is most common between dusk and dawn.
                Precautions include remaining in well-screened areas and using
                    mosquito nets, clothing that covers most of the body, insect
                    repellent containing DEET on exposed areas, and pyrethrum-
                    containing insect spray for environs and clothing.
        2. Chemoprophylaxis (see Table 1 for doses)
            a. Travel to areas with no chloroquine-resistant P. falciparum:
                    Chloroquine beginning 1-2 weeks before travel and 4 weeks
                    after leaving risk area.
                    Alternative: Hydroxychloroquine (for persons who do not
                    tolerate chloroquine).

b. Travel to areas with chloroquine-resistant P. falciparum:
    Mefloquine, 250 mg as a single dose taken weekly beginning one week
    before travel; prophylaxis is continued weekly during travel in malarious
    areas and for four weeks after leaving such areas.
    <u>Alternatives</u>: Doxycycline beginning 1-2 days before travel
    and for 4 weeks after leaving risk area. Chloroquine advocated for
    persons with contraindication to mefloquine and doxycycline,
    especially pregnant females and children. If chloroquine is
    used, the traveler should take a single dose (Table 2) of
    Fansidar to take for prompt use with a febrile illness if
    professional medical care is not available.
c. Contraindications to mefloquine: pregnant women and travelers with a
    history of epilepsy or psychiatric disorders; rare serious side effects are
    psychosis and seizures.
3. Primaquine: This drug may be given after the traveler has left the
    risk area to prevent relapses due to P. vivax and P. ovale.
    Primaquine prophylaxis is usually given during the last 2 weeks
    of the 4 week period of prophylaxis after exposure. Indications is
    not clear, but best advised when the traveler has prolonged
    exposure, such as missionaries and Peace Corp volunteers. (Primaquine is now
    available from Winthrop Pharmaceuticals and is no longer available from the
    CDC).

Distribution of Malaria and Chloroquine-resistant *Plasmodium falciparum*, 1991

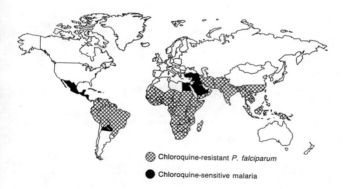

⊗ Chloroquine-resistant *P. falciparum*

● Chloroquine-sensitive malaria

Health Information for International Travel 1992; US Department of Health and Human
Services, June 1992, pg 99.

Doses of antimalarial agents for treatment and prophylaxis

TABLE 1. Drugs used in the prophylaxis of malaria

Drug	Adult dose
Chloroquine phosphate* (Aralen)	300 mg base (500 mg salt) orally, once/week *(Travelers to Africa should also take Proguanil and should carry Fansidar (3 tabs) for empiric treatment of a febrile illness if professional medical care is not available.)*
Hydroxychloroquine sulfate (Plaquenil)	310 mg base (400 mg salt) orally, once/week
Mefloquine (Lariam)	228 mg base (250 mg salt) orally, once/week
Doxycycline*	100 mg orally, once/day
Proguanil	200 mg orally, once/day in combination with weekly chloroquine (not available in U.S.; obtain in Canada, Europe and many African countries)
Primaquine	15 mg base (26.3 mg salt) orally, once/day for 14 days

*   Alternatives to Mefloquine for travel to countries where drug resistant
      P. falciparum is endemic

TABLE 2. Drug used in the presumptive treatment of malaria

Drug	Adult dose
Pyrimethamine-sulfadoxine (Fansidar*)	3 tablets (75 mg pyrimethamine and 1500 mg sulfadoxine), orally as a single dose

Treatment of Malaria

(See pages 137-138) revised guidelines for quinidine gluconate for severe P. falciparum infection (MMWR 40 RR-4:21, 1991).

1. Quinidine gluconate has replaced quinine dihydrochloride as the preferred agent for parenteral treatment of severe infections caused by P. falciparum.
2. Indications for parenteral treatment: a) prominent vomiting, b) signs or symptoms of neurologic dysfunction, or c) peripheral asexual parasitemia (parasite index) of ≥5% of red blood cells.
3. Administration: loading dose of 10 mg (6.2 mg quinidine base)/kg given over 1-2 hrs; then constant infusion with 0.02 mg/kg/min (quinidine gluconate).
4. Monitor in ICU with attention to hydration, blood glucose, EKGs and quinidine levels. Slow infusion if levels >6 mcg/mL, QT >0.6 sec or QRS widened to >25% of baseline.
5. Continue IV treatment until parasitic index is <1% and/or oral meds tolerated. Treatment is continued (oral plus parenteral) for 3-7 days; additional tetracycline (250 mg po q 6h x 7 days) is recommended.

TREATMENT OF FUNGAL SYSTEMIC INFECTIONS

Adapted from NIAID Mycosis Study Group Reports (Ann Intern Med 98:13,1983; Ann Intern Med 103:861,1985; Chest 93:848,1987), recommendations of the American Thoracic Society (Amer Rev Respir Dis 138:1078,1988), consultants of the Medical Letter 32:58,1990, and Mayo Clin Proc 67:69, 1992

Fungus	Form	Preferred Treatment	Dose, alternative agent(s), comment
Aspergillus	Bronchopulmonary	Corticosteroids	
	Aspergilloma (fungus ball)	Usually none	Massive hemoptysis - surgical resection with perioperative amphotericin. Progressive invasive disease - amphotericin B IV, 30-40 mg/kg
	Invasive pulmonary or extrapulmonary	Amphotericin B IV	Total dose: 30-40 mg/kg Most patients require rapid advance in daily dose to 0.5-1.0 mg/kg; for neutropenic patients the usual dose is 1.0-1.5 mg/kg Flucytosine or rifampin sometimes added, but efficacy is not established Itraconazole appears promising: 100-400 mg/day
Blastomyces	Acute pulmonary (immunocompetent)	Usually none	
	Acute pulmonary - severe or progressive	Itraconazole po Ketoconazole po	200-400 mg/day 400 mg/day; with unfavorable clinical response - increase to 600-800 mg/day Alternative: Amphotericin B IV, 30-40 mg/kg
	Chronic pulmonary	Itraconazole po Ketoconazole po	200-400 mg/day 400 mg/day, up to 600-800 mg/day
	Disseminated (immunocompetent without renal or CNS involvement)	Itraconazole po Ketoconazole po	200-400 mg/day 400 mg/day, up to 600-800 mg/day
	Disseminated with GU involvement	Itraconazole po Ketoconazole po	200-400 mg/day 600-800 mg/day Alternative: Amphotericin B IV, 30-40 mg/kg (continued)

Fungus	Form	Preferred Treatment	Dose, alternative agent(s), comment
Blastomyces (continued)	Disseminated Immunosuppressed or CNS involvement	Amphotericin B IV Itraconazole po	Total dose: 30-40 mg/kg 200-400 mg/day
Candida	Localized - mucocutaneous		
	Oral (thrush)	Nystatin S&S Clotrimazole troche Ketoconazole po Fluconazole po	500,000 units 3-5x/day x 10-14 days 10 mg troches 3-5x/day x 10-14 days 200 mg po bid, 5-7 days 200 mg, then 100 mg/day (50 mg/day is also effective) AIDS: Continue any of above regimens indefinitely or use prn
	Vaginal	Miconazole topical Nystatin topical Clotrimazole topical Ketoconazole po Fluconazole po Itraconazole po	Intravaginal cream (2%) or suppository (100 mg) qd x 7 days Intravaginal cream or tablet (100,000 units) bid x 7 days Intravaginal cream (1%) or tablet (100 mg) qd x 7 days (available without prescription) 200 mg po bid x 5-7 days 150 mg po x 1 400 mg po, 200 mg/day x 2 days
	Cutaneous - intertrigo balanitis, paronychia	Nystatin, ciclopirox, clotrimazole, miconazole,	Topical treatment, keep area dry and clean with maximal exposure to air
	Chronic mucocutaneous	Ketoconazole po	200 mg po bid x 3-12 months Alternative: Intermittent amphotericin B ± topical anti-Candida agent or fluconazole
	Esophageal	Fluconazole	100 mg po qd (up to 400 mg/day) x > 3wks (and >2 wks post-resolution of symptoms) Alternative: Amphotericin B (0.2-0.4 mg/kg/day) x 7-14 days or ketoconazole, 200 mg po bid x 10-21 days AIDS: Maintenance fluconazole 100-200 mg po qd (continued)

112

Fungus	Form	Preferred Treatment	Dose, alternative agent(s), comment
Candida (*continued*)	Peritoneal (peritoneal dialysis)	Amphotericin B topical or IV ± flucytosine	Topical treatment: 2-4 ug/L in dialysate fluid Flucytosine: 50-100 mg/L dialysate fluid Catheter may require removal
	Peritoneal - (post op, perforated viscus, etc)	Amphotericin B IV Fluconazole	Total dose: 3-10 mg/kg (Indications to treat are often unclear) 200-400 mg/day
	Urinary	No treatment or amphotericin B topically	Remove catheter or use for bladder instillations of amphotericin B: 50 mg/L in D5W and infuse 1 L/day via closed triple lumen catheter x 5 days Alternative: Flucytosine: 25/mg/kg po qid or fluconazole: 200 mg po/day Fungus ball: Surgical removal and amphotericin B IV
	Bloodstream Septicemia	Amphotericin B IV	Total dose: 3-10 mg/kg Remove or change IV lines Line sepsis: Remove line and treat with amphotericin B (≥3 mg/kg) ± flucytosine
		Fluconazole	400 mg, then 200 mg/day
	Disseminated or metastatic (deep organ infection)	Amphotericin B IV ± flucytosine po	Total dose: 20-40 mg/kg (0.3-0.8 mg/kg/day) 150 mg/kg/day (flucytosine) Indications for flucytosine: Normal marrow and renal function or clinical deterioration with amphotericin B Alternative: Fluconazole: 200-400 mg/day (best results with peritonitis, UTI, and hepatosplenic abscesses for patients who refuse or cannot tolerate amphotericin B)

(continued)

113

Fungus	Form	Preferred Treatment	Dose, alternative agent(s), comment
Candida (continued)	Endocarditis	Amphotericin B IV ± flucytosine po	Total dose: 30-40 mg/kg 150 mg/kg/day (flucytosine) Surgery required
Chromoblastomycosis		Flucytosine po	100 mg/kg/day x 8-12 wks Alternatives: Ketoconazole po 400 mg/day x 3-6 mo, thiabendazole, intra-lesional amphotericin B or combination of flucytosine and one of these; Itraconazole promising, 100-200 mg/day Small lesions usually respond to flucytosine; large lesions should be surgically excised with perioperative flucytosine
Coccidioides	Pulmonary - acute	Usually none	
	Pulmonary - severe, cavitary or progressive infiltrate	Ketoconazole po Amphotericin B IV Itraconazole po	400-600 mg/day x 6-18 mo. 7-20 mg/kg (amphotericin) 400 mg/day x 6-18 mo Fluconazole: Preliminary experience with 200 mg/day is promising
	Pulmonary cavitary disease - giant cavities (>5 cm), sub-pleural location, serious hemoptysis and secondary infection	Surgical excision	Perioperative amphotericin B often advocated (500 mg)
	Disseminated (non-meningeal, immunocompetent)	Amphotericin B IV	Total dose: 30-40 mg/kg (amphotericin) Alternative is ketoconazole in dose of 400-800 mg/day x 6-18 mo. or longer, but response rates are low, relapse rates in responders is high *Note: Itraconazole: Preliminary results with 400 mg/day x 12 mo are promising* (Lancet 340:648, 1992).
	Disseminated - immuno-suppressed non-meningeal	Amphotericin B IV	Total dose: 30-40 mg/kg Fluconazole: Preliminary results with 400 mg/day are promising. Itraconazole: 400 mg/day is promising

(continued)

Fungus	Form	Preferred Treatment	Dose, alternative agent(s), comment
Coccidioides (continued)	Meningitis	Amphotericin B IV and topically	Total dose: 30-40 mg/kg IV Intrathecal: 0.5-0.7 mg 2x/wk Alternative: Miconazole or ketoconazole (1200-2400 mg/day) ± intrathecal Amphotericin B
Cryptococcus	Pulmonary - stable and immunocompetent	Usually none	Exclude extrapulmonary disease: culture blood, urine and CSF; follow x-rays q 1-2 mo. x 1 yr
	Pulmonary - progressive and/or immunosuppressed host	Amphotericin B IV ± flucytosine	Total dose: 15-20 mg/kg (amphotericin) Alternative for immunocompetent host with progressive pulmonary or extrapulmonary non-meningeal is ketoconazole 200-800 mg po/day
	Extrapulmonary non-meningeal	Amphotericin B ± flucytosine	Total dose: 2-3 gm (amphotericin B) Alternative for immunocompetent patient is ketoconazole 400 mg/day or fluconazole 200 mg/day (up to 400 mg/day) or itraconazole 400 mg/day
	Disseminated including meningeal without AIDS	Amphotericin B ± flucytosine	Standard: Amphotericin (0.3 mg/kg/day) + flucytosine (150 mg/kg/day) x 6 weeks Four week regimen: Immunocompetent host without neurologic complications, pretreatment CSF WBC > 20/mm3 + Ag < 1:32; and post-therapy CSF Ag < 1:8 + neg India ink
	Meningitis AIDS patients	Amphotericin B, 0.5-0.7 mg/kg/day ± flucytosine, (100 mg/kg/day) until 15 mg/kg Amphotericin B + neg CSF culture. Amphotericin B (0.7 mg/kg/day) x 10-14 days, then fluconazole (400 mg/day po) x 8-10 wks, then fluconazole (200 mg/day)	Fluconazole 200-400 mg/day (considered safe for initial treatment only if mental status is normal) Maintenance treatment with fluconazole (200 mg/day) required for all patients. Maintenance dose of amphotericin B (for fluconazole failures) is 1 mg/kg/wk or itraconazole 200-400 mg/day

(continued)

115

Fungus	Form	Preferred Treatment	Dose, alternative agent(s), comment
Histoplasma	Pulmonary - acute ± erythema nosodum	Usually none	Severe/acute: Some recommend amphotericin B (500 mg over 2-3 wks) + corticosteroids or ketoconazole (400 mg/day) x 6 mo.
	Pulmonary - chronic	Itraconazole po Ketoconazole po	200-400 mg/day x 6-12 mo. 400 mg/day x 6-12 mo. (up to 800 mg/day) Amphotericin B (30-40 mg/kg) for patients who are seriously ill, or immunosuppressed (AIDS patients) or fail ketoconazole
	Pulmonary - cavitary Stable, minimal Sx, thin wall cavity	None	
	Persistent, thick walled cavity (>2 mm) or progressive sx	Itraconazole po Ketoconazole po	200-400 mg/day x 6-12 mo. 400 mg/day x 6-12 mo. (up to 800 mg/day) Alternative: Amphotericin B IV, 30-40 mg/kg Surgery for intractable hemoptysis despite medical Rx
	Disseminated - immuno-competent, without CNS involvement	Itraconazole po Ketoconazole po	200-400 mg/day x 6-12 mo. 400 mg/day x 6-12 mo. (up to 800 mg/day) Patients with severe illness, AIDS or immunosuppression should receive amphotericin B
	Disseminated - CNS involvement or immunosuppressed	Amphotericin B IV	Total dose: 30-40 mg/kg AIDS: Amphotericin in dose of 0.5-1.0 gm, then maintenance itraconazole po 400 mg/day or amphotericin B IV 1.0-1.5 mg/kg/wk
	Mediastinal granuloma or fibrosis	Surgical resection if symptomatic	Invasive disease into airways, esophagus, etc (rare): Treat with ketoconazole, itraconazole or amphotericin B
	Ocular	Laser photocoagulation Intraocular steroids Retinal irradiation	Appears to be immune-mediated disease

(continued)

116

Fungus	Form	Preferred Treatment	Dose, alternative agent(s), comment
Paracoccidioides	Pulmonary or mucocutaneous	Ketoconazole po Itraconazole po	200-400 mg/day x 6-12 mo. 100 mg/day x 6 mo. Alternative: Amphotericin B IV, 30-35 mg/kg (preferred for severe disease) or sulfonamides;
Phycomycetes Absidia Mucor (Mucormycosis) Rhizopus	Pulmonary and extrapulmonary including rhinocerebral	Amphotericin B IV	Total dose: 30-40 mg/kg Most patients require rapid increase to daily dose of 0.5-1.0 mg/kg Rhinocerebral: Surgical debridement required
Pseudoallescheria boydii	Sinusitis, endophthalmitis	Ketoconazole po or miconazole IV	200-600 mg/day x 1-12 mo. 200-1200 mg q8h
Sporothrix (Sporotrichosis)	Lymphocutaneous	SSKI po Heat	1 ml (1 gm/ml) tid increasing to 12-15 ml/day x 6-8 wks Alternative: Ketoconazole, 400-800 mg/day or fluconazole, 400 mg/day or itraconazole, 100 mg/day
	Extracutaneous	Amphotericin B IV	Total dose: 30-35 mg/kg (0.5 mg/kg/day) Alternative: Ketoconazole, 400-800 mg/day or fluconazole, 400 mg/day or itraconazole, 100 mg/day

TREATMENT OF DERMATOPHYTIC FUNGAL INFECTIONS

Condition	Agents	Location	Treatment
Tinea corporis (Ringworm)	T. rubrum T. mentagrophytes M. canis E. floccosum	Circular, erythema well demarcated with scaly, vesicular or pustular border Non-hairy skin Pruritic	Topical agents: Miconazole, clotrimazole, econazole, naftifine, ciclopirox bid or ketoconazole, oxiconazole, sulconazole qd for ≥ 4 wks. If no response: griseofulvin x 4 wks
Tinea cruris (Jock itch)	E. floccosum T. rubrum T. mentagrophytes	Erythema and scaly Groin and upper thighs Pruritic	Topical agents as above. Loose fitting clothes. Absorbant powder. Unresponsive cases: griseofulvin x 2-4 wks
Tinea pedis (Athlete's foot)	T. rubrum T. mentagrophytes E. floccosum	Foot, esp fissures between toes; scaly, vesicles, pustules ± nail involvement	Topical agents as above. Keep feet dry and cool. Unresponsive cases: griseofulvin 6-8 wks. Nail involvement: oral griseofulvin or ketoconazole 6-24 mo (until new nail) or itraconazole (100 mg/day) x 3-6 mo.
Tinea capitis (Ringworm -- scalp	T. tonsurans T. mentagrophytes T. verrucosum M. canis	Scaling and erythematous area on scalp with broken hairs and localized alopecia	Griseofulvin x 4-8 wks + 2.5% selenium sulfide shampoo 2x/wk. Alternative to griseofulvin is ketoconazole
Tinea versicolor	Malassezia furfur	Scaling oval macular and patchy lesions on upper trunk and arms; dark or light, fail to tan	Topical 2.5% selenium sulfide applied as thin layer over entire body x 1-2 hrs or overnight for 1-2 wks, then monthly x 3; wash off. Alternatives: Topical clotrimazole, econazole, ketoconazole, naftifine or haloprogin or oral ketoconazole

118

TREATMENT OF VIRAL INFECTIONS

A. Herpesvirus Group (Adapted from: Medical Letter 32:73,1990)

Virus	Regimen	Comment
HERPES SIMPLEX		
Genital-primary	<u>Acyclovir</u>: Oral - 200 mg 5 x daily x 10 days; IV - 15 mg/kg/day x 5 days	Mild lesions and symptoms are usually not treated (NEJM 308:916, 1983)
Genital-recurrent	<u>Acyclovir</u>: 200 mg po 5 x daily x 5 days	Initiate during prodrome or at first sign of lesions
Genital-prophylaxis	<u>Acyclovir</u>: 200 mg po, 2-5 x/day or 400 mg po bid	Indicated only with ≥ 6 recurrences/yr. Good efficacy and good safety profile with treatment up to 5 yrs (JAMA 265:747, 1991) Contraindicated in pregnancy
Perirectal	<u>Acyclovir</u>: 400 mg po 5 x daily x 10 days	
Encephalitis	<u>Acyclovir</u>: IV - 10 mg/kg q8h x 10-14 days	(NEJM 314:144, 1986)
Mucocutaneous progressive	<u>Acyclovir</u>: IV - 5-10 mg/kg q8h 7-14 days; oral - 200-400 mg po 5 x/day x 7-14 days or 400 mg 5x/day	AIDS patients often require preventative therapy with acyclovir 200-400 mg po 3-5 x/day indefinitely
Burn wound	<u>Acyclovir</u>: IV - 5 mg/kg q8h x 7 days; oral - 200 mg 5 x/day x 7-14 days	
Prophylaxis - high risk patients	<u>Acyclovir</u>: IV - 5 mg/kg q8h; oral - 200 mg 3-5 x/daily	Organ and bone marrow transplant recipients; treat seropositive patients for 1-3 mo. post-transplant (NEJM 320:1381, 1989)
Keratitis	<u>Trifluridine</u>: Topical (1%) 1 drop q2h up to 9 drops/day (3%) ointment	Ophthalmologist should supervise treatment
Acyclovir - resistant strains	<u>Foscarnet</u>: IV 60 mg/kg q8h	Thymidine kinase deficient strains, usually from immunosuppressed patients unresponsive to acyclovir

(continued)

Virus	Regimen	Comment
VARICELLA-ZOSTER		
Chickenpox, Adult	<u>Acyclovir</u>: 800 mg po 5x/day x 7-10 days	Must treat within 24 hrs of exantham; efficacy established (Ann Intern Med 117:358, 1992)
Chickenpox, Children	<u>Acyclovir</u>: 20 mg/kg up to 800 mg/po q6h x 5 days	Must treat within 24 hrs of exantham; no reduction in serologic response noted; considered cost effective due to decrease in parent work-time lost (NEJM 325:1539, 1991)
Pneumonia	<u>Acyclovir</u>: IV - 10-12 mg/kg q8h x 7 days; oral - 800 mg 5 x daily x 10 days	Efficacy not clearly established, but appears best if treatment is initiated within 36 hrs of admission (RID 12:788, 1990)
Dermatomal Immuno-suppressed	<u>Acyclovir</u>: IV 10-12 mg/kg q8h x 7 days	Indications to treat are greater for severe disease, early disease or zoster in immunosuppressed host (NEJM 308:1448, 1983; Am J Med 85 Suppl 2A:84, 1988)
Normal host	<u>Acyclovir</u>: Oral 800 mg 5 x daily x 7-10 days	Acyclovir and/or corticosteroids (prednisone 40 mg/day x 7 days, then taper over 3 wks) may reduce post-herpetic neuralgia. Steroids usually reserved for persons >40 years. Acyclovir should be started ≤ 4 days from onset or while lesions are still forming. Post-herpetic neuralgia: Amitriptyline
Ophthalmic zoster	<u>Acyclovir</u>: Oral 600-800 mg 5 x daily x 10 days	Consult ophthalmologist (Ophthalmology 93:763, 1986)
Disseminated zoster or varicella (immuno-suppressed host)	<u>Acyclovir</u>: IV 10-12 mg/kg q8h x 7 days	Alternatives are Foscarnet (60 mg/kg q8h) or vidarabine (10 mg/kg/day IV) x 5-7 days (NEJM 308:1448, 1983; NEJM 314:208, 1986)
Acyclovir resistant strains	<u>Foscarnet</u>: 60 mg/kg q8h IV	
Exposure (zoster or chickenpox)		
Immunosuppressed	<u>Varicella-zoster</u> immune globulin	(Ann Intern Med 108:221, 1988)
Susceptible health care workers	None	Must refrain from patient contact from days 10-21
Prophylaxis in transplant recipients	<u>Acyclovir</u>: 5 mg/kg IV q8h or 200 mg po q6h day 8-35	(Lancet 2:706, 1983; NEJM 320: 1381, 1989)

(continued)

Virus	Regimen	Comment
CYTOMEGALOVIRUS Immunocompetent	None	
Immunosuppressed Retinitis	Ganciclovir: Induction - 5 mg/kg IV bid x 14-21 days. Maintenance - 5 mg/kg IV qd Foscarnet: Induction - 60 mg/kg IV q8h x 14-21 days Maintenance - 90 mg/kg IV qd	Efficacy of ganciclovir and foscarnet established. Comparative trial in AIDS patients showed equal effectiveness vs CMV; Foscarnet recipients lived an average of 3 mo. longer possibly due to current AZT treatment and/or anti-HIV activity of foscarnet (NEJM 326:213, 1992). Most recommend foscarnet if AZT is to be continued or there is leukopenia; most recommend ganciclovir for elderly patients and those with renal failure. Failure with progressive CMV retinitis is treated by reinduction or use of the alternative agent
Colitis, enteritis esophagitis, viremia, mucocutaneous lesions, encephalitis, neuritis	As above (Ganciclovir preferred for non-AIDS patients)	Efficacy in these settings is less well established including indications for treatment and need for life-long maintenance
Pneumonitis AIDS patients		Up to 50% of BAL specimens yield CMV; most have alternative cause of pneumonitis; indications for treatment in absence of alternative pathogen are not clear
Marrow transplant recipients	Ganciclovir: 7.5-10 mg/kg/day IV x 20 days ± maintenance: 5 mg/kg 3-5 x/wk for 8-20 doses with or without CMV hyperimmune globulin or IV gamma globulin 500 mg/kg qod x 10 doses or 400 mg/kg on days 1, 4, 8 and 200 mg/kg on day 14	Ganciclovir-IVIG efficacy best supported for marrow recipients (Ann Intern Med 109:777, 1988; 109:783, 1988; Transplantation 46:905 1988; JID 158:488, 1988) Ganciclovir monotherapy: Response rates: marrow - 22-50%; solid organs - 50-100% (reviews of 14 reports - Pharmacotherapy 12:300, 1992). IVIG monotherapy: Mortality 79% (JID 156:641, 1987)
Solid organ transplants	Ganciclovir: 7.5-10 mg/kg/day x 10-20 days	Response rates in heart, liver and renal transplant recipients in 14 reports: 67/85 (79%) (Pharmacotherapy 12:300, 1992). Maintenance therapy used in 2 of 14 reports

(continued)

Virus	Regimen	Comment
Pneumonitis (continued)		
Prophylaxis Marrow	Acyclovir: 500 mg/M² q8h day 5-30 ± maintenance with 800 mg po qid to day 180 (HSV prophylaxis concurrently)(NEJM 318:70, 1988)	Indications: 1) CMV pos autograft and allograft recipients; 2) seronegative allograft recipients of seropos donor; 3) asymptomatic patients with CMV pos BAL on day 35.
	Acyclovir: 200 mg po q6h day 8-35 (HSV prophylaxis concurrently) (NEJM 2:706, 1983)	Acyclovir: Value in prophylaxis vs HSV and VZV established; for CMV data are conflicting with some
	Ganciclovir: 5 mg/kg IV bid 5 days/ wk starting days 35-120 in patients with CMV pos BAL. Patients also received IV gamma globulin q2wks to day 180 (NEJM 324:1005, 1991; NEJM 325:1601, 1991)	negative reports (Br J Cancer 59: 434, 1989) Ganciclovir: Major complication is neutropenia
	Ganciclovir: 2.5 mg/kg IV q8h 7 days pretx, 6 mg/kg 3x/wk when ANC >500 to day 70 (Blood 76, Suppl 574a, 1990)	CMV poor blood products: Benefit may be restricted to seroneg donor and recipient
	Foscarnet: 40 mg/kg IV q8h days 7-30, then 60 mg/kg IV qd to day 75 (JID 166:473, 1992)	
Organ transplant recipients	Acyclovir: 800 mg po 5x/day (Ann Intern Med 114:598, 1991) Ganciclovir: 5 mg/kg IV q12h day to 14, then 6 mg/kg 5 days/wk to day 28 (NEJM 326:1182, 1992).	Indications: Best results are with ganciclovir in CMV seropositive heart recipients. Results with CMV-IVIG and oral acyclovir are disappointing (Transplant Proc 23:1170, 1991, and 23:1498, 1991).
EPSTEIN-BARR VIRUS		
Oral hairy leukoplakia	Acyclovir: 800 mg po 5x/day	Efficacy established. Relapse rates high
EBV associated lymphomas	No antiviral agent	Acyclovir confers no benefit (NEJM 311:1163, 1984)
Infectious mononucleosis	No antiviral agent	Prednisone (80 mg/d x 2-3 days, then taper over 2 wks) advocated for impending airway closure and prolonged course with high fever or persistent morbidity (JAMA 256: 1051, 1986)

B. **Influenza A: Amantadine**
1. Recommendations (Advisory Council on Immunization Practices: MMWR 37:361,1988; 39:RR-7, 1-15 and 41:RR9, 12, 1992)
    a. Prophylaxis: 70-90% effective in preventing influenza A infection.
    Highest priority - Control presumed influenza A outbreaks in institutions with high risk persons; administer to all residents regardless of vaccination status as soon as possible after outbreak recognized and as long as there is influenza activity in community. This form of prophylaxis should also be offered to unvaccinated staff who provide care for high risk patients.

Other recommendations - 1) As adjunct to late vaccination of high risk persons (2 weeks required for vaccine response); **2)** Unvaccinated persons providing care to high risk persons in the home or in care facilities; continue until vaccine induces immunity (2 wks) or continue throughout epidemic if employee cannot be vaccinated or; **3)** Consider for vaccinated health care personnel if outbreak involves strain not covered in the vaccine; **4)** Immunodeficient persons who are expected to have a poor antibody response to the vaccine, especially high risk persons with contraindications to influenza vaccine.

    b. <u>Treatment</u>: Amantadine can reduce the severity and duration of influenza, but is not known to prevent complications in high risk patients. Consequently, no specific recommendation is made. If given, it should be started within 48 hrs of the onset of symptoms and should be discontinued when clinically warranted, usually within 3-5 days. In closed populations, persons who have influenza and are treated should be separated from those receiving amantadine for prophylaxis.

    c. Amantidine resistant strains of influenza A may emerge with amantadine treatment and may be transmitted to others.

2. <u>Dose</u> (MMWR 37:373,1988)

    a. <u>Prophylaxis</u>: 100 mg/day (all adults)

    b. <u>Treatment</u>: Age 10-64 - 200 mg/day in one or two doses; Age > 65 yrs - 100 mg/day as single daily dose; Seizure disorder - 100 mg/day

    c. Creatinine clearance in ml/min/1.73 M^2 (<u>use 1/2 dose when 100 mg/day indicated</u>).
       > 80: 200 mg/day
       60-80: 200 mg alternating with 100 mg/day
       40-60: 100 mg/day
       30-40: 200 mg twice weekly
       20-30: 100 mg three times weekly
       10-20: 200 mg alternating with 100 mg weekly

3. <u>Side effects</u> (dose related): Anxiety, insomnia, dizziness, drunk feeling, slurred speech, ataxia, depression, lightheadedness, inability to concentrate. Incidence is 5-10% for healthy young adults taking 200 mg/day; lower prophylactic dose presumably decreases side effects and retains efficacy. Less frequent side effects include seizures and confusion; seizures and behavioral change are most common in the elderly, those with poor renal function and patients with a pre-existing seizure disorder or psychiatric condition. Dose reduction reduces frequency.

4. <u>Information source (CDC)</u>: Technical Information Services, Center for Prevention Services, Mailstop E06, CDC, Atlanta, GA 30333, (404) 639-1819.

C. HIV: Antiretroviral therapy

Agent	Indication (FDA)	Dose	Side Effects
AZT (Retrovir, Zidovudine)	CD 4 count <500/cu mm	Usual dose: 500 mg po q4h while awake (500 mg/d) or 200 mg po tid (600 mg/d). Lowest effective dose: 300 mg/d. HIV associated dementia: 1000-1200 mg/d HIV associated ITP: 1000-1200 mg/d	Major: Marrow toxicity with severe anemia or leukopenia that is related to dose, duration of treatment and stage of disease. Monitor therapy with CBC and suspend treatment for Hgb <7.5 gm% or ANC <750/mm^3. Frequency is 3%/yr in asymptomatic patients and 40%/yr with AIDS. Other: Headache, insomnia, myalgias and nausea (usually resolve with continued use) Cardiomyopathy: Late stage disease Myopathy: Long-term use Contraindications: Toxicity with Hg<7.5gm% or absolute neutrophil count (ANC) <750/mm^3; concurrent use with ganciclovir
ddI (dideoxyinosine, Videx)	Adults with advanced HIV infection and prolonged prior treatment with AZT	Must take 2 tabs for buffering action >60 kg: 200 mg bid <60 kg: 125 mg bid	Major: 1) Pancreatitis in 5-9%, which is fatal in 6% (0.35% of all recipients); rates are higher in patients with advanced HIV infection (AIDS or CD4 <100) and with conditions associated with pancreatitis. 2) Peripheral neuropathy 5-12% related to cumulative dose. Other: Diarrhea in 30-35%. Rare: leuokpenia, anemia, hepatic failure, cardiomyopathy
ddC (dideoxytidine HIVID Zalcitabine)	Two criteria: 1)CD4 cell count <300/cu mm. 2) Prior treatment with AZT alone showing "clinical or immunologic deterioration." FDA approved only for use in combination with AZT	0.750 mg tid	Major: Peripheral neuropathy in 17-31% related to cumulative dose. Other: Pancreatitis (1%), oral or esophageal ulcers, cardiomyopathy, nausea, vomiting, diarrhea, rash, fever, headache, fatigue, arthralgias, mialgias

D. Hepatitis Viruses

Interferon alpha-2b (Medical Letter 32:1-2,1990 and 32:76-77,1990)

Chronic hepatitis C: Four studies showed interferon alfa-2b (2-3 million units SC 3x/wk x 6 mo) produced a statistically significant improvement in ALT; the three using 3 million units 3x/wk showed normal or near-normal ALT levels in about 50% of treated patients compared to 10% of controls. About 50% of responders relapsed within 6 months after treatment was discontinued (NEJM 321:1501,1506,1989). Enrollment criteria in these trials required compensated liver disease (no encephalopathy, ascites, variceal bleed; pro time <3 sec prolonged; bilirubin <2 mg/dl). Indications for treatment and therapeutic regimen to use are controversial. Some authorities suggest criteria include 1) Positive HCV serology, 2) exclusion of autoimmune hepatitis, 3) symptomatic hepatitis, 4) liver biopsy (best results with chronic persistent hepatitis; chronic active hepatitis or cirrhosis are relative contraindications). Initial treatment is 3 million units 3x/wk, treatment is continued for at least 3 months to determine response according to serum aminotransferase levels and treatment is continued for 6-12 months in responders. Some responders may require life-long treatment with 1-2 doses/week. Responders often show transient increases in ALT so that decision to retreat should be delayed 1-3 months.

<u>Hepatitis B</u>: Initial studies show interferon alfa-2b (5 million units SC daily x 4 mo) led to sustained loss of HBV DNA and HBeAg in one-third and return of liver function tests to normal in 40% (Perrillo RP et al, New Engl J Med 323:295, 1990). Enrollment criteria in these trials were compensated liver disease, chronic HBV (HBsAg >6 mo.) elevated ALT and evidence of HBV replication (HBeAg). Follow-up at 3-7 yrs shows prolonged remission in 20 of 23 who responded, 3 had reappearance of HBsAg within 1 yr, and 13 became negative for HBsAg (Korenman J et al Ann Intern Med 114:629,1991). Indications for treatment are arbitrary: most use the criteria in the trials including compensated liver disease, liver biopsy showing chronic hepatitis, ALT levels ≥ 2x normal and presence of HBeAg.

   a.   Recommended regimen is 5 million units/day or 10 million units 3x/wk x 4 mo. Lower doses are less effective and higher doses are usually too toxic.

   b.   Response rates: 30-40%. Predictors of response are e antigen (HBeAg), high AST (>100 U/L), persistence of HBV DNA at low initial levels (<100 pg/ml) and biopsy showing increased necroinflammation.

   c.   Monitoring: Clinical and laboratory review at 2-4 wk intervals. Lab monitoring should include CBC, platelet count, liver function tests, TSH, and albumin prior to treatment and at treatment weeks 1,2,4,8,12 and 16. HBsAg and HBeAg should be measured at baseline, end of treatment and at 3 and 6 months.

<u>Preparations of Interferons</u>:

alpha-2a	"Roferon A" Hoffmann-LaRoche
alfa-2b	"Intron A" Schering Corp.
alfa-nl	"Wellferon" Burroughs-Wellcome

<u>Adverse reactions</u>: About 50% experience flu-like symptoms of fever, malaise, myalgias and headache; Sx often respond to acetaminophen and decrease with continued treatment. Later side effects include fatigue, muscle aches, irritability, autoimmune reactions, granulocytopenia and thrombocytopenia, psychiatric symptoms, thyroid disorders and alopecia. Most side effects are dose related. Adverse reactions sufficiently severe to interfere with daily activities in 20-50% receiving 30 million units/week. Severe psychological reactions are more common in those with prior CNS disease or psychiatric problems. Long term effects are unknown and treatment requires subcutaneous injections. Wholesale cost to pharmacist is $25/3 million units.

TREATMENT OF MYCOBACTERIAL INFECTIONS

I. **TREATMENT OF TUBERCULOSIS:** Official statement of the American Thoracic Society and the Centers for Disease Control (Amer Rev Resp Dis 134:355-363,1986;136:492-496,1987, AMA Drug Evaluation, Section 15 pp 1:1-1:7,1990, MMWR 41RR-10, 1992)

New guidelines to be issued by CDC, ATS and IDSA in late 1992 include 2 major changes to the guideline summarized below:
  1) All patients should receive initial treatment with four drugs unless they are from a geographic area in which resistance is nil.
  2) All patients should have observed treatment until the patient can demonstrate compliance.

Classification of drugs:
  Major: INH and rifampin
  Adjunctive: Pyrazinamide, ethambutol, streptomycin
  Second line: Ethionamide, capreomycin, kanamycin, amikacin, cycloserine, PAS
  Experimental: Fluoroquinolones, clofazimine, amoxicillin-clavulante, clarithromycin azithromycin

A. Treatment of tuberculosis in adults
  1. TB without HIV infection
      Option 1: INH, rifampin, pyrazinamide and ethambutol or streptomycin is continued until susceptibility to INH and rifampin is demonstrated. These four drugs are continued 8 weeks followed by INH and rifampin for 16 weeks given daily, 2x/week or 3x/week (See B for doses). Continue treatment at least 6 months total and at least 3 months beyond culture conversion.
      Option 2: INH, rifampin, pyrazinamide and ethambutol or streptomycin daily for 2 weeks, then 2x/wk for 6 wks, then INH and rifampin for 16 weeks.
      Option 3: INH, rifampin, pyrazinamide, ethambutol or streptomycin with directly observed treatment 3x/wk for 6 months.

  2. Tuberculosis with HIV infection: Options 1, 2, and 3 are appropriate, but treatment must continue a total of at least 9 months and at least 6 months beyond culture conversion. (In general, TB is treated 50% longer in patients with HIV infection.)

  3. Tuberculosis with resistant strains (or contraindication to first line agent)
      a. Resistant to INH or rifampin: Treatment with INH or rifampin, ethambutol pyrazinamide plus streptomycin x 6 mo (non-AIDS) or 9 mo (AIDS). (Some advocate INH or rifampin, ethambutol and pyrazinamide x 18 mo.)
      b. Resistant to INH and rifampin: Treat with multiple drug regimen including at least two agents active in vitro x 18-24 mo.
  Note: *1) Intermittent therapy: Treatment 2x/wk appears to be as effective as 3x/wk; need for daily drugs for ≥2 wks at inception of treatment is not established.*
          2) Aminoglycoside: Streptomycin preferred and may be given intravenously; capreomycin, kanamycin or amikacin may be preferred on basis of in vitro sensitivity tests; cost of amikacin is about 100 x that of streptomycin
          3) Utility of inclusion of INH (or rifampin) in regimen despite in vitro resistance is debated
          4) When resistance suspected, give 3 drugs not previously used pending in vitro sensitivity tests; never add a single drug when resistance suspected.
          5) Hospitalized patients with multiply resistant strains should not be discharged home until sputum smear is negative.

126

B. Recommended first line agents (Table 1)

(Amer Rev Resp Dis 134:355-363,1986 and Medical Letter 34:10,1992, MMWR 41:RR-10, pg 14, 1992)

Agent	Forms	Daily dose (maximum)	Twice/Thrice* weekly dose (maximum)	Cost/mo. (daily regimen)	Adverse reactions	Comment
Isoniazid	Tabs: 100 mg, 300 mg Syrup: 50 mg/5 ml Vials: 1 gm (IM)	5 mg/kg po or IM (300 mg)**	15 mg/kg (900 mg)*	$ 0.60	Elevated hepatic enzymes, peripheral neuropathy, hepatitis, *** hypersensitivity	Peripheral neuropathy is uncommon with dose of 5 mg/kg. Puridoxine (50 mg/day) suggested for those with diabetes, HIV, uremia, alcoholism, malnutrition, pregnancy or seizure disorder
Rifampin	Caps: 150 mg, 300 mg Vials: 600 mg (IV)	10-20 mg/kg po (600 mg)** IV (600 mg)	10 mg/kg (600 mg)*	$118.00	Orange discoloration of secretions & urine, nausea, vomiting, fever, hepatitis, *** purpura (rare)	May be given as 10 mg/ml suspension or intravenously. Accelerates clearance of methadone, coumadin, corticosteroids, estrogens, digitalis, ketoconazole, cyclosporine, dilantin, oral hypoglycemics (see Drug Interactions, pp. 79 and 80)
Pyrazinamide	Tabs: 500 mg	15-30 mg/kg po (2 gm)**	50-70 mg/kg	$121.00	Hepatitis,*** hyperuricemia, arthralgias, rash, GI intolerance	Hyperuricemia is common, gout is rare
Streptomycin	Vials: 1 gm, 4 gm	15 mg/kg IM (1 gm)** pts > 40 yrs: 10 mg/kg IM (500-750 mg)**	25-30 mg/kg pts > 40 yrs: 20 mg/kg	$118.00	Ototoxicity and possible nephrotoxicity	Decrease dose for renal failure
Ethambutol	Tabs: 100 mg, 400 mg	15-25 mg/kg po (2.5 gm)**	50 mg/kg (2x/wk) 25-30 mg/kg (3x/wk)	$106.00	Optic neuritis, skin rash	25 mg/kg/day 1st 1-2 months or if strain is INH resistant. Decrease dose for renal failure

* Dosage for treatment 2x/week and 3x/week are the same except for ethambutol.

** Usual dose for adults.

***All patients receiving INH, rifampin and/or pyrazinamide should be instructed to report immediately any symptoms of hepatitis: anorexia, nausea, vomiting, jaundice, malaise, fever >3 days or abdominal tenderness.

127

C. Second line antituberculous drugs (Table 2)

Agent	Forms	Daily dose (maximum)	Adverse reactions	Monitoring
Capreomycin	Vials: 1 gm	15-30 mg/kg IM (1 gm)*	Auditory, vestibular, and renal toxicity	Audiometry, vestibular function, renal function
Kanamycin	Vials: 75 mg, 500 mg and and 1 gm	13-30 mg/kg IM (1 gm)*	Auditory, vestibular (rare), and renal toxicity	Audiometry, vestibular function, renal failure
Ethionamide	Tabs: 250 mg	15-20 mg/kg PO (1 gm)*	Gastrointestinal intolerance, hepatotoxicity, hypersensitivity	Hepatic enzymes
PAS	Tabs: 500 mg, 1 gm	12 gm	Gastrointestinal intolerance, hepatotoxicity, sodium load, hypersensitivity	
Cycloserine	Caps: 250 mg	1 gm	Psychosis, rash, convulsions	Assess mental status

* Usual daily dose of adult

D. Monitoring Treatment (Table 3)

1. Drug toxicity
    a. Baseline tests: Hepatic enzymes, bilirubin, serum creatinine or BUN, CBC, platelet count or estimate.
        Pyrazinamide: uric acid; ethambutol: visual acuity.
        Frequency of INH hepatitis by age: 25 yrs - 1%; 35 yrs - 6%; 45 yrs - 11%; 55 yrs - 18%; 65 yrs - 11% (Goldberg MJ. Med Clin N Amer 72:661,1988).

    b. During treatment: Clinical monitoring with assessment at least once monthly; laboratory monitoring is not recommended except for symptoms suggesting toxicity. The purpose of monthly monitoring is to determine compliance, determine symptoms of neuropathy (paresthesias) and determine symptoms of hepatotoxicity (anorexia, nausea, vomiting, dark urine, jaundice malaise, fever >3 days or abdominal tenderness).

2. Evaluation of response: Sputum examination (smear and culture): Twice monthly until conversion is documented. Positive sputum at 3 months: Review compliance and drug susceptibility.

128

Table 3: Monitoring treatment (MMWR 41:RR-10, pg 15, 1992)

	Month 1	Month 2	Month 3 to completion
Medical evaluation	At least twice	Twice monthly	Once monthly if asymptomatic and smear/culture negative
Bacteriology*	Initially 3-6 sputum samples for diagnosis. Susceptibility testing of all strains	Sputum smear and culture 2x/month until sputum smear negative and patient asymptomatic	Sputum smear and culture 2x/month until sputum smear negative* and patient asymptomatic, then monthly
Drug monitoring**	Baseline lab studies in patients >35 years of age. Question and observe for evidence of toxicity; test if they occur	Question and observe for evidence of toxicity; test if they occur	Question and observe for evidence of toxicity; test if they occur

* Cultures should be obtained at least monthly until negative. This is the most reliable method for detecting treatment failure. Sputum conversion should occur within 3 months. Patients with treatment failure need to be evaluated for compliance and drug resistance
** Toxicity monitoring should be individualized based on drugs used, age and other factors such as alcohol consumption and concurrent drugs

E. Special considerations

1. Extrapulmonary tuberculosis

    a. Nine-month two-drug regimen recommended for sensitive strains; consider longer treatment for lymphadenitis, bone and joint tuberculosis.

    b. Six-month regimen is "probably effective."

    c. Some authorities recommend corticosteroids for tuberculosis pericarditis and meningitis. (See Recommendations of IDSA, pg 169)

2. Pregnancy and lactation

    a. INH plus rifampin; ethambutol should be added for suspected resistant strains.

    b. Streptomycin is only antituberculous drug with established fetal toxicity (interferes with ear development and causes congenital deafness); kanamycin and capreomycin presumably share this toxic potential.

    c. Breast feeding should not be discouraged.

3. Treatment failures (persistent positive cultures after 5-6 months)

   a. Susceptibility tests on current isolate while continuing same regimen or augmenting this with two additional drugs.

   b. Sensitive strain: Consider treatment under direct observation.
      Resistant strain: At least 2 active drugs x 18-24 mo.

4. Relapse after treatment

   a. INH + rifampin regimen previously: Organism at time of relapse is usually sensitive if the original strain was. Therefore, give same regimen initially, measure susceptibility, modify the regimen accordingly and consider observed treatment.

   b. Regimen not containing INH and rifampin: Presume new isolate is resistant to agents used. See 3b above.

5. Multiply resistant strains of M. tuberculosis

   a. Definition: Resistance to INH and rifampin

   b. Epidemiology: Sporadic cases are usually acquired in third world countries, reflect non-compliance with standard treatment regimens for active tuberculosis or represent acquisition from one of these sources. Epidemics have been reported primarily through airborne spread from undiagnosed cases in AIDS patients in correctional facilities, shelters, nursing homes, crack houses and health care facilities in New York, New Jersey and Miami (NEJM 324:1644, 1991; NEJM 326:1514, 1992)

   c. Incidence (MMWR 41:RR-11, 1992): Susceptibility data for first quarter 1991

	U.S.	NYC
Resistance to INH or rifampin	14%	33%
Resistance to INH and rifampin	3%	19%

   d. Treatment (Medical Letter 34:10, 1992; NEJM 324:289, 1991): Regimens that include at least two drugs active in vitro for 18-24 mo. This combination often includes pyrazinamide, ethambutol, streptomycin and ciprofloxacin (750 mg po bid) or ofloxacin (400 mg po bid); other drugs besides standard first and second line agents include imipenem and amikacin. Strains resistant to INH and rifampin are often also resistant to ethambutol and streptomycin; about half are resistant to pyrazinamide.

   e. Outcome: Cure rates in all persons are <60%; mortality rates ascribed to tuberculosis in AIDS patients with multiply resistant strains are 72-89% and the median survival rate is 4-16 weeks. In 172 patients without AIDS the sputum conversion rate with multidrug regimens given under observation was about 65% and many convertors subsequently relapsed; the overall success rate was 56% (M. Goble et al, data presented at ICAAC, Anaheim, CA, Oct, 1992).

II.   **PREVENTATIVE TREATMENT FOR TUBERCULOSIS INFECTION IN THE U.S.**
(Recommendations of the Advisory Committee for Elimination of Tuberculosis,
MMWR 39:#RR-8, pp 9-15, 1990)

A.   **Indications**

1.   High risk groups (persons in any category should be treated regardless
of age unless previously treated).

   a.   Persons with HIV infection with PPD ≥ 5 mm and persons at risk for
HIV whose serologic status is unknown but HIV is suspected.

   b.   Close contacts of newly diagnosed cases with PPD ≥ 5 mm. Children and
adolescents with neg PPD who have been close contacts with infectious
persons within past 3 months are candidates until there is a negative
repeat PPD at 12 weeks post contact.

   c.   Recent seroconverters with PPD ≥ 10 mm increase within 2 yr period for
persons < 35 yrs and ≥ 15 mm increase for persons over 35 years.

   d.   Persons with x-ray showing fibrotic lesions likely to represent healed TB
and PPD ≥ 5 mm.

   e.   Intravenous drug abusers known to be HIV seronegative and PPD
≥ 10 mm.

   f.   Persons with medical conditions that have been associated with increased
risk of TB and PPD ≥ 10 mm: silicosis; diabetes mellitus (esp if poorly
controlled); corticosteroid treatment (≥ 15 mg/day prednisone for over 2-
3 wks); other immunosuppressive treatment; hematologic and
lymphoproliferative diseases such as leukemia and Hodgkin's disease; end
stage renal disease, and conditions associated with rapid weight loss or
chronic malnutrition including gastrectomy, jejunoileal by-pass and weight
loss of 10% or more below ideal body weight.

2.   Persons under 35 years with PPD ≥ 10 mm.

   a.   Foreign born persons from high prevalence countries.

   b.   Medically underserved low-income populations including blacks,
Hispanics and Native Americans.

   c.   Residents of long term care facilities.

B.   **Preventative treatment**

1.   Usual regimen: Isoniazid, 300 mg/day for 6-12 months.

   a.   Persons with HIV infection and those with stable chest x-rays compatible
with past TB should be treated for 12 months.

   b.   Others: 6-12 months

2.   Directly observed therapy: Isoniazid in dose of 15 mg/kg (up to 900 mg) twice
weekly.

3.   Multiply resistant strains: Decision to treat should be based on extent of exposure,
host factors and in vitro sensitivities of the contact strain. Health care workers
with HIV infection are 40 x more likely to develop active disease. Recommended
regimens depending on sensitivity test results are pyrazinamide + fluoroquinolone
or pyrazinamide + ethambutol. Duration is 12 mo. for HIV infected persons and
6 mo. for all others.

C. **Monitoring**: Patients should be monitored in person by trained personnel at monthly intervals. Black and Hispanic women, especially postpartum, may be at greatest risk for serious or fatal reaction and should be monitored more frequently. Purpose of monitoring is to evaluate compliance and evaluate toxicity: peripheral neuropathy and hepatotoxicity.

III. **SCREENING FOR TUBERCULOSIS**
(Recommendations of Advisory Committee for Elimination of Tuberculosis, MMWR 39:#RR-8, pp 1-8, 1990)

A. **Background**
1. It is estimated that > 90% of patients with active tuberculosis have harbored M. tuberculosis for over 1 year.
2. The estimated number of persons in the U.S. with latent infection is 10-15 million.
3. Preventative treatment with isoniazid is 90-95% effective when compliance is good.

B. **Populations to be screened**
1. Persons with HIV infection.
2. Close contacts with persons known or suspected to have tuberculosis.
3. Persons with medical risks known to increase the risk of disease if infection has occurred.
4. Foreign born persons from countries with high prevalence of TB.
5. Medically underserved low income populations, e.g., blacks, Hispanics and Native Americans.
6. Alcoholics and IV drug abusers.
7. Residents of long term care facilities including correctional facilities, nursing homes, mental institutions, etc.

C. **Screening**
1. PPD: 5 units given intracutaneously is the preferred test.
2. Persons with signs or symptoms of pulmonary tuberculosis should have chest x-ray regardless of skin test results.

D. **PPD-Tuberculin anergy and HIV infection** (MMWR 40RR-5, 27, 1991)
1. Anergy with delayed-type hypersensitivity (DTH) skin test antigens in persons with HIV infection is inversely related to CD4 cell counts. Anergy to each of 2 or 3 skin test antigens (Candida albicans, mumps and tetanus) is <10% with healthy persons and HIV infected persons with CD4 counts >500 mm^3; it is >80% for HIV infected persons with CD4 counts <50/mm^3.
2. Recommendations for DTH testing
    a. Persons with HIV infection should have concurrent anergy testing in conjunction with PPD testing.
    b. Degree of immunosuppression should not influence decisions regarding anergy testing.
    c. Recommended testing is with two DTH skin test antigens, i.e., Candida, mumps or tetanus toxoid (Multitest CMI not recommended).
    d. Interpretation: Any induration to DTH antigens is considered positive at 48-72 hrs.
3. Treatment recommendations for persons with HIV infection.
    a. PPD >5 mm induration: INH prophylasis*. Some believe 2 mm of induration should be the cutoff (JAMA 267:369, 1992), but this has not been generally accepted (JAMA 267:409, 1992)

132

b. PPD negative plus anergy: INH prophylaxis* for those who are contacts of persons with TB and those with a risk of ≥10% of TB: IVDU's, prisoners, homeless persons, migrant workers and the persons born in Asia, Africa and Latin America.

* INH x ≥ 1 year; must have x-ray and clinical evaluation to exclude active TB.

IV. ATYPICAL MYCOBACTERIA (See Wolinsky E, CID 15:1, 1992)

Agent	Condition	Treatment
M. kansasii	Pulmonary Osteomyelitis Disseminated	3 drugs x 18 mo: INH, rifampin and ethambutol or these three agents for 12 mo. plus streptomycin (1 gm IM 2x/wk) x 3 mo.* Also consider ciprofloxacin, clarithromycin
M. avium complex (MAC)	Immunocompetent host: Pulmonary Lymphadenitis Osteomyelitis	3-5 drugs: INH, rifampin, ethambutol x 18-24 mo. plus streptomycin x 2-4 mo.* Also consider clarithromycin, ciprofloxacin, clofazimine, cycloserine, ethionamide lymphadenitis and amikacin. Use of INH is controversial
	Immunosuppressed host: Disseminated disease (AIDS etc)	3-5 drugs: Rifampin, ethambutol, clofazimine, clarithromycin, ciprofloxacin, amikacin or kanamycin. Alternative is clarithromycin + ethambutol or clofazimine. Clofazimine usually reserved for extra-pulmonary disease
M. marinum	Skin soft tissue	Ethambutol + rifampin ± streptomycin*, minocycline or doxycycline* or sulfa-trimethoprim*. Also consider ciprofloxacin. Surgery often required for deep infections
M. xenopi	Pulmonary	3 drugs: Rifampin, INH + ethambutol* ± streptomycin. Also consider ethionamide, cycloserine, clarithromycin, ciprofloxacin
M. malmoense	Pulmonary	Same as MAC (Rifampin, INH + ethambutol)
M. simiae	Pulmonary	Same as MAC (often refractory)
M. scrofulaceum	Lymphadenitis Disseminated	Same as MAC (usually very resistant, with lymphadenitis-resection)
M. fortuitum	Pulmonary Disseminated Skin/soft tissue iatrogenic infections	Amikacin, ciprofloxacin + sulfonamide*. Also consider clofaximine, clarithromycin (or erythromycin), doxycycline, imipenem, cefoxitin, ciprofloxacin
M. bovis	Pulmonary	Same as M. tuberculosis, but resistant to pyrazinamide
M. szulgai	Pulmonary and extrapulmonary	Same as M. kansasii

(continued)

Agent	Condition	Treatment
M. haemophilum	Skin/soft tissue	Rifampin, clofazimine, doxycycline, sulfa-trimethoprim
M. chelonae ss abscessus	Skin/soft tissue esp post-op augmentation mammoplasty, median sternotomy and other iatrogenic infections	Amikacin* + cefoxitin. Also consider clofazimine, clarithromycin
M. chelonea ss chelonea	Same	Tobramycin or amikacin + cefoxitin*. Also consider clofazimine, clarithromycin, doxycycline, erythromycin
M. smegmatis	Soft tissue, bone, etc.	Ethambutol, amikacin, ciprofloxacin sulfonamides, clofazimine, imipenem

* Regimens with established efficacy

DRUGS FOR TREATMENT OF PARASITIC INFECTIONS
(Reprinted from The Medical Letter on Drugs and Therapeutics 34:18-25,1992 with permission)

Infection	Drug	Adult Dosage*	Pediatric Dosage*
AMEBIASIS (Entamoeba histolytica)			
asymptomatic			
Drug of choice:	Iodoquinol[1]	650 mg tid x 20d	30-40 mg/kg/d in 3 doses x 20d
OR	Paromomycin	25-30 mg/kg/d in 3 doses 7d	25-30 mg/kg/d in 3 doses 7d
Alternative:	Diloxanide furoate[2]	500 mg tid x 10d	20 mg/kg/d in 3 doses x 10d
mild to moderate intestinal disease			
Drugs of choice:	Metronidazole[3]	750 mg tid x 10d	35-50 mg/kg/d in 3 doses x 10d
OR	Tinidazole[4]	2 grams/d x 3d	50 mg/kg (max. 2 grams) qd x 3d
	followed by iodoquinol[1]	650 mg tid x 20d	30-40 mg/kg/d in 3 doses x 20d
OR	paromomycin	25-30 mg/kg/d in 3 doses x 7d	25-30 mg/kg/d in 3 doses x 7d
severe intestinal disease			
Drugs of choice:	Metronidazole[3]	750 mg tid x 10d	35-50 mg/kg/d in 3 doses x 10d
OR	Tinidazole[4]	600 mg bid 5d	50 mg/kg (max. 2 grams) qd x 3d
	followed by iodoquinol[1]	650 mg tid x 20d	30-40 mg/kg/d in 3 doses x 20d
OR	paromomycin	25-30 mg/kg/d in 3 doses x 7d	25-30 mg/kg/d in 3 doses x 7d
Alternatives:	Dehydroemetine[2,5]	1 to 1.5 mg/kg/d (max. 90 mg/d) IM for up to 5d	1 to 1.5 mg/kg/d (max. 90 mg/d) IM in 2 doses for up to 5d
	followed by iodoquinol[1]	650 mg tid x 20d	30-40 mg/kg/d in 3 doses x 20d
hepatic abscess			
Drugs of choice:	Metronidazole[3]	750 mg tid x 10d	35-50 mg/kg/d in 3 doses x 10d
OR	Tinidazole[4]	800 mg tid x 5d	60 mg/kg (max. 2 grams) qd x 3d
	followed by iodoquinol[1]	650 mg tid x 20d	30-40 mg/kg/d in 3 doses x 20d
Alternatives:	Dehydroemetine[2,5]	1 to 1.5 mg/kg/d (max. 90 mg/d) IM for up to 5d	1 to 1.5 mg/kg/d (max. 90 mg/d) IM in 2 doses for up to 5d
	followed by chloroquine phosphate	600 mg base (1 gram)/d x 2d, then 300 mg base (500 mg)/d x 2-3 wks	10 mg base/kg (max. 300 mg base)/d x 2-3 wks
	plus iodoquinol[1]	650 mg tid x 20d	30-40 mg/kg/d in 3 doses x 20d
AMEBIC MENINGOENCEPHALITIS, PRIMARY			
Naegleria			
Drug of choice:	Amphotericin B[6,7]	1 mg/kg/d IV, uncertain duration	1 mg/kg/d IV, uncertain duration
Acanthamoeba			
Drug of choice:	see footnote 8		
***Ancylostoma duodenale*, see HOOKWORM**			
ANGIOSTRONGYLIASIS			
Angiostrongylus cantonensis			
Drug of choice:	Mebendazole[7,9,10]	100 mg bid x 5d	100 mg bid x 5d
Angiostrongylus costaricensis			
Drug of choice:	Thiabendazole[7,9]	75 mg/kg/d in 3 doses x 3d[11] (max. 3 grams/d)	75 mg/kg/d in 3 doses x 3d[11] (max. 3 grams/d)
ANISAKIASIS (Anisakis)			
Treatment of choice:	Surgical or endoscopic removal		
ASCARIASIS (Ascaris lumbricoides, roundworm)			
Drug of choice:	Mebendazole	100 mg bid x 3d	100 mg bid x 3d
OR	Pyrantel pamoate	11 mg/kg once (max. 1 gram)	11 mg/kg once (max. 1 gram)
OR	Albendazole	400 mg once	400 mg once
BABESIOSIS (Babesia)			
Drugs of choice:[12]	Clindamycin[7]	1.2 grams bid parenteral or 600 mg tid oral x 7d	20-40 mg/kg/d in 3 doses x 7d
	plus quinine	650 mg tid oral x 7d	25 mg/kg/d in 3 doses x 7d

Infection	Drug	Adult Dosage*	Pediatric Dosage*
BALANTIDIASIS (Balantidium coli)			
Drug of choice:	Tetracycline[7]	500 mg qid x 10d	40 mg/kg/d in 4 doses x 10d (max. 2 grams/d)[13]
Alternatives:	Iodoquinol[1,7]	650 mg tid x 20d	40 mg/kg/d in 3 doses x 20d
	Metronidazole[3,7]	750 mg tid x 5d	35-50 mg/kg/d in 3 doses x 5d
BAYLISASCARIASIS (Baylisascaris procyonis)			
Drug of choice:	See footnote 14		
BLASTOCYSTIS hominis infection			
Drug of choice:	See footnote 15		
CAPILLARIASIS (Capillaria philippinensis)			
Drug of choice:	Mebendazole[7]	200 mg bid x 20d	200 mg bid x 20d
Alternatives:	Albendazole	200 mg bid x 10d	200 mg bid x 10d
	Thiabendazole[7]	25 mg/kg/d in 2 doses x 30d	25 mg/kg/d in 2 doses x 30d
Chagas' disease, see TRYPANOSOMIASIS			
Clonorchis sinensis, see FLUKE infection			
CRYPTOSPORIDIOSIS (Cryptosporidium)			
Drug of choice:	See footnote 16		
CUTANEOUS LARVA MIGRANS (creeping eruption)			
Drug of choice:[17]	Thiabendazole	Topically and/or 50 mg/kg/d in 2 doses (max. 3 grams/d) x 2-5d[11]	Topically and/or 50 mg/kg/d in 2 doses (max. 3 grams/d) x 2-5d[11]
Cysticercosis, see TAPEWORM infection			
DIENTAMOEBA fragilis infection			
Drug of choice:	Iodoquinol[1]	650 mg tid x 20d	40 mg/kg/d in 3 doses x 20d
OR	Paromomycin	25-30 mg/kg/d in 3 doses x 7d	25-30 mg/kg/d in 3 doses x 7d
OR	Tetracycline[7]	500 mg qid x 10d	40 mg/kg/d in 4 doses x 10d (max. 2 grams/d)[13]
Diphyllobothrium latum, see TAPEWORM infection			
DRACUNCULUS medinensis (guinea worm) infection			
Drug of choice:	Metronidazole[3,7,18]	250 mg tid x 10d	25 mg/kg (max. 750 mg/d) in 3 doses x 10d
Alternative:	Thiabendazole[7,18]	50-75 mg/kg/d in 2 doses x 3d[11]	50-75 mg/kg/d in 2 doses x 3d[11]
Echinococcus, see TAPEWORM infection			
Entamoeba histolytica, see AMEBIASIS			
ENTAMOEBA polecki infection			
Drug of choice:	Metronidazole[3,7]	750 mg tid x 10d	35-50 mg/kg/d in 3 doses x 10d
ENTEROBIUS vermicularis (pinworm) infection			
Drug of choice:	Pyrantel pamoate	11 mg/kg once (max. 1 gram); repeat after 2 weeks	11 mg/kg once (max. 1 gram); repeat after 2 weeks
OR	Mebendazole	A single dose of 100 mg; repeat after 2 weeks	A single dose of 100 mg; repeat after 2 weeks
OR	Albendazole	400 mg once, repeat in 2 weeks	400 mg once, repeat in 2 weeks
Fasciola hepatica, see FLUKE infection			
FILARIASIS			
Wuchereria bancrofti, Brugia malayi			
Drug of choice:[19]	Diethylcarbamazine[20]	Day 1: 50 mg, oral, p.c.	Day 1: 1 mg/kg, oral, p.c.
		Day 2: 50 mg tid	Day 2: 1 mg/kg tid
		Day 3: 100 mg tid	Day 3: 1-2 mg/kg tid
		Days 4 through 21:	Days 4 through 21:
		6 mg/kg/d in 3 doses[21]	6 mg/kg/d in 3 doses[21]
Loa loa			
Drug of choice:	Diethylcarbamazine[20]	Day 1: 50 mg, oral, p.c.	Day 1: 1 mg/kg, oral, p.c.
		Day 2: 50 mg tid	Day 2: 1 mg/kg tid
		Day 3: 100 mg tid	Day 3: 1-2 mg/kg tid
		Days 4 through 21:	Days 4 through 21:
		9 mg/kg/d in 3 doses[21]	9 mg/kg/d in 3 doses[21]
Mansonella ozzardi			
Drug of choice:	See footnote 19		
Mansonella perstans			
Drug of choice:[22]	Mebendazole[7]	100 mg bid x 30d	
Tropical Pulmonary Eosinophilia (TPE)			
Drug of choice:	Diethylcarbamazine	6 mg/kg/d in 3 doses x 21d	6 mg/kg/d in 3 doses x 21d
Onchocerca volvulus			
Drug of choice:	Ivermectin[7]	150 µg/kg oral once, repeated every 6 to 12 months	150 µg/kg oral once, repeated every 6 to 12 months

136

Infection	Drug	Adult Dosage*	Pediatric Dosage*
FLUKE, hermaphroditic, infection			
Clonorchis sinensis (Chinese liver fluke)			
Drug of choice:	Praziquantel	75 mg/kg/d in 3 doses	75 mg/kg/d in 3 doses
Fasciola hepatica (sheep liver fluke)			
Drug of choice:[23]	Bithionol[2]	30-50 mg/kg/d on alternate days x 10-15 doses	30-50 mg/kg on alternate days x 10-15 doses
Fasciolopsis buski (intestinal fluke)			
Drug of choice:	Praziquantel[7]	75 mg/kg/d in 3 doses x 1d	75 mg/kg/d in 3 doses x 1d
	OR Niclosamide[7]	a single dose of 4 tablets (2 g), chewed thoroughly	11-34 kg: 2 tablets (1 g) >34 kg: 3 tablets (1.5 g)
Heterophyes heterophyes (intestinal fluke)			
Drug of choice:	Praziquantel[7]	75 mg/kg/d in 3 doses x 1d	75 mg/kg/d in 3 doses x 1d
Metagonimus yokogawai (intestinal fluke)			
Drug of choice:	Praziquantel[7]	75 mg/kg/d in 3 doses x 1d	75 mg/kg/d in 3 doses x 1d
Nanophyetus salmincola			
Drug of choice:	Praziquantel[7]	60 mg/kg/d in 3 doses x 1d	60 mg/kg/d in 3 doses x 1d
Opisthorchis viverrini (liver fluke)			
Drug of choice:	Praziquantel	75 mg/kg/d in 3 doses x 1d	75 mg/kg/d in 3 doses x 1d
Paragonimus westermani (lung fluke)			
Drug of choice:	Praziquantel[7]	75 mg/kg/d in 3 doses x 2d	75 mg/kg/d in 3 doses x 2d
Alternative:	Bithionol[2]	30-50 mg/kg on alternate days x 10-15 doses	30-50 mg/kg on alternate days x 10-15 doses
GIARDIASIS (*Giardia intestinalis*, formerly *G. lamblia*)			
Drug of choice:	Quinacrine HCl	100 mg tid p.c. x 5d	6 mg/kg/d in 3 doses p.c. x 5d (max. 300 mg/d)
Alternatives:	Metronidazole[3,7]	250 mg tid x 5d	15 mg/kg/d in 3 doses x 5d
	Tinidazole[4]	2 grams once	50 mg/kg once (max. 2 grams)
	Furazolidone	100 mg qid x 7-10d	
	Paromomycin[24]	25-30 mg/kg/d in 3 doses x 7d	6 mg/kg/d in 4 doses x 7-10d
GNATHOSTOMIASIS (*Gnathostoma spinigerum*)			
Treatment of choice:	Surgical removal		
	OR Mebendazole[7]	200 mg q3h x 6d	
HOOKWORM infection (*Ancylostoma duodenale, Necator americanus*)			
Drug of choice:	Mebendazole	100 mg bid x 3d	100 mg bid x 3d
	OR Pyrantel pamoate[7]	11 mg/kg (max. 1 gram) x 3d	11 mg/kg (max. 1 gram) x 3d
	OR Albendazole	400 mg once	400 mg once
Hydatid cyst, see TAPEWORM infection			
Hymenolepis nana, see TAPEWORM infection			
ISOSPORIASIS (*Isospora belli*)			
Drug of choice:	Trimethoprim-sulfamethoxazole[7,25]	160 mg TMP, 800 mg SMX qid x 10d, then bid x 3 wks	
LEISHMANIASIS (*L. mexicana, L. tropica, L. major, L. braziliensis, L. donovani* [Kala-azar])			
Drug of choice:[26]	Stibogluconate sodium[2]	20 mg Sb/kg/d IV or IM x 20-28d[27]	20 mg Sb/kg/d IV or IM x 20-28d[27]
	OR Meglumine antimoniate	20 mg Sb/kg/d x 20-28d[27]	20 mg Sb/kg/d x 20-28d[27]
Alternatives:[28]	Amphotericin B[7]	0.25 to 1 mg/kg by slow infusion daily or every 2d for up to 8 wks	0.25 to 1 mg/kg by slow infusion daily or every 2d for up to 8 wks
	Pentamidine isethionate[7]	2-4 mg/kg IM for up to 15 doses[27]	2-4 mg/kg IM for up to 15 doses[27]
	Topical treatment[29]		
LICE infestation (*Pediculus humanus, capitis, Phthirus pubis*)[30]			
Drug of choice:	1% Permethrin[31]	Topically	Topically
	OR 0.5% Malathion	Topically	Topically
Alternatives:	Pyrethrins with piperonyl butoxide	Topically[32]	Topically[32]
	Lindane	Topically[32]	Topically[32]
MALARIA, Treatment of (*Plasmodium falciparum, P. ovale, P. vivax,* and *P. malariae*)			
All *Plasmodium* except Chloroquine-Resistant *P. falciparum*			
ORAL			
Drug of choice:	Chloroquine phosphate[33,34]	600 mg base (1 gram), then 300 mg base (500 mg) 6 hrs later, then 300 mg base (500 mg) at 24 and 48 hrs	10 mg base/kg (max. 600 mg base), then 5 mg base/kg 6 hrs later, then 5 mg base/kg at 24 and 48 hrs
- PARENTERAL			
Drug of choice:[35]	Quinidine gluconate[7,36]	10 mg/kg loading dose (max. 600 mg) in normal saline slowly over 1 hr, followed by continuous infusion of 0.02 mg/kg/min for 3 days maximum	Same as adult dose
	OR Quinine dihydrochloride[37]	20 mg salt/kg loading dose in 10 ml/kg 5% dextrose over 4 hrs, followed by 10 mg salt/kg over 2-4 hrs q8h (max. 1800 mg/d) until oral therapy can be started	Same as adult dose

Infection	Drug	Adult Dosage*	Pediatric Dosage*
Chloroquine-resistant _P. falciparum_[38]			
ORAL			
Drugs of choice:[38]	Quinine sulfate[40,41] plus	650 mg tid x 3d	[†]25 mg/kg/d in 3 doses x 3d
	pyrimethamine- sulfadoxine[42]	3 tablets at once on last day of quinine	<1 yr: ¼ tablet 1-3 yrs: ½ tablet 4-8 yrs: 1 tablet 9-14 yrs: 2 tablets
OR	plus tetracycline[7,13]	250 mg qid x 7d	20 mg/kg/d in 4 doses x 7d[13]
OR	plus clindamycin[7]	900 mg tid x 3d	20-40 mg/kg/d in 3 doses x 3d

MALARIA, Treatment of Chloroquine-resistant _P. falciparum_ (continued)

ORAL _(continued)_			
Alternatives:	Mefloquine[43,44] Halofantrine[47]	1250 mg once[45] 500 mg q6h x 3 doses	25 mg/kg once[46] (<45 kg) 8 mg/kg q6h x 3 doses (<40 kg)
PARENTERAL			
Drug of choice:	Quinidine gluco- nate[7,36]	same as above	same as above
OR	Quinine dihydro- chloride[37]	same as above	same as above
Prevention of relapses: _P. vivax_ and _P. ovale_ only			
Drug of choice:	Primaquine phosphate[48]	15 mg base (26.3 mg)/d x 14d or 45 mg base (79 mg)/wk x 8 wks	0.3 mg base/kg/d x 14d

MALARIA, Prevention of[49]

Chloroquine-sensitive areas			
Drug of choice:	Chloroquine phos- phate[50]	300 mg base (500 mg salt) orally, once/week beginning 1 week be- fore and continuing for 4 weeks after last exposure	5 mg/kg base (8.3 mg/kg salt) once/week, up to adult dose of 300 mg base
Chloroquine-resistant areas[38]			
Drug of choice:[51]	Mefloquine[44,50,52]	250 mg oral once/week[53]	15-19 kg: ¼ tablet 20-30 kg: ½ tablet 31-45 kg: ¾ tablet >45 kg: 1 tablet
OR	Doxycycline[7,50,54]	100 mg daily	>8 years of age: 2 mg/kg/d orally, up to 100 mg/day
OR	Chloroquine phosphate[50] plus	as above	as above
	pyrimethamine- sulfadoxine[42] for presumptive treat- ment[55]	Carry a single dose (3 tablets) for self-treatment of febrile illness when medical care is not im- mediately available	<1 yr: ¼ tablet 1-3 yrs: ½ tablet 4-8 yrs: 1 tablet 9-14 yrs: 2 tablets
	or plus proguanil[56] (in Africa south of the Sahara)	200 mg daily during exposure and for 4 weeks afterwards	<2 yrs: 50 mg daily 2-6 yrs: 100 mg daily 7-10 yrs: 150 mg daily 10 yrs: 200 mg daily

* The letter d stands for day.

MICROSPORIDIOSIS

Enterocytozoon bieneusi			
Drug of choice:	none[57]		
Encephalitozoon hellem			
Drug of choice:	none[58]		

Mites, see SCABIES

MONILIFORMIS moniliformis infection			
Drug of choice:	Pyrantel pamoate[7]	11 mg/kg once, repeat twice, 2 wks apart	11 mg/kg once, repeat twice, 2 wks apart

Naegleria species, see AMEBIC MENINGOENCEPHALITIS, PRIMARY

Necator americanus, see HOOKWORM infection

Onchocerca volvulus, see FILARIASIS

Opisthorchis viverrini, see FLUKE infection

Paragonimus westermani, see FLUKE infection

Pediculus capitis, humanus, Phthirus pubis, see LICE

Pinworm, see ENTEROBIUS

Infection	Drug	Adult Dosage*	Pediatric Dosage*
PNEUMOCYSTIS carinii pneumonia[59]			
Drug of choice:	Trimethoprim-sulfamethoxazole	TMP 15-20 mg/kg/d, SMX 75-100 mg/kg/d, oral or IV in 3 or 4 doses x 14-21d	Same as adult dose
Alternatives:	OR Pentamidine	3-4 mg/kg IV qd x 14-21 days	Same as adult dose
	Trimethoprim[7] plus dapsone[7,60]	5 mg/kg PO q6h x 21 days 100 mg PO qd x 21 days	
	Primaquine[7,48] plus clindamycin[7]	15 mg base PO qd x 21 days 600 mg IV q6h x 21 days, or 300-450 mg PO q6h x 21 days	
	Trimetrexate plus folinic acid	45 mg/m² IV qd x 21 days 20 mg/m² PO or IV qd x 21 days	
Primary and secondary prophylaxis			
Drug of Choice:	Trimethoprim-sulfamethoxazole	1 DS[61] tab PO qd, bid, or 3x/week	
Alternatives:	Dapsone[7,60]	25-50 mg PO qd, or 100 mg PO 2 x week	
	Aerosol pentamidine	300 mg inhaled monthly via *Respirgard II nebulizer*	
Roundworm, see ASCARIASIS			
SCABIES (Sarcoptes scabiei)			
Drug of choice:	5% Permethrin	Topically	Topically
Alternatives:	Lindane[32]	Topically	Topically
	10% Crotamiton	Topically	Topically
SCHISTOSOMIASIS (Bilharziasis)			
S. haematobium			
Drug of choice:	Praziquantel	40 mg/kg/d in 2 doses x 1d	40 mg/kg/d in 2 doses x 1d
S. japonicum			
Drug of choice:	Praziquantel	60 mg/kg/d in 3 doses x 1d	60 mg/kg/d in 3 doses x 1d
S. mansoni			
Drug of choice:	Praziquantel	40 mg/kg/d in 2 doses x 1d	40 mg/kg/d in 2 doses x 1d
Alternative:	Oxamniquine[62]	15 mg/kg once[43]	20 mg/kg/d in 2 doses x 1d[63]
S. mekongi			
Drug of choice:	Praziquantel	60 mg/kg/d in 3 doses x 1d	60 mg/kg/d in 3 doses x 1d
Sleeping sickness, see TRYPANOSOMIASIS			
STRONGYLOIDIASIS (Strongyloides stercoralis)			
Drug of choice:[64]	Thiabendazole	50 mg/kg/d in 2 doses (max. 3 grams /d) x 2d[11,65]	50 mg/kg/d in 2 doses (max. 3 grams/d) x 2d[11,65]
	OR Ivermectin[2]	200 µg/kg/d x 1-2d	
	OR Albendazole	400 mg qd x 3d	400 mg qd x 3d
TAPEWORM infection — Adult (intestinal stage)			
Diphyllobothrium latum (fish), *Taenia saginata* (beef), *Taenia solium* (pork), *Dipylidium caninum* (dog)			
Drug of choice:	Praziquantel[7]	10-20 mg/kg once	10-20 mg/kg once
	OR Niclosamide[7]	A single dose of 4 tablets (2 grams), chewed thoroughly	11-34 kg: a single dose of 2 tablets (1 gram); >34 kg: a single dose of 3 tablets (1.5 grams)
Hymenolepis nana (dwarf tapeworm)			
Drug of choice:	Praziquantel[7]	25 mg/kg once	25 mg/kg once
Alternative:	Niclosamide	A single daily dose of 4 tablets (2 g), chewed thoroughly, then 2 tablets daily x 6d	11-34 kg: a single dose of 2 tablets (1 g) x 1d, then 1 tablet (0.5 grams) /d x 6d; >34 kg: a single dose of 3 tablets (1.5 g) x 1d, then 2 tablets (1 gram)/d x 6d
— Larval (tissue stage)			
Echinococcus granulosus (hydatid cyst)			
Drug of choice:	Albendazole[66]	400 mg bid x 28 days, repeated as necessary	15 mg/kg/d x 28 days, repeated as necessary
Echinococcus multilocularis			
Treatment of choice:	See footnote 67		
Cysticercus cellulosae (cysticercosis)			
Drug of choice:[68]	Praziquantel[7]	50 mg/kg/d in 3 doses x 15d	50 mg/kg/d in 3 doses x 15d
	OR Albendazole	15 mg/kg/d in 3 doses x 8d, repeated as necessary	15 mg/kg/d in 3 doses x 8d, repeated as necessary
Alternative:	Surgery		
Toxocariasis, see VISCERAL LARVA MIGRANS			
TOXOPLASMOSIS (Toxoplasma gondii)[69]			
Drugs of choice:	Pyrimethamine[70]	25-100 mg/d x 3-4 wks	2 mg/kg/d x 3d, then 1 mg/kg/d (max. 25 mg/d) x 4 wks[71]
	plus sulfadiazine	1-2 grams qid x 3-4 wks	100-200 mg/kg/d x 3-4 wks
Alternative:	Spiramycin	3-4 grams/d[72]	50-100 mg/kg/d x 3-4 wks

Infection	Drug	Adult Dosage*	Pediatric Dosage*
Drugs of choice:	Steroids for severe symptoms		
	plus mebendazole[7,73]	200-400 mg tid x 3d, then 400-500 mg tid x 10d	

TRICHOMONIASIS (*Trichomonas vaginalis*)

Drug of choice:[74]	Metronidazole[3]	2 grams once or 250 mg tid orally x 7d	15 mg/kg/d orally in 3 doses x 7d
OR	Tinidazole[4]	2 grams once	50 mg/kg once (max. 2 grams)

TRICHOSTRONGYLUS infection

Drug of choice:	Pyrantel pamoate[7]	11 mg/kg once (max. 1 gram)	11 mg/kg once (max. 1 gram)
Alternative:	Mebendazole[7]	100 mg bid x 3d	100 mg bid x 3d
OR	Albendazole	400 mg once	400 mg once

TRICHURIASIS (*Trichuris trichiura*, whipworm)

Drug of choice:	Mebendazole	100 mg bid x 3d	100 mg bid x 3d
OR	Albendazole	400 mg once[75]	400 mg once[75]

TRYPANOSOMIASIS

T. cruzi (South American trypanosomiasis, Chagas' disease)

Drug of choice:	Nifurtimox[2,76]	8-10 mg/kg/d orally in 4 doses x 120d	1-10 yrs: 15-20 mg/kg/d in 4 doses x 90d; 11-16 yrs: 12.5-15 mg/kg/d in 4 doses x 90d
Alternative:	Benznidazole[77]	5-7 mg/kg/d x 30-120d	

TRYPANOSOMIASIS (continued)

T. brucei gambiense; T. b. rhodesiense (African trypanosomiasis, sleeping sickness)
hemolymphatic stage

Drug of choice:	Suramin[2]	100-200 mg (test dose) IV, then 1 gram IV on days 1,3,7,14, and 21	20 mg/kg on days 1,3,7,14, and 21
OR	Eflornithine	see footnote 78	
Alternative:	Pentamidine isethionate[7]	4 mg/kg/d IM x 10d	4 mg/kg/d IM x 10d

late disease with CNS involvement

Drug of choice:	Melarsoprol[2,79]	2-3.6 mg/kg/d IV x 3 doses; after 1 wk 3.6 mg/kg per day IV x 3 doses; repeat again after 10-21 days	18-25 mg/kg total over 1 month; initial dose of 0.36 mg/kg IV, increasing gradually to max. 3.6 mg/kg at intervals of 1-5d for total of 9-10 doses
OR	Eflornithine	see footnote 78	
Alternatives:	Tryparsamide	One injection of 30 mg/kg (max. 2g) IV every 5d to total of 12 injections; may be repeated after 1 month	
	plus suramin[2]	One injection of 10 mg/kg IV every 5d to total of 12 injections; may be repeated after 1 month	

VISCERAL LARVA MIGRANS[80]

Drug of choice:[81]	Diethylcarbamazine[7]	6 mg/kg/d in 3 doses x 7-10d	6 mg/kg/d in 3 doses x 7-10d
Alternatives:	Thiabendazole	50 mg/kg/d in 2 doses x 5d (max. 3 grams/d)[11]	50 mg/kg/d in 2 doses x 5d (max. 3 grams /d)[11]
	Mebendazole[7]	100-200 mg bid x 5d[82]	

Whipworm, see TRICHURIASIS

Wuchereria bancrofti, see FILARIASIS

* The letter d stands for day.

1. Dosage and duration of administration should not be exceeded because of possibility of causing optic neuritis; maximum dosage is 2 grams/day.

2. In the USA, this drug is available from the CDC Drug Service, Centers for Disease Control, Atlanta, Georgia 30333; telephone: 404-639-3670 (evenings, weekends, and holidays: 404-639-2888).

3. Metronidazole is carcinogenic in rodents and mutagenic in bacteria; it should generally not be given to pregnant women, particularly in the first trimester.

4. A nitro-imidazole similar to metronidazole, but not marketed in the USA; tinidazole appears to be at least as effective as metronidazole and better tolerated. Ornidazole, a similar drug, is also used outside the USA.

5. Contraindicated in pregnancy

6. One patient with a *Naegleria* infection was successfully treated with amphotericin B, miconazole, and rifampin (JS Seidel et al, N Engl J Med, 306:346, 1982).

7. An approved drug, but considered investigational for this condition by the U.S. Food and Drug Administration

8. Strains of *Acanthamoeba* isolated from fatal granulomatous amebic encephalitis are usually sensitive *in vitro* to pentamidine, ketoconazole (*Nizoral*), 5-fluorocytosine, and (less so) to amphotericin B (RJ Duma et al, Antimicrob Agents Chemother, 10:370, 1976). For treatment of keratitis caused by *Acanthamoeba*, concurrent topical use of 0.1% propamidine isethionate (*Brolene* – Rhône-Poulenc Rorer, Canada) plus neosporin, or oral itraconazole (*Sporanox* – Janssen) plus topical miconazole, has been successful (MB Moore and JP McCulley, Br J Ophthalmol, 73:271, 1989; Y Ishibashi et al, Am J Ophthalmol, 109:121, 1990).

9. Effectiveness documented only in animals

10. Most patients recover spontaneously without antiparasitic drug therapy. Analgesics, corticosteroids, and careful removal of CSF at frequent intervals can relieve symptoms (J Koo et al, Rev Infect Dis, 10:1155, 1988). Albendazole, levamisole (*Ergamisol*), or ivermectin has also been used successfully in animals.

11. This dose is likely to be toxic and may have to be decreased.

12. Azithromycin (*Zithromax*) 150 mg/kg plus quinine has been effective in experimental animals. Concurrent use of pentamidine and trimethoprim-sulfamethoxazole has been reported to cure an infection with *B. divergens* (D Raoult et al, Ann Intern Med, 107:944, 1987).

13. Not recommended for children less than eight years old.

14. Drugs that could be tried include diethylcarbamazine, levamisole, and fenbendazole (KR Kazacos, J Am Vet Med Assoc, 195:894, 1989) and ivermectin. Steroid therapy may be helpful, especially in eye or CNS infection. Ocular baylisascariasis has been treated successfully using laser therapy to destroy intraretinal larvae.

15. Clinical significance of these organisms is controversial; but metronidazole 750 mg tid x 10d or iodoquinol 650 mg tid x 20d anecdotally have been reported to be effective (RA Miller and BH Minshew, Rev Infect Dis, 10:930, 1988; PW Doyle et al, J Clin Microbiol, 28:116, 1990).

16. Infection is self-limited in immunocompetent patients. In AIDS patients with large-volume intractable diarrhea, octreotide (*Sandostatin*) 300-500 µg tid subcutaneously may control the diarrhea, but not the infection (DJ Cook et al, Ann Intern Med, 108:708, 1988). Paromomycin may be helpful in some patients (K Clezy et al, AIDS, 5:1146, 1991; J Gathe, Jr et al, Int Conf AIDS, 6:384, 1990).

17. Albendazole 200 mg bid x 3 days has also been reported to be effective (SK Jones et al, Br J Dermatol, 122:99, 1990).

18. Not curative, but decreases inflammation and facilitates removing the worm. Mebendazole 400-800 mg/d for 6d has been reported to kill the worm directly.

19. A single dose of ivermectin, 25-200 µg/kg, has been reported to be effective for treatment of microfilaremia due to W. bancrofti and M. ozzardi (EA Ottesen et al, N Engl J Med, 322:1113, 1990; M Sabry et al, Trans R Soc Trop Med Hyg, 85:640, 1991; TB Nutman et al, J Infect Dis, 156:662, 1987).

20. Antihistamines or corticosteroids may be required to decrease allergic reactions due to disintegration of microfilariae in treatment of filarial infections, especially those caused by *Loa loa*. Diethylcarbamazine should be administered with special caution in heavy infections with *Loa loa* because it can provoke an encephalopathy (B Carme et al, Am J Trop Med Hyg, 44:684, 1991). Apheresis has been reported to be effective in lowering microfilarial counts in patients heavily infected with loiasis. Diethylcarbamazine, 300 mg once weekly, has been recommended for prevention of loiasis (TB Nutman et al, N Engl J Med, 319:752, 1988).

21. For patients with no microfilaremia in the blood or skin, full doses can be given from day one.

22. Ivermectin may also be effective.

23. Unlike infections with other flukes, *hepatica* infections may not respond to praziquantel. Limited data, however, indicate that triclabendazole (*Fasinex*), a veterinary fasciolide, is safe and effective in a single oral dose of 10 mg/kg (L Loutan et al, Lancet, 2:383, 1989).

141

24. Not absorbed; may be useful for treatment of giardiasis in pregnant women.

25. In sulfonamide-sensitive patients, such as some patients with AIDS, pyrimethamine 50-75 mg daily has been effective (LM Weiss et al, Ann Intern Med, 109:474, 1988). In immunocompromised patients, it may be necessary to continue therapy indefinitely.

26. Limited data indicate that ketoconazole, 400 to 600 mg daily for four to eight weeks, may be effective for treatment of cutaneous and mucosal leishmaniasis (RE Saenz et al, Am J Med, 89:147, 1990).

27. May be repeated or continued. A longer duration may be needed for some forms of visceral leishmaniasis.

28. Recent studies indicate that stibogluconate (pentavalent antimony)-resistant L. donovani may respond to recombinant human gamma interferon in addition to antimony (R Badaro et al, N Engl J Med, 322:16, 1990), pentamidine followed by a course of antimony (CP Thakur et al, Am J Trop Med Hyg, 45:435, 1991), or ketoconazole (JP Wali et al, Lancet, 336:810, 1990). Recently, liposomal encapsulated amphotericin B (AmBisome, Vestar, San Dimas, CA) was used successfully to treat multiple-drug-resistant visceral leishmaniasis (RN Davidson et al, Lancet, 337:1061, 1991).

29. Application of heat 39° to 42°C directly to the lesion for 20 to 32 hours over a period of 10 to 12 days has been reported to be effective in cutaneous L. tropica (FA Neva et al, Am J Trop Med Hyg, 33:800, 1984).

30. For infestation of eyelashes with crab lice, use petrolatum.

31. FDA-approved only for head lice

32. Some consultants recommend a second application one week later to kill hatching progeny. Seizures have been reported in association with the use of lindane. Do not use higher than recommended doses and avoid warm baths before application (M Tenenbein, J Am Geriatr Soc, 39:394, 1991). Prolonged use of lindane has been associated with aplastic anemia (AE Rauch et al, Arch Intern Med, 150:2393, 1990).

33. If chloroquine phosphate is not available, hydroxychloroquine sulfate is as effective; 400 mg of hydroxychloroquine sulfate is equivalent to 500 mg of chloroquine phosphate.

34. In P. falciparum malaria, if the patient has not shown a response to conventional doses of chloroquine in 48-72 hours, parasitic resistance to this drug should be considered. P. vivax with decreased susceptibility to chloroquine has been reported from Papua New Guinea (KH Rieckmann et al, Lancet, 2:1183, 1989) and from Indonesia (IK Schwartz et al, N Engl J Med, 324:927, 1991). Intramuscular injection of chloroquine can be painful and has been reported to cause abscesses.

35. A recent study found artemether, a Chinese drug, effective for parenteral treatment of severe malaria in children (NJ White et al, Lancet, 339:317, 1992).

36. Some experts consider quinidine more effective than quinine. EKG monitoring is necessary to detect arrhythmias. Oral drugs should be substituted as soon as possible.

37. Not available in the USA. P. falciparum infections with a high parasitemia may require a loading dose of 20 mg/kg (NJ White et al, Am J Trop Med Hyg, 32:1, 1983). IV administration of quinine dihydrochloride can be hazardous; constant monitoring of the pulse and blood pressure is necessary to detect arrhythmia or hypotension. Use of parenteral quinine may also lead to severe hypoglycemia; blood glucose should be monitored. Oral drugs should be substituted as soon as possible.

38. Chloroquine-resistant P. falciparum infections have been reported in all areas that have malaria except Central America north of Panama, Mexico, Haiti, the Dominican Republic, and the Middle East (including Egypt). In pregnancy, chloroquine prophylaxis has been used extensively and safely, but the safety of other prophylactic antimalarial agents in pregnancy is unclear. Therefore, travel during pregnancy to chloroquine-resistant areas should be discouraged. For chloroquine-resistant parasitemia > 10%, exchange transfusion has been used (KD Miller et al, N Engl J Med, 321:65, 1989; M Saddler et al; F Vachon et al; KD Miller et al, N Engl J Med, 322:58, 1990).

39. Chloroquine-resistant falciparum malaria acquired outside of Southeast Asia, East Africa, Bangladesh, Oceania and the Amazon basin is likely to respond to quinine (or quinidine) plus pyrimethamine-sulfadoxine. In pregnancy, quinine (or quinidine) plus clindamycin is a reasonable alternative.

40. Although quinine will usually control an attack of resistant falciparum malaria, in a substantial number of infections from Southeast Asia, Bangladesh, Oceania, East Africa, and the Amazon region it fails to prevent recurrence. In these regions, there may be pyrimethamine-sulfadoxine resistance, and addition of tetracycline or clindamycin may decrease the rate of recurrence.

41. In Southeast Asia, there is a relative increase in resistance to quinine and the usual treatment dose should be extended to seven days.

42. Fansidar tablets contain 25 mg of pyrimethamine and 500 mg of sulfadoxine.

43. At this dosage, adverse effects including nausea, vomiting, diarrhea, dizziness, disturbed sense of balance, toxic psychosis, and seizures can occur. Mefloquine is teratogenic in animals. It should not be given together with quinine or quinidine, and caution is required in using quinine or quinidine to treat patients with malaria who have taken mefloquine for prophylaxis. The pediatric dosage has not been approved by the FDA.

44. In the USA, a 250-mg tablet of mefloquine contains 228 mg of mefloquine base. Outside the USA, each 274-mg tablet contains 250 mg base.

45. Outside the USA, the manufacturer recommends dividing the 1250-mg dose into 750 mg followed 6-8 hours later by 500 mg (D Kingston, Med J Aust, 153:235, 1990).

46. NJ White, Eur J Clin Pharm, 34:1, 1988

47. May be effective in multiple-drug-resistant falciparum malaria (ed., Lancet, 2:537, 1989). Failures in treatment of multiple-drug-resistant malaria have, however, been reported (GD Shanks et al, Am J Trop Med Hyg, 45:488, 1991). For patients with minimal previous exposure to malaria, a second course of therapy is recommended one week after the first course.

48. Primaquine phosphate can cause hemolytic anemia, especially in patients whose red cells are deficient in glucose-6-phosphate dehydrogenase. This deficiency is most common in Blacks, Orientals, and Mediterranean peoples. Patients should be screened for G-6-PD deficiency before treatment. Primaquine should not be used during pregnancy.

49. At present, no drug regimen guarantees protection against malaria. If fever develops within a year (particularly within the first two months) after travel to malarious areas, travelers should be advised to seek medical attention. Insect repellents, insecticide-impregnated bed nets, and proper clothing are important adjuncts for malaria prophylaxis.

50. For prevention of attack after departure from areas where P. vivax and P. ovale are endemic, which includes almost all areas where malaria is found (except Haiti), some experts in addition prescribe primaquine phosphate 15 mg base (26.3 mg)/d or, for children, 0.3 mg base/kg/d during the last two weeks of prophylaxis. Others prefer to avoid the toxicity of primaquine and rely on surveillance to detect cases when they occur, particularly when exposure was limited or doubtful. See also footnote 48.

51. For prophylaxis where both chloroquine and pyrimethamine/sulfadoxine resistance coexist, mefloquine is the usual drug of choice. In mefloquine-resistant areas, such as Thailand, doxycycline is recommended.

52. The pediatric dosage has been approved by the FDA, and the drug has not been approved for use during pregnancy. Women should take contraceptive precautions while taking mefloquine and for two months after the last dose. Mefloquine is not recommended for children weighing less than 15 kg, or for patients taking beta-blockers, calcium-channel blockers, or other drugs that may prolong or otherwise alter cardiac conduction. Patients with a history of seizures or psychiatric disorders and those whose occupation requires fine coordination or spatial discrimination should probably avoid mefloquine (Medical Letter, 32:13, 1990).

53. Beginning one week before travel and for four weeks after leaving.

54. Beginning one day before travel and continuing weekly for the duration of stay and for four weeks after leaving. The FDA considers use of tetracyclines as antimalarials to be investigational. Use of tetracyclines is contraindicated in pregnancy and in children less than eight years old. Physicians who prescribe doxycycline as malaria chemoprophylaxis should advise patients to use an appropriate sunscreen (Medical Letter, 31:59, 1989) to minimize the possibility of a photosensitivity reaction and should warn women that Candida vaginitis is a frequent adverse effect.

55. Resistance to Fansidar should be anticipated in Southeast Asia, Bangladesh, Oceania, the Amazon basin, and in east Africa. Use of Fansidar is contraindicated in patients with a history of sulfonamide or pyrimethamine intolerance. In pregnancy at term and in infants less than two months old, pyrimethamine-sulfadoxine may cause hyperbilirubinemia.

56. Proguanil (Paludrine – Ayerst, Canada; ICI, England), which is not available in the USA but is widely available overseas, is recommended mainly for use in Africa south of the Sahara. Failures in prophylaxis with chloroquine and proguanil have, however, been reported in travelers to Kenya (AJ Barnes, Lancet, 338:1338, 1991)

57. In a limited number of patients with severe diarrhea, albendazole 400 mg bid for 4-6 weeks was reported to produce remission (C Blanshard et al, Int Conf AIDS, 7:248, 1991). Octreotide (Sandostatin, Sandoz) has provided symptomatic relief (JP Cello et al, Ann Intern Med, 115:705, 1991).

58. A keratopathy in an AIDS patient was treated successfully with surgical debridement, topical antibiotics, and itraconazole (Sporanox – Janssen) (RW Yee et al, Ophthalmology, 98:196, 1991).

59. AIDS patients should be treated for 21 days. In moderate or severe PCP with room air PO₂ ≤70 mmHg or Aa gradient ≥35 mmHg prednisone should also be used (Medical Letter, 33:101, 1991).

60. Assay for G-6-PD deficiency recommended at start of therapy.

61. Each double-strength tablet contains 160 mg TMP and 800 mg SMX

62. Contraindicated in pregnancy. Neuropsychiatric disturbances and seizures have been reported in some patients (H Stokvis et al, Am J Trop Med Hyg, 35:330, 1986).

63. In east Africa, the dose should be increased to 30 mg/kg, and in Egypt and South Africa, 30 mg/kg/d x 2d. Some experts recommend 40-60 mg/kg over 2-3 days in all of Africa (KC Shekhar, Drugs, 42:379, 1991).

64. In immunocompromised patients it may be necessary to continue therapy or use other agents.

65. In disseminated strongyloidiasis, thiabendazole therapy should be continued for at least five days.

143

66. With a fatty meal to enhance absorption. Some patients may benefit from or require surgical resection of cysts (RK Tompkins, Mayo Clin Proc, 66:1281, 1991). Praziquantel may also be useful preoperatively or in case of spill during surgery.

67. Surgical excision is the only reliable means of treatment, although some reports have suggested use of albendazole or mebendazole (JF Wilson et al, Am J Trop Med Hyg, 37:162, 1987; A Davis et al, Bull WHO, 64:383, 1986).

68. Corticosteroids should be given for two to three days before and during drug therapy. Any cysticercoidal drug may cause irreparable damage when used to treat ocular or spinal cysts, even when corticosteroids are used.

69. In ocular toxoplasmosis, corticosteroids should also be used for anti-inflammatory effect on the eyes.

70. Pyrimethamine is teratogenic in animals. To prevent hematological toxicity from pyrimethamine, it is advisable to give leucovorin (folinic acid), about 10 mg/day, either by injection or orally. Some clinicians use pyrimethamine 50 to 100 mg daily after a loading dose of 200 mg with a sulfonamide to treat CNS toxoplasmosis in patients with AIDS and, when sulfonamide sensitivity developed, have given clindamycin 1.8 to 2.4 g/d in divided doses instead of the sulfonamide. In AIDS patients, chronic suppressive treatment with lower dosage should continue indefinitely (Medical Letter, 34:95, 1991; B Danneman et al, Ann Intern Med, 116:33, Jan 1, 1992).

71. Congenitally infected newborns should be treated with pyrimethamine every two or three days and a sulfonamide daily for about one year (JS Remington and G Desmonts in JS Remington and JO Klein, eds, Infectious Disease of the Fetus and Newborn Infant, 3rd ed, Philadelphia/Saunders, 1990, page 89).

72. For treatment during pregnancy, continue the drug until delivery.

73. Albendazole or flubendazole (not available in the USA) may also be effective for this indication.

74. Sexual partners should be treated simultaneously. Outside the USA, ornidazole has also been used for this condition. Metronidazole-resistant strains have been reported; higher doses of metronidazole for longer periods are sometimes effective against these strains (J Lossick, Rev Infect Dis, 12:S665, 1990).

75. In heavy infection it may be necessary to extend therapy for 3 days.

76. The addition of gamma interferon to nifurtimox for 20 days in a limited number of patients and in experimental animals appears to have shortened the acute phase of Chagas' disease (RE McCabe et al, J Infect Dis, 163:912, 1991).

77. Limited data

78. In T. b. gambiense infections, eflornithine is highly effective in both the hemolymphatic and CNS stages. Its effectiveness in T. b. rhodesiense infections has been variable. Some clinicians have given 400 mg/kg/d IV in 4 divided doses for 14 days, followed by oral treatment with 300 mg/kg/d for 3-4 wks (F Doua et al, Am J Trop Med Hyg, 37:525, 1987).

79. In frail patients, begin with as little as 18 mg and increase the dose progressively. Pretreatment with suramin has been advocated for debilitated patients. Corticosteroids have been used to prevent arsenical encephalopathy (J Pepin et al, Lancet, 1:1246, 1989).

80. For severe symptoms or eye involvement, corticosteroids can be used in addition.

81. Ivermectin or albendazole may also be effective (D Stürchler et al, Ann Trop Med Parasitol, 83:473, 1989).

82. One report of a cure using 1 gram tid for 21 days has been published (A Bekhti, Ann Intern Med, 100:463, 1984).

144

ADVERSE EFFECTS OF SOME ANTIPARASITIC DRUGS*

ALBENDAZOLE (Zentel)
Occasional: diarrhea; abdominal pain; migration of ascaris through mouth and nose
Rare: leukopenia; alopecia; increased serum transaminase activity

BENZNIDAZOLE (Rochagan)
Frequent: allergic rash; dose-dependent polyneuropathy; gastrointestinal disturbances; psychic disturbances

BITHIONOL (Bitin)
Frequent: photosensitivity reactions; vomiting; diarrhea; abdominal pain; urticaria
Rare: leukopenia; toxic hepatitis

CHLOROQUINE HCl and CHLOROQUINE PHOSPHATE (Aralen, and others)
Occasional: pruritus; vomiting; headache; confusion; depigmentation of hair; skin eruptions; corneal opacity; weight loss; partial alopecia; extraocular muscle palsies; exacerbation of psoriasis, eczema, and other exfoliative dermatoses; myalgias; photophobia
Rare: irreversible retinal injury (especially when total dosage exceeds 100 grams); discoloration of nails and mucus membranes; nerve-type deafness; peripheral neuropathy and myopathy; heart block; blood dyscrasias; hematemesis

CROTAMITON (Eurax)
Occasional: rash; conjunctivitis

DEHYDROEMETINE
Frequent: cardiac arrhythmias; precordial pain; muscle weakness; cellulitis at site of injection
Occasional: diarrhea; vomiting; peripheral neuropathy; heart failure; headache; dyspnea

DIETHYLCARBAMAZINE CITRATE USP (Hetrazan)
Frequent: severe allergic or febrile reactions in patients with microfilaria in the blood or the skin; GI disturbances
Rare: encephalopathy

DILOXANIDE FUROATE (Furamide)
Frequent: flatulence
Occasional: nausea; vomiting; diarrhea
Rare: diplopia; dizziness; urticaria; pruritus

EFLORNITHINE (Difluoromethylornithine, DFMO, Ornidyl)
Frequent: anemia; leukopenia
Occasional: diarrhea; thrombocytopenia; seizures
Rare: hearing loss

FLUBENDAZOLE – similar to mebendazole

FURAZOLIDONE (Furoxone)
Frequent: nausea; vomiting
Occasional: allergic reactions, including pulmonary infiltration, hypotension, urticaria, fever, vesicular rash; hypoglycemia; headache
Rare: hemolytic anemia in G-6-PD deficiency and neonates; disulfiram-like reaction with alcohol; MAO-inhibitor interactions; polyneuritis

HALOFANTRINE (Halfan)
Occasional: diarrhea; abdominal pain; pruritus

IODOQUINOL (Yodoxin)
Occasional: rash; acne; slight enlargement of the thyroid gland; nausea; diarrhea; cramps; anal pruritus
Rare: optic atrophy; loss of vision, peripheral neuropathy after prolonged use in high dosage (for months); iodine sensitivity

IVERMECTIN (Mectizan)
Occasional: Mazzotti-type reaction seen in onchocerciasis, including fever, pruritus, tender lymph nodes, headache; and joint and bone pain
Rare: hypotension

LINDANE (Kwell; and others)
Occasional: eczematous rash; conjunctivitis
Rare: convulsions; aplastic anemia

MALATHION (Ovide)
Occasional: local irritation

MEBENDAZOLE (Vermox)
Occasional: diarrhea; abdominal pain; migration of ascaris through mouth and nose
Rare: leukopenia; agranulocytosis; hypospermia

MEFLOQUINE (Lariam)
Frequent: vertigo; lightheadedness; nausea; other gastrointestinal disturbances; nightmares; visual disturbances; headache
Occasional: confusion
Rare: psychosis; hypotension; convulsions; coma

MEGLUMINE ANTIMONIATE (Glucantime) Similar to stibogluconate sodium

MELARSOPROL (Arsobal)
Frequent: myocardial damage; albuminuria; hypertension; colic; Herxheimer-type reaction; encephalopathy; vomiting; peripheral neuropathy
Rare: shock

METRONIDAZOLE (Flagyl, and others)
Frequent: nausea; headache; dry mouth; metallic taste
Occasional: vomiting; diarrhea; insomnia; weakness; stomatitis; vertigo; paresthesias; rash; dark urine; urethral burning; disulfiram-like reaction with alcohol
Rare: seizures; encephalopathy; pseudomembranous colitis; ataxia; leukopenia; peripheral neuropathy; pancreatitis

NICLOSAMIDE (Niclocide)
Occasional: nausea; abdominal pain

NIFURTIMOX (Lampit)
Frequent: anorexia; vomiting; weight loss; loss of memory; sleep disorders; tremor; paresthesias; weakness; polyneuritis
Rare: convulsions; fever; pulmonary infiltrates and pleural effusion

ORNIDAZOLE (Tiberal)
Occasional: dizziness; headache; gastrointestinal disturbances
Rare: reversible peripheral neuropathy

OXAMNIQUINE (Vansil)
Occasional: headache; fever; dizziness; somnolence; nausea; diarrhea; rash; insomnia; hepatic enzyme changes; ECG changes; EEG changes; orange-red discoloration of urine
Rare: seizures; neuropsychiatric disturbances

PAROMOMYCIN (Humatin)
Frequent: GI disturbances
Rare: eighth-nerve damage (mainly auditory); renal damage

PENTAMIDINE ISETHIONATE (Pentam 300, NebuPent)
Frequent: hypotension; hypoglycemia often followed by diabetes mellitus; vomiting; blood dyscrasias; renal damage; pain at injection site; GI disturbances
Occasional: may aggravate diabetes; shock; hypocalcemia; liver damage; cardiotoxicity; delirium; rash
Rare: Herxheimer-type reaction; anaphylaxis; acute pancreatitis; hyperkalemia

PERMETHRIN *(Nix, Elimite)*
Occasional: burning; stinging; numbness; increased pruritus; pain; edema; erythema; rash

PRAZIQUANTEL *(Biltricide)*
Frequent: malaise; headache; dizziness
Occasional: sedation; abdominal discomfort; fever; sweating; nausea; eosinophilia; fatigue
Rare: pruritus; rash

PRIMAQUINE PHOSPHATE USP
Frequent: hemolytic anemia in G-6-PD deficiency
Occasional: neutropenia; GI disturbances; methemoglobinemia in G-6-PD deficiency
Rare: CNS symptoms; hypertension; arrhythmias

PROGUANIL *(Paludrine)*
Occasional: oral ulceration; hair loss; scaling of palms and soles
Rare: hematuria (with large doses); vomiting; abdominal pain; diarrhea (with large doses)

PYRANTEL PAMOATE *(Antiminth)*
Occasional: GI disturbances; headache; dizziness; rash; fever

PYRETHRINS and PIPERONYL BUTOXIDE *(RID, others)*
Occasional: allergic reactions

PYRIMETHAMINE USP *(Daraprim)*
Occasional: blood dyscrasias; folic acid deficiency
Rare: rash; vomiting; convulsions; shock; possibly pulmonary eosinophilia

QUINACRINE HCl USP *(Atabrine)*
Frequent: dizziness; headache; vomiting; diarrhea
Occasional: yellow staining of skin; toxic psychosis; insomnia; bizarre dreams; blood dyscrasias; urticaria; blue and black nail pigmentation; psoriasis-like rash
Rare: acute hepatic necrosis; convulsions; severe exfoliative dermatitis; ocular effects similar to those caused by chloroquine

QUININE DIHYDROCHLORIDE and SULFATE
Frequent: cinchonism (tinnitus, headache, nausea, abdominal pain, visual disturbance)
Occasional: deafness; hemolytic anemia; other blood dyscrasias; photosensitivity reactions; hypoglycemia; arrhythmias; hypotension; drug fever
Rare: blindness; sudden death if injected too rapidly

SPIRAMYCIN *(Rovamycine)*
Occasional: GI disturbances
Rare: allergic reactions

STIBOGLUCONATE SODIUM *(Pentostam)*
Frequent: muscle pain and joint stiffness; nausea; transaminase elevations; T-wave flattening or inversion
Occasional: weakness; colic; liver damage; bradycardia; leukopenia
Rare: diarrhea; rash; pruritus; myocardial damage; hemolytic anemia; renal damage; shock; sudden death

SURAMIN SODIUM *(Germanin)*
Frequent: vomiting; pruritus; urticaria; paresthesias; hyperesthesia of hands and feet; photophobia; peripheral neuropathy
Occasional: kidney damage; blood dyscrasias; shock; optic atrophy

THIABENDAZOLE *(Mintezol)*
Frequent: nausea; vomiting; vertigo
Occasional: leukopenia; crystalluria; rash; hallucinations; olfactory disturbance; erythema multiforme; Stevens-Johnson syndrome
Rare: shock; tinnitus; intrahepatic cholestasis; convulsions; angioneurotic edema

TINIDAZOLE *(Fasigyn)*
Occasional: metallic taste; nausea; vomiting; rash

TRIMETREXATE (with "leucovorin rescue")
Occasional: rash; peripheral neuropathy; bone marrow depression; increased serum aminotransferase concentrations

TRYPARSAMIDE
Frequent: nausea; vomiting
Occasional: impaired vision; optic atrophy; fever; exfoliative dermatitis; allergic reactions; tinnitus

Table 1: HIV INFECTION AND AIDS

INDICATOR CONDITIONS IN CASE DEFINITION OF AIDS (1987-92, ADULTS)

Candidiasis, of esophagus, trachea, bronchi or lungs
Coccidioidomycosis, extrapulmonary *
Cryptococcosis, extrapulmonary
Cryptosporidiosis with diarrhea > 1 month
Cytomegalovirus of any organ other than liver, spleen or lymph nodes
Herpes simplex with mucocutaneous ulcer > 1 month or bronchitis,
    pneumonitis, esophagitis
Histoplasmosis, extrapulmonary*
HIV-associated dementia*: Disabling cognitive and/or motor dysfunction
    interfering with occupation or activities of daily living
HIV-associated wasting*: Involuntary weight loss > 10% of baseline plus
    chronic diarrhea (≥ 2 loose stools/day ≥ 30 days) or chronic weakness and
    documented enigmatic fever ≥ 30 days
Isosporosis with diarrhea > 1 mo*
Kaposi sarcoma in patient under 60 yrs (or over 60 yrs*)
Lymphoma of brain in patient under 60 yrs (or over 60 yrs*)
Lymphoma, non-Hodgkins of B cell or unknown immunologic phenotype and
    histology showing small, noncleaved lymphoma or immunoblastic sarcoma
<u>Mycobacterium</u> <u>avium</u> or <u>M</u>. <u>kansasii</u>, disseminated
<u>Mycobacterium</u> <u>tuberculosis</u>, disseminated*
Nocardiosis*
<u>Pneumocystis</u> <u>carinii</u> pneumonia
Progressive multifocal leukoencephalopathy
Salmonella septicemia (non-typhoid), recurrent*
Strongyloidosis, extraintestinal
Toxoplasmosis of internal organ

---

*   Requires positive HIV serology

Table 2: PROPOSED EXPANDED AIDS SURVEILLANCE CASE DEFINITION FOR ADOLESCENTS AND ADULTS

	Clinical Categories		
	A	B	C*
CD4 cell Categories	Asymptomatic, or PGL or Acute HIV Infection	Symptomatic** (not A or C)	AIDS Indicator Condition (1987)
1) >500/cu mm	A 1	B 1	C 1
2) 200-499/cu mm	A 2	B 2	C 2
3) <200/cu mm	A 3	B 3	C 3

*   All patients in the shaded categories would be reported as having AIDS based on the prior AIDS-indicator conditions (Table 1) and/or a CD4 cell count <200/cu mm.

**   Includes but is not limited to bacterial infections (pneumonia, meningitis, endocarditis or sepsis); vulvovaginal candidiasis persistent >1 month and poorly responsive to treatment; thrush, oral hairy leukoplakia; severe cervical dysplasia or carcinoma; shingles with two episodes or >1 dermatome; ITP; listeriosis; nocardiosis; PID; peripheral neuropathy; constitutional symptoms such as fever (38.5°C or diarrhea for >1 month).

TABLE 3: SEROPREVALENCE RATES OF HIV IN THE U. S.

Category	Reference	Rate	Comment
Gay men	Am J Epid 126:568,1987 J AIDS 2:77,1989	14-50%	Average in MACS (5000 participants) was 36% at entry with 1% annual seroconversion rate
IV drug abusers	JAMA 261:2677,1989	1-60%	Review of 92 studies showed great variation by location: NYC: 34-61%; New Jersey: 17-29%; Boston: 28%; Puerto Rico: 45-59%; Detroit: 8-12%; San Francisco: 5-16%; Miami: 5%; New Orleans: 1%; Atlanta: 10%; Denver: 1-5%; Los Angeles: 2-5%; Minn: 1%; Annual seroconversion rate in Baltimore: 5%
Methadone clinic clients	NEJM 326:375,1992	9.2%	Eight city surveys with rates ranging from 0.7% (Seattle) to 28.6% (Newark)
Hemophilia	JAMA 253:3409,1985	Type A-70% Type B-35%	Applies to hemophiliacs who received clotting factors before 1985
Regular sex partners of HIV-infected persons	Arch Intern Med 149:645,1989 Amer J Med 85:472,1988 JAMA 266:1664,1991	0-58%	Average is 20-25% for wives of hemophiliac men with HIV infection; discordant couple study shows efficiency of transmission 20x greater for male–female transmission
Prostitutes	MMWR 36:157,1987 JAMA 263:60,1990	0-57%	Great variation by location and confounding variable of IVDU: Newark: 57%; Wash. DC: 50%; Miami: 19%; San Francisco: 6%; LA: 4%; Atlanta: 1%; Las Vegas: 0
Hospital admissions	NEJM 323:213,1990	0.1-7.8%	Average is 1.3%
College students	NEJM 323:1538,1990	0.2%	
Childbearing women	JAMA 265:1704,1991	0.15%	Highest rates were NYC: 0.58%; Wash DC: 0.55%; NJ: 0.49%; Florida: 0.45%
STD Clinic clients	STD 19:235,1992 NEJM 326:375,1992	0.5-11%	Summary of 176,439 sera from 98 STD clinics; median - 2.3%
Applicants to military	MMWR 37:67,1988 JAIDS 3:1168,1990 JAMA 265:1709,1991	0.13%	Annual seroconversion rate is 0.04%
Blood donors		0.02%	
General population	Science 253:37,1991 MMWR 30 RR-16,1990	0.4%	Based on assumed validity of one million HIV infected persons in U.S. Annual seroconversion rate based on assumption of 60,000 new infections/year is 0.02%

TABLE 4: CARE PLAN

	All patients	CD4 300-500/cu mm	CD4 100-300/cu mm	CD4< 150
Antiretroviral		AZT[a] or ddI[b]	AZT[a] or ddI[a] AZT + ddI[b] AZT + ddC[b]	AZT[a] or ddI[a] AZT + ddI[b] AZT + ddC[b]

Opportunistic infection (Prophylaxis)	Pneumovax
	PPD + : INH[a]
	Influenza vaccine[a]
			PCP prophylaxis[a]	PCP prophylaxis[a]
				Cryptococcus[b]:
				  Ketoconazole or
				  Fluconazole
				M. avium:
				  rifabutin[a] or
				  clarithromycin
				Toxoplasmosis[a]
				  TMP-SMX or
				  dapsone plus
				  pyrimethamine

[a] Efficacy established. PCP prophylaxis advocated for patients with CD4 cell count < 200/cu mm or prior PCP.

[b] Efficacy not established; clinical trials being conducted. Benefit of ddC + AZT versus AZT alone shown for CD4 cell counts as surrogate marker (Ann Intern Med 116:13,1992); efficacy of AZT + ddI is not established.
Toxoplasmosis: TMP-SMX (4-7 DS/week) appears to be effective (Ann Intern Med 117:106,1992); for patients unable to take TMP-SMX with CD4 cell count < 100-150/cu mm plus positive toxoplasmosis serology, some advocate dapsone (50 mg/day) plus pyrimethamine (50 mg/week).

TABLE 5: ANTIRETROVIRAL AGENTS: NUCLEOSIDE ANALOGS

	AZT	ddI	ddC
Indications: FDA labeling	CD4 < 500	Advanced HIV infection + prolonged therapy with AZT	CD4 count < 300 + clinical or immunologic deterioration with AZT treatment
Usual dose	500-600 mg/day	> 60 kg: 200 mg bid < 60 kg: 125 mg bid	0.75 mg tid
Oral bioavailability	60%	Tablet: 40% Tablet is 20-25% higher than powder	85%
Serum half life	1.1 hr	1.6 hr	1.2 hr
Intracellular half life	3 hr	12 hr	3 hr
CNS penetration (% serum levels)	60%	20%	20%
Elimination	Metabolized to AZT glucuronide (GAZT)	Renal excretion - 50%	Renal excretion - 70%
Major toxicity	Marrow suppression: Anemia and/or Granulocytopenia	Pancreatitis (Peripheral neuropathy)	Peripheral neuropathy (Pancreatitis)

Table 6. MANAGEMENT OF OPPORTUNISTIC INFECTIONS IN PATIENTS WITH HIV INFECTION

	Preferred	Alternative	Comment
PROTOZOA			
Pneumocystis carinii			
Acute infection	Trimethoprim (15 mg/kg/day) + sulfamethoxazole (75 mg/kg/day) po or IV x 21 days in 3-4 daily doses	Pentamidine (4 mg/kg/day) IV (or IM) x 21 days;	Some recommend trimethoprim-sulfamethoxazole/dapsone in dose of 20 mg/kg/day (trimethoprim)
		Trimethoprim (15 mg/kg/day) po or IV + dapsone* (100 mg/day) x 21 days (100 mg/day) x 21 days	Side effects to sulfonamide (rash, fever, leukopenia, hepatitis, etc.) most common at 1-2 wks.
		Atovaquone*** 750 mg po with food x 21 days (mild to moderate disease)	
		Clindamycin (600 mg IV q6h or 300-450 mg po q6h) + primaquine* (15 mg based po/day) x 21 days	Patients with moderately severe or severe disease (pO$_2$ <70 mmHg) should receive corticosteroids (prednisone, 40 mg bid x 5 days, then 40 mg qd x 5 days, then 20 mg/day to completion of treatment). Side effects include CNS toxicity, thrush, H. simplex infection, tuberculosis and other OIs
		Atovaquone*** (750 mg po tid with food) x 21 days available by: 1) treatment IND for persons with mild-moderately severe PCP in patients intolerant of sulfa and 2) open label for severe PCP for persons intolerant or unresponsive to TMP-SMX + pentamidine	
Prophylaxis	Trimethoprim (2.5-5 mg/kg) + sulfamethoxazole po as 1 DS qd or 3x/wk	Aerosolized pentamidine (300 mg) q month (300 mg) q month via Respirgard II nebulizer	Prophylaxis is indicated for any HIV infected patient with a history of Pneumocystis pneumonia or a CD4 count < 200/cu mm
		Dapsone* 25-100 mg po/day or 100 mg 2x/wk (usually 50 mg po/day)	
		Pyrimethamine (25 mg) + sulfadoxine (500 mg)1-2x/wk (1-2 Fansidar/wk)	Serious reactions including death from Stevens-Johnson syndrome have been reported with Fansidar; efficacy not established
		Pentamidine (4 mg/kg) IM or IV q 2 wks	Efficacy not established

152

(continued)

	Preferred	Alternative	Comment
Toxoplasma encephalitis Acute infection	Pyrimethamine (100-200 mg loading dose, then 50-100 mg/day) po x 6 wks + folinic acid (10 mg/day) po + sulfadiazine or trisulfapyrimidines (4-8 gm/day) po for at least 6 wks	Pyrimethamine + folinic acid (prior doses) + clindamycin (600 mg) IV q6-8h for at least 6 wks	All patients who respond to primary therapy should receive life-long suppressive therapy. Repeat MRI or CT scan at 2 weeks
		Atovaquone*** 750 mg 4x/day po with food	Relative merits of alternative regimens for patients who have become intolerant to or have failed pyrimethamine + sulfadiazine, are unknown
		Azithromycin*** (1800 mg po 1st day, then 1200 mg po/day x 6 wks, then 600 mg/day) or Atovaquone*** for patients who fail or were intolerant of standard treatment; both preferably used in combination with pyrimethamine	Corticosteroids if significant edema/mass effect (Decadron, 4 mg po or IV q6h)
Suppressive therapy	Pyrimethamine (25-50 mg) po q d plus folinic acid (5 mg/day) or sulfadiazine or trisulfapyrimidines (2-4 gm/day) po qid	Pyrimethamine (25-50 mg) po qd plus clindamycin (300-450 mg) po q6-8h	Suppressive treatment for toxoplasmosis will also prevent PCP
Prophylaxis	Trimethoprim-sulfamethoxazole (1DS 4x/wk - 1 DS qd) or Dapsone* (50 mg/day) + pyrimethamine(50 mg/wk)	Pyrimethamine (25 mg) po qd (see comment)	Possibly effective agents include atovaquone, trimethoprim-sulfa, azithromycin, clarithromycin and trimetrexate
			Sometimes advocated for patients with positive toxoplasmosis serology + CD4 count <150/mm^3
			Pyrimethamine (25 mg 3x/wk) is ineffective; efficacy of 25 mg po qd is not established
Cryptosporidia	Symptomatic treatment with nutritional supplements and anti-diarrheal agents (Lomotil, Loperamide, paregoric, etc)	Octreotide (Sandostatin) 50-200 µg SC or IV at 1 mcg/hr	Efficacy of spiramycin, paromomycin and octreotide not established; other possibly effective agents: DFMO, bovine colostrum and transfer factor. Non-steroidal anti-inflammatory agents sometimes useful.
		Paromomycin 250 mg po qid	
		Azithromycin*** (1200 mg po 1st day, then 600 mg/day x 27 days, then 300 mg/day)	Nutritional supplements often required; for severe cases: Vivonex, TEN or parenteral hyperalimentation

153

(continued)

	Preferred	Alternative	Comment
Isospora Acute infection	Trimethoprim (5 mg/kg) + sulfamethoxazole po bid (2 DS po bid or 1 DS tid) po x 2-4 wks	Pyrimethamine (50-75 mg/day) + folinic acid, (5-10 mg/day) x 1 mo	Duration of high dose therapy is not well defined
Suppressive treatment	Trimethoprim (2.5-5.0 mg/kg) + sulfamethoxazole (1-2 DS/day) po	Pyrimethamine (25 mg) + sulfadoxine (500 mg) po q wk (1 Fansidar/wk); pyrimethamine, 25 mg + folinic acid 5 mg/day	Duration is not well defined
FUNGI **Candida** Thrush Initial infection	Ketoconazole** (200-400 mg) po qd; Nystatin (500,000 units) gargled 5x/day; clotrimazole oral troches (10 mg) 5x/day or fluconazole (50-100 mg) po qd	Amphotericin B (0.3-0.5 mg/kg) IV/day;	Treat until symptoms resolve (7-10 days) and then begin maintenance therapy Amphotericin B usually reserved for patients who fail with alternative regimens
Maintenance (optional or prn)	Nystatin (above doses), clotrimazole (above doses) or ketoconazole** (200 mg) po qd	Fluconazole (50-100 mg) po qd	Possible salutary advantage for fluconazole and ketoconazole for maintenance treatment is prevention of cryptococcal infection
Vaginitis	Intravaginal miconazole suppository (100 mg) or cream (2%) x 7 days; clotrimazole cream (1%) or troche (100 mg) qd x 7	Ketoconazole** (200 mg) po qd or bid x 5-7 days Fluconazole (150 mg) x 1	May require continuous treatment to prevent relapse: Ketoconazole** (200 mg) po qd or fluconazole (50-100 mg) po qd
Esophagitis Initial infection	Fluconazole (100-200 mg) po qd; up to 400 mg/day x 2-3 wks	Ketoconazole** (200-400 mg) po bid x 2-3 wks Amphotericin B (0.3-0.5 mg/kg IV/day) ± flucytosine (100 mg/kg/day) x 5-7 days	
Maintenance	Fluconazole (50-100 mg) po qd	Ketoconazole** (200 mg) po qd Nystatin (above dose) or clotrimazole (above doses)	
Cryptococcal meningitis Initial treatment	Amphotericin B (0.5-0.8 mg/kg/day IV) with or without 5-flucytosine (100-150 mg/kg/day in 4 doses) to complete 1 gm of amphotericin B (some continue amphotericin B until therapeutic response or for 10-14 days	Fluconazole (200 mg po bid) x 6-10 wks Itraconazole (200 mg) po bid (see comment)	Fluconazole is acceptable as initial treatment only for patients with normal mental status. Other favorable prognostic findings are crypt antigen < 1:32 and CSF WBC > 20/mm³[1] (continued)

154

	Preferred	Alternative	Comment
Initial treatment	Amphotericin B (0.7 mg/kg/day) ± 5 FC (100 mg/day po) x 2-3 wks, then fluconazole (400 mg/day) x 8-10 wks, then 200 mg/day indefinitely		Cryptococcal antigen is nearly always detected in CSF, and in blood of 95% of patients; it is less useful in monitoring response to treatment
Maintenance therapy	Fluconazole (200 mg) po qd up to 400 mg/day	Amphotericin B (1 mg/kg/wk)	Life long maintenance treatment required for all patients
Histoplasmosis			
Disseminated Initial treatment	Amphotericin B (0.5-1.0 mg/kg/day IV) x 4-8 wks; total dose = 1-2.5 gm		
	Itraconazole (200 mg) po bid		
Maintenance	Itraconazole (200 mg) po bid	Ketoconazole** (200 mg) po bid	
	Amphotericin B 1.0-1.5 mg/kg/wk		
Coccidioidomycosis			
Initial treatment	Amphotericin B (0.5-1.0 mg/kg IV/day x ≥ 8 wks) (2-2.5 gm total dose)	Fluconazole (200 mg) po bid	Intrathecal amphotericin B usually added for coccidioidomycosis meningitis
Maintenance	Amphotericin B (1 mg/kg/wk) or fluconazole (400 mg qd)	Ketoconazole** (400-800 mg) po qd	
		Itraconazole (200 mg) po qd	
MYCOBACTERIA			
M. tuberculosis			
Treatment	All patients should receive <u>observed treatment</u> with <u>4 agents</u>: INH (300 mg po/day) + rifampin (600 mg po/day) + pyrazinamide (20-30 mg/kg po/day) + ethambutol (15-25 mg/kg/day) or streptomycin (1.0 gm IM/day). Treat daily x2 weeks (above doses), then daily or intermittent (2-3x/wk): INH (900 mg), rifampin (600 mg), PZA (50-70 mg/kg) and ethambutol (100 mg/kg/wk) or streptomycin 20-30 mg/kg) x6 wks.	Second line drugs: Ethionamide, capreomycin, kanamycin, amikacin, cycloserine, PAS Experimental drugs: Fluoroquinolones, imipenem, clofazimine, clarithromycin	Observed treatment preferred for all patients Intermittent treatment: 2x/wk appears as effective as 3x/wk Duration of treatment: Usually 50% longer in patients with HIV infection; for sensitive strains -- 9 mo or 6 mo post-sputum conversion INH: Should supplement with pyroxidime (50 mg/day) in AIDS patients

(continued)

155

	Preferred	Alternative	Comment
Treatment	Subsequent treatment based on sensitivity tests: Sensitivity to INH + rifampin: continue INH and rifampin alone to complete 9-12 mo (6 mo post-sputum conversion)		Aminoglycoside: Streptomycin preferred and may be given IV; capreomycin, kanamycin or amikacin may be preferred based on in vitro sensitivity tests; amikacin cost is 100x streptomycin ($60/day vs 4$/day)
	Resistant to INH or rifampin (or inability to take INH or rifampin): INH or rifampin + PAZ + ethambutol or streptomycin x18 mo or 12 mo post-sputum conversion		Suspected resistance: Give 3 drugs never seen pending in vitro sensitivity tests; never add a single drug
	Resistant to INH and rifampin: Treat with at least two drugs active in vitro x 18-24 mo		Fluoroquinolones: Ciprofloxacin (750 mg po bid) or ofloxacin (400 mg po bid) often used for resistant strains
Prophylaxis	INH (300 mg po qd) ± pyridoxine (50 mg po/qd)	Rifampin (600 mg po qd)	INH prophylaxis for ≥ 1 yr is indicated for all HIV infected patients with positive PPD (≥ 5mm induration) or anergy and high risk category or simply HIV + high risk (high risk=IV drug use, homeless, migrant farm worker); for INH intolerance or INH-induced hepatitis (transaminase > 5 x normal) some advocate rifampin (600 mg/day)
			For skin test conversion following contact with multiply resistant strain: Decision for prophylaxis depends on host and in vitro sensitivity of contact strain; may use fluoroquinolones (ciprofloxacin or ofloxacin) plus pyrazinamide or ethambutol
			Pyridoxine (50 mg/day) advocated for alcoholics, pregnant patients and malnourished patients

(continued)

	Preferred	Alternative	Comment
M. avium-intracellulare			
Treatment	Choose 3-5 from the following: Clofazimine (100-200 mg po/day), rifampin (600 mg po/day), ethambutol (25 mg/kg po/day x 6 wks, then 15 mg/kg), ciprofloxacin (750 mg po bid), amikacin (7.5 mg/kg IM or IV q12h, then 7.5 mg/kg/day for ≤ 2 months), clarithromycin (1 gm po bid) or azithromycin (600-900 mg po qd)	Other combinations include ethionamide, rifabutin (in place of rifampin), cycloserine, pyrazinamide, imipenem	INH should be included if M. tuberculosis is considered likely; but this drug adds little with M. avium infections; role of in vitro susceptibility tests is controversial
	Clarithromycin + clofazimine or ethambutol (above doses)		
Prophylaxis	Clarithromycin (500 mg po bid) Rifabutin (300 mg po qd)		Prophylaxis sometimes advocated for patients with CD4 counts < 100 or < 150/mm³
M. kansasii	INH (300 mg po/day) + rifampin 600 mg po/day) + ethambutol (15-25 mg/kg po/day) x 12 mo ± streptomycin (1 gm IM 2x/wk) x 3 mo	Also consider ciprofloxacin (750 mg po bid) and clarithromycin (500 mg-1 gm po bid)	Usual treatment is 12 months
VIRUSES			
Herpes simplex			
Initial treatment			
Mild	Acyclovir (200 mg po 5x/day) at least 10 days (until lesions crusted)		Failure to respond: double oral dose or give IV
Severe	Acyclovir (15 mg/kg IV/day) at least 7 days	Foscarnet (40 mg/kg IV q8h) x 3 wks Topical trifluridine 1% solution q8h	If fails to respond to acyclovir give 30 mg/kg/day IV and test sensitivity of isolate to acyclovir; resistant HSV, high dose IV acyclovir (12-15 mg/kg IV q8h or by continuous infusion) or foscarnet
Maintenance	Acyclovir (400 mg po bid or 200 mg) 3-5x/day	Foscarnet (40 mg/kg IV/day)	Alternative is to treat each episode
Visceral	Acyclovir (30 mg/kg IV/day) at least 10 days	Foscarnet (60 mg/kg IV q8h) x ≥ 10 days	

157

(continued)

	Preferred	Alternative	Comment
Herpes zoster			
Dermatomal	Acyclovir (30 mg/kg IV/day) or 800 mg po 5x/day at least 7 days (until lesions crust)	Foscarnet (40 mg/kg IV q8h)	Some authorities recommend avoidance of corticosteroids; postherpetic neuralgia is less common in young patients; no maintenance therapy is recommended
			Foscarnet for preferred acyclovir-resistant cases
Disseminated ophthalmic nerve involvement or visceral	Acyclovir (30-36 mg/kg IV/day) at least 7 days	Foscarnet (40-60 mg/kg IV q8h)	No maintenance therapy recommended
Cytomegalovirus			
Retinitis			
Initial treatment	Foscarnet (60 mg/kg IV q8h) x 14-21 days		Ganciclovir and foscarnet appear comparably effective vs CMV; possible advantage of foscarnet is that it prolongs survival by an average of 3 mo; this may reflect concurrent use of AZT or synergy of foscarnet + AZT vs HIV
	Ganciclovir (5 mg/kg IV bid) x 14-21 days		Foscarnet requires infusion pump
			Alternative options with antiretroviral agents are: ganciclovir + ddI or ganciclovir + AZT with G-CSF for neutropenia
Maintenance	Foscarnet (90 mg/kg IV/day)		Maintenance therapy required life long
	Ganciclovir (5 mg/kg IV/day)		
Enteritis, colitis esophagitis, encephalitis, neuritis, pneumonitis, viremia plus fever and/or wasting, cutaneous lesions	Ganciclovir (5 mg/kg) IV bid x 14-21 days		Efficacy not clearly established for disseminated CMV other than retinitis; CMV is rare cause of pulmonary disease in AIDS patients. Ganciclovir preferred if renal failure; foscarnet preferred if neutropenia or AZT used concurrently
	Foscarnet (60 mg/kg IV q8h) x 14-21 days		Indications for maintenance therapy not established, but advocated by some authorities for CMV colitis, neuritis, encephalitis and recurrent esophagitis (continued)

158

	Preferred	Alternative	Comment
BACTERIA			
S. pneumoniae	Penicillin	Erythromycin Cephalosporins	Traditional therapy usually adequate
H. influenzae	Cefuroxime/cefamandole Ampicillin/amoxicillin	Trimethoprim-sulfamethoxazole Cephalosporins - 3rd gen	Traditional therapy usually adequate
Nocardia	Sulfadiazine (4-8 gm po or IV/day) to maintain sulfa level at 15-20 mcg/ml	Trimethoprim-sulfa (4-6 DS/day) Minocycline (100 mg bid)	Other suggested regimens: Imipenem + amikacin Sulfonamide + amikacin or minocycline
Pseudomonas aeruginosa	Aminoglycoside + antipseudomonad penicillin (ticarcillin, piper- acillin or mezlocillin)	Aminoglycoside + antipseudomonad cephalosporin (ceftazidime or cefoperazone) or imipenem	Antibiotic selection requires in vitro sensitivity data
Rhodococcus equi	Vancomycin (2 gm IV/day) ± rifampin (600 mg po qd), cipro- floxacin (750 mg po bid) or imipenem (0.5 gm IV qid) x 2-4 wks	Erythromycin (2-4 gm IV/day)	Ciprofloxacin (750 mg po bid) may be used for long term maintenance, but resistance is likely to develop
Rochalimaea quintana (bacillary angiomatosis)	Erythromycin (250-500 mg po qid) x 2-8 wks	Doxycycline (100 mg po bid)	
Salmonella			
Acute	Ampicillin (8-12 gm IV/day x 1-4 wks) then amoxicillin (500 mg po tid) to complete 2-4 wk course	Trimethoprim (5-10 mg/kg/day) + sulfamethoxazole IV or po x 2-4 wks	Relapse common
	Ciprofloxacin (500-750 mg po bid) x 2-4 wks	Cephalosporins - 3rd gen	
Maintenance	Amoxicillin (250 mg) po bid	Ciprofloxacin (500 mg po qd or bid)	Indications for maintenance therapy, specific regimens and duration not well defined
		Trimethoprim-sulfamethoxazole (2.5 mg/kg trimethoprim or 1 DS) po bid	
Staph. aureus	Antistaphylococcal penicillin (nafcillin, oxacillin) ± gentamicin (1 mg/kg IV q8h) or rifampin (600 mg/day)	Cephalosporin: 1st gen ± gentamicin or rifampin	MRSA stains must be treated with vancomycin
		Vancomycin (1 gm IV bid) ± gentamicin or rifampin	Oral agent: cephalexin

159

- Patients with severe forms of G6PD deficiency are at risk for hemolytic anemia when given oxident drugs such as dapsone, sulfonamides and primaquine. Some advocate screening all potential ricipients, some restrict screening to persons at greatest risk (black males, men of Mediterranean decent, from India or from the Far East, e.g., endemic malaria areas); some simply observe for evidence of hemolysis that usually occurs in first several days of treatment and often resolves with continued administration. Patients with the Mediterranean variant are at risk for severe hemolysis.

** Ketoconazole requires gastric acid for absorption; this may be enhanced by administration with orange juice, coke or 0.2 N HCl.

*** Azithromycin is FDA approved, but not for this indication. It is available from Pfizer Labs at (203) 441-5941. Clarithromycin is FDA approved, but not for this indication. It is available from Abbott at (800) 688-9118.

Table 7. TREATMENT OF MISCELLANEOUS AND NON-INFECTIOUS DISEASE COMPLICATIONS OF HIV INFECTION CLASSIFIED BY ORGAN SYSTEM*

Condition	Treatment	Comment
Cardiac		
Cardiomyopathy	Digitalis, diuretic and cautious use of vasodilators; Discontinue nucleoside (AZT, ddI or ddC) x 4 wks	Echo is best screening test. If patient does not respond to nucleoside withdrawal: Biopsy shows endocarditis: myocarditis: Solumedrol, 100-125 mg IV/day x 3 days, then prednisone 1 mg/kg/day with taper over 1 mo. If bx shows microbial agent (CMV, M avium, cryptococcus): treat
Pulmonary		
Lipid interstitial pneumonitis	AZT	Relatively rare in adult patients
	Prednisone	Indications and optimal dose of corticosteroid treatment not established; most initiate this treatment after initial observation shows progression; maintenance prednisone sometimes required
Renal		
Nephropathy (HIV-associated; Nephropathy-HIVAN)	Hemodialysis (utility of dialysis in preventing rapid progression of HIVAN is not established)	Must distinguish from: 1) heroin-associated nephropathy, which has a far better prognosis, and 2) acute tubular necrosis
Neurologic		
Peripheral neuropathy (painful peripheral neuropathy)	Nortriptyline, 10 mg hs (see comment). Capsaicin-containing ointments (Zostrix, etc) for topical application; Lidocaine 10-30% ointment for topical use.	Increase dose by 10 mg q 5 days to maximum of 50 mg hs
Myopathy	Discontinue AZT x 3 wks. Nonsteroidal anti-inflammatory agents. Prednisone, 40-60 mg/day (severe cases)	Indication for treatment is proximal muscle weakness + elevated creatine kinase. Often unclear if due to HIV or AZT so use "drug holiday"
HIV-associated dementia	AZT, 1000-1200 mg/day	Benefit of higher dose for CNS complications is not established; monitor therapy with neurocognitive tests
	ddI, 200-300 mg po bid (efficacy not established)	Nimodipine (calcium channel blocker) 30 mg q4h (experimental for this indication)
Hematologic		
Idiopathic thrombocyto-penia (ITP)	Prednisone, 60-100 mg/day	Relapses common with attempts to taper or discontinue steroids
	AZT, 1000-1200 mg/day	Utility of usual doses of AZT not established; initial reports showing benefit employed 1200 mg/day

(continued)

161

Condition	Treatment	Comment
ITP - continued	IV gamma globulin (1 gm/kg) x 3 (days, 1, 2 & 15), then every 2-3 wks	Failure to respond common with repeated courses
	Splenectomy	Not advocated by many authorities
	Splenic irradiation	Experience limited
Anemia	Transfusions and/or erythropoietin (r-HuEPO) 50-100 U/kg 2x/wk SC; increase dose 25 U/kg if response is inadequate at 4-8 wks and again at 4-8 wk intervals; maximal dose is 300 U/kg; titrate maintenance dose	Discontinue AZT for hemoglobin < 7.5 gm%
		EPO recommended only if baseline EPO level is < 500 U/mL
Neutropenia	Neupogen (G-CSF) or Prokine (GM-CSF) 1 μg/kg/day SC; usual maintenance dose is 0.13 μg/kg/day (0.1-1.0 μg/kg/day)	Usual cause is AZT; ganciclovir or HIV per se. Low doses (1 mcg/kg/day) of G-CSF and GM-CSF usually adequate and higher doses are often poorly tolerated; monitor with CBC and dif 2x/wk and titrate up to 10 μg/kg; reduce dose 50% q week for maintenance to keep ANC > 750-1500/ml
Tumors Kaposi's sarcoma	Topical liquid nitrogen	Restrict to few lesions that are small
	Intralesional vinblastin (0.01-0.02 mg/lesion) q 2wks x ≤ 3	Restrict to few lesions
	Alpha interferon, (9-20 mil units/d ± maintenance	Documented benefit of alpha interferon only for patients with CD4 count > 200/mm³; neutropenia common with AZT; Use G-CSF or substitute ddI
	Radiation	Skin - well tolerated; oral lesion - mucositis common
	Laser	Laser, radiation or vinblastine injection preferred for oral lesions
	Chemotherapy; adriamycin, bleomycin and either vincristine or vinblastine; etoposide (VP-16) monotherapy	Preferred for patients with widespread skin involvement (> 25 lesions), edema and/or symptomatic visceral organ involvement (especially lung KS)
Lymphoma	Regimens containing cyclophosphamide, adriamycin, vincristine and corticosteroids ± cranial radiation	
	CNS lymphoma - cranial radiation ± chemotherapy	

(continued)

Condition	Treatment	Comment
Dermalogic		
Bacillary angiomatosis	Erythromycin, 250-500 mg po qid x 2-8 wks	Alternative: Doxycycline, 100 mg bid
Molluscum contagiosum	Freeze; surgical extirpation	
Dermatophytic fungi	Skin - Topical miconazole or clotrimazole. Refractory cases--griseofulvin, 330-660 mg po/day or ketoconazole, 200 mg po/day x 1-3 mo. Nails - griseofulvin, 660 mg/day x 6-15 mo	Ointments (miconazole and clotrimazole) are non-prescription
Seborrhea	Skin - Steroid cream (hydrocortisone 1%) or topical ketoconazole; scalp - shampoos containing zirconium sulfide, salicylic acid or coal tar	
Gastrointestinal		
Anorexia	Megace, 80 mg qid	May use up to 800 mg/day
Nausea/vomiting	Compazine, 5-10 mg po q6-8h; Tigan, 250 mg po q6-8h; Dramamine, 50 mg po q6-8h; Ativan 0.025-0.05 mg/kg IV or IM; Haloperidol, 1-5 mg bid po or IM, Ondansetron (Zofran) 0.2 mg/kg IV or IM	Phenothiazines (Compazine, etc.), haloperidol, benzamides (Tigan, Reglan, etc.) may cause dystonia Must consider medications as cause
Mouth		
Aphthous ulcers	Mouth rinses with Miles solution, Dyclone, Benadryl or viscous Lidocaine (2%) Intralesional or topical corticosteroids; Prednisone, 40 mg po/day x 1-2 weeks, then taper (severe or refractory cases)	Miles solution - 60 mg hydrocortisone, 20 cc mycostatin, 2 gm tetracycline and 120 cc viscous Lidocaine
Oral hairy leukoplakia	Acyclovir, 800 mg po 5 x/day x 2-3 wks	Most lesions are asymptomatic and do not require treatment Relapses are common when acyclovir is discontinued and may require acyclovir maintenance therapy
Gingivitis/periodontitis	Metronidazole, 250 mg po tid or 500 mg po bid x 7-14 days and chlorhexidine gluconate (0.12% as Peridex) for oral rinse bid	

163

(continued)

Condition	Treatment	Comment
Esophagus		
Candida	See Table 6 (pg 154)	For patients with complete response, discontinue after induction therapy and use maintenance only if there is relapse
Cytomegalovirus	Ganciclovir, 5 mg/kg IV bid x 14-21 days or foscarnet 60 mg/kg IV q8h x 14-21 days	
Herpes simplex	Acyclovir, 400-1000 mg po 5x/day or 5 mg/kg IV tid x 7-10 days	
Aphthous ulcer	Prednisone, 40 mg/day po x 2 wks, then slow taper	
Diarrhea		
Specific microbial agent	See Table 6 (pg 154)	
Bacterial overgrowth	Doxycycline (100 mg po bid), metronidazole (750 mg po bid) amoxicillin-clavulanate (500 mg po qid)	Diagnosis requires quantitative culture of small bowel aspirate or hydrogen breath test
Symptomatic treatment	Lomotil/loperamide/paregoric, etc.	Utility of bismuth salts (Pepto-Bismol), indomethacin and octreotide not known
Wasting	Polymeric formulas: Ensure, Sustical, Enrich, Magnacal, etc.	Polymeric formulas: Non-prescription, about $1.50/can; 10 cans/day required for total caloric needs
	Elemental formulas: Vivonex TEN	Elemental diet for severe malabsorption states usually crypto-sporidia or severe CMV infection; parenteral hyperalimentation and feeding gastrostomy rarely used
Psychiatric and sleep disorders		
Anxiety	Lorazepan (Ativan) 0.5-1 mg bid	Benzodiazepine agonist, Class IV; limit to 2-3 days
	Buspirone (BuSpar) 5 mg tid	Nonbenzodiazepine-nonbarbiturate; dependence liability negligible; increase dose 5 mg q 2-4 day to effective daily dose of 15-30 mg
Depression	Fluoxetine (Prozac) 20 mg qd	Major side effects are nausea, nervousness, insomnia, weight loss, dry mouth, constipation; insomnia may be treated with Desyrel, 25-50 mg hs
	Nortriptyline 10 mg - 25 mg hs, then increase	Tricyclic; increase dose after 25 mg 3-4 x/day; if > 100 mg/day follow serum levels with 50-150 mg/ml
Delirium	Haldol (0.5-1 mg) hs	

(continued)

Condition	Treatment	Comment
Insomnia	Diphenhydramine (Benedryl), 25 mg hs	Non-prescription
	Trazodone (Desyrel), 25-50 mg po hs	Preferably for < 1 week
	Chloral hydrate, 500 mg po hs	Class IV; preferably < 1 week
Apathy	Ritalin 5-10 mg tid	Not effective with severe dementia; seizure potential
Pain	ASA, acetaminophen, 325-650 mg q4h	Acute pain is best relieved with opioides. Chronic pain is best treated with nonopioid initially (ASA, acetaminophen, ibuprofen, nortriptyline)
	Non-steroidal anti-inflammatory agents (Motrin, 200-400 mg q6h; Naprosyn, 250-375 mg bid)	
	Codeine, 30-60 mg q4-6h po SC or IM	Dependence liability for opioides
	Meperidine, 50-150 mg q3-4h po, SC, IM, IV	Side effects of opioides: Sedation, constipation, respiratory depression, nausea and vomiting
	Methadone, 2.5-10 mg q6-8h po, SC, IM	
	Dilaudid, 2-8 mg q6-8h po, SC, IM Morphine, 5-20 mg SC, IM or rectal	
Terminal Illness	Morphine or other opioides orally or parenterally; MS Contin (continuous release morphine) po 15, 30, 60 or 100 mg, usual dose is 15-60 mg po q12h	Tolerance will develop within 1 week for opioides; PCA pump is consequently preferred for some patients to reduce cumulative dose
	Patient controlled analgesia (PCA) for morphine	
	Methadone (above doses)	

165

Table 8.   Occupational exposure to HIV (MMWR 39:1,1990)

<u>Definition</u>

   <u>Exposure</u>: Needlestick or cut with sharp object, contact with mucous membranes or contact with skin (especially if chapped, abraded or dermatitis, contact is prolonged and/or involves extensive area with blood or tissue).

   <u>Body fluid of source</u>: (1) Blood or body fluid, (2) other body fluids to which universal precautions apply: cerebrospinal fluid, synovial fluid, pleural fluid, peritoneal fluid, pericardial fluid and amniotic fluid, or (3) laboratory specimens containing HIV. (All seroconversions in non-laboratory health care workers have involved blood or bloody fluid). Saliva, urine and stool are not considered potential sources of HIV.

   <u>Source</u>: Source must be evaluated for hepatitis B virus and HIV. If source has AIDS, is known to be seropositive or refuses testing, the worker is evaluated clinically and serologically for HIV. Some states allow testing source without consent.

   <u>Serology</u>: Worker is tested serologically at 0, 6 weeks (optional), 12 weeks and 6 months post-exposure. The worker is advised to report any acute illness, especially if it resembles acute HIV infection (fever, rash, myalgia, lymphadenopathy, dysphagia, hepatosplenomegaly and leukopenia with atypical lymphocytes). Most health care workers who have acquired HIV from needlestick injuriers have noted this infectious mononucleosis-like illness at 1-3 wks post-exposure.

   <u>Precautions</u>: During the follow-up, especially the first 6-12 weeks, the worker should refrain from donating blood or sperm and should abstain from sexual intercourse or use appropriate measures to prevent HIV transmission.

<u>Prophylactic AZT: Relevant issues</u>

1. The <u>risk</u> of HIV transmission with the usual type of needlestick injury from an HIV infected source is about 0.4% (1/250).

2. Data from <u>animal studies</u> are inadequate to support or refute the potential efficacy of AZT; studies in the SCID-hu mouse model showed delayed viremia without prevention of infection (McCune et al, Science 247:564,1990. Pretreatment with AZT before SIV challenge failed to prevent transmission.

3. Four anecdotal cases of patients with blood exposures showed AZT initiated within 45 minutes and 6 hrs did not prevent seroconversion (Lange JM et al, NEJM 322:1375, 1990; Looke DFM et al, Lancet 335:1280, 1990

4. <u>Side effects</u> of AZT in health care workers receiving 1200 mg/day for 6 weeks showed 29% had anemia (Hgb 9.5-12 gm/dL) and 14% discontinued the drug due to reversible subjective complaints (headache, nausea, myalgias) (MMWR 39:1,1990). Teratogenic and carcinogenic potential in humans are unknown, although prolonged administration of AZT to rats and mice resulted in vaginal carcinomas in 8% at 22 months (MMWR 31:1,1990). Men and women receiving AZT should avoid conception.

(continued)

AZT Prophylaxis: Protocol of the NIH, CDC and San Francisco General Hospital

Criteria for inclusion

1. Exposure to the following body fluids: blood, semen, vaginal secretions and bloody body fluids; tissue that has not been inactivated or fluids or tissue containing HIV in research labs.

2. Type of exposure: Occupational contact with specimens above by percutaneous inoculation, e.g., needlestick or cut with sharp object, contact with mucous membranes or non-intact skin.

3. Patient source: Patient source has AIDS or ARC, positive HIV serology or positive HIV culture. Some include patients with unknown serostatus and high risk: IV drug abuse, gay male, hemophiliac or regular sexual partner of person with HIV infection.

4. Women must not be pregnant or breast feeding.

5. Must agree to use effective method of birth control during treatment and 4 weeks thereafter.

6. Treatment must be initiated within 72 hrs of exposure. (Rapid initiation within minutes or a few hours is highly desired if prevention of transmission is the major goal; it is possible that AZT will modify the course of HIV infection if given in the first weeks of infection that are associated with high grade viremia. (NEJM 324:954,1991)

7. Informed consent that includes counseling concerning methods to minimize risk to sexual contacts, lack of documented efficacy of this treatment, the possibility that treatment will delay seroconversion, side effects of AZT including possible teratogenic and carcinogenic effects and costs of treatment (wholesale price of about $1.44/100 mg tab).

Regimen: 200 mg 6x/day for 3 days (1200 mg/day); then 100 mg or 200 mg 5x/day for 25 days.

Monitoring

1. HIV serology at 0 (baseline), 6 wks, 3 mo, 6 mo and 12 mo. (The serology at 12 mo is desired to detect delayed seroconversion that may result from AZT treatment.)

2. CBC and SMA-12 at 2, 4 and 6 wks.

SEPSIS AND SEPSIS SYNDROME

A. Definitions (R. Bone, Ann Intern Med 115:457, 1991)*

Disorder	Requirements for Clinical Diagnosis
Bacteremia[T]	Positive blood cultures
Sepsis	Clinical evidence suggestive of infection *plus* signs of a systemic response to the infection (all of the following): • Tachypnea (respiration >20 breaths/min [if patient is mechanically ventilated >10L/min]) • Tachycardia (heart rate >90 beats/min) • Hyperthermia or hypothermia (core or rectal temperature >38.4°C [101°F] or <35.6°C [96.1°F])
The sepsis syndrome (may also be considered *incipient septic shock* in patients who later become hypotensive)	Clinical diagnosis of sepsis outlined above, *plus* evidence of altered organ perfusion (one or more of the following): • PaO$_2$/FIo$_2$ no higher than 280 (in the absence of other pulmonary or cardiovascular disease) • Lactate level above the upper limit of normal • Oliguria (documented urine output < 0.5 mL/kg body weight for at least 1 hour in patients with catheters in place) • Acute alteration in mental status Positive blood cultures are not required[TT]
Early septic shock	Clinical diagnosis of sepsis syndrome outlined above, *plus* hypotension (systolic blood pressure below 90 mm Hg or a 40 mm Hg decrease below baseline systolic blood pressure) that lasts for less than 1 hour and is responsive to conventional therapy (intravenous fluid administration or pharmacologic intervention)
Refractory septic shock	Clinical diagnosis of sepsis syndrome outlined above, *plus* hypotension (systolic blood pressure below 90 mm Hg or a 40 mm Hg decrease below baseline systolic blood pressure) that lasts for more than 1 hour despite adequate volume resuscitation and that requires vasopressors or higher doses of dopamine (> 6 μ/kg per hour)

* Adapted from Kreger BE et al, Amer J Med 68:344, 1980.
[T] The related term *septicemia* is imprecise and should be abandoned.
[TT] The sepsis syndrome may result from infection with gram-positive or gram-negative bacteria, pathogenic viruses, fungi, or rickettsia; however, an identical physiologic response may result from such noninfectious processes as severe trauma or pancreatitis. Blood cultures may or may not be positive.

B. Antibiotic selection (Medical Letter 34:49, 1992)

1. <u>Initial treatment</u>: Aminoglycoside (gentamicin, tobramycin, netilmicin or amikacin) <u>plus</u> one of the following:

   - Third generation cephalosporin (cefotaxime, ceftizoxime, cefoperazone, ceftriaxone or ceftazidine) <u>or</u>
   - Antipseudomonad penicillin (ticarcillin, piperacillin or mezlocillin) <u>or</u>
   - Ticarcillin-clavulanic acid <u>or</u>
   - Imipenem

2. <u>Suspected methicillin resistant S. aureus</u>: Add vancomycin ± rifampin

3. <u>Intra-abdominal sepsis</u>: Any of the following:

   - Metronidazole or clindamycin <u>plus</u> Amingolycoside
   - Ticarcillin-clavulanic acid ± aminoglycoside
   - Ampicillin-sulbactam ± aminoglycoside
   - Imipenem ± aminoglycoside
   - Cefoxitin ± aminoglycoside
   - Cefotetan ± aminoglycoside

4. <u>Biliary tract</u>: Cephalosporin ± aminoglycoside ± anti-anaerobic agent (such as metronidazole)

5. <u>Neutropenia</u>: Aminoglycoside <u>plus</u> one of the following:

   - Ticarcillin, ticarcillin-clavulanic acid, mezlocillin, piperacillin, ceftazidine or imipenem
   - With or without vancomycin (see JID 163:951, 1991)

GUIDELINES FOR USE OF SYSTEMIC GLUCOCORTICOSTEROIDS
IN MANAGEMENT OF SELECTED INFECTIONS
(Adapted from Infectious Diseases Society of America, J Infect Dis 165:1-13, 1992)

1. Immunosuppression is related to several variables

   a. Dose: Usually > 0.3 mg/kg/day, especially if > 1 mg/kg/day (prednisone)
   b. Duration: < 5 days has minimal effect
   c. Concurrent drugs: Cytotoxic agents

2. Recommendations

Condition	Recommend*	Comment
Systemic		
Gram-negative sepsis and shock	E/I	Exceptions: Adrenal insufficiency and typhoid fever with shock. Four clinical trials showed no benefit in septic shock (NEJM 317:653, 1987; 317:659, 1987)
Toxic shock syndrome	C/III	Possible benefit if given in first few days (JAMA 252: 3399, 1984)
Typhoid fever	C/I	Controlled trial showed survival benefit with chloramphenicol + Decadron (3 mg/kg) vs chloro alone (NEJM 310:82, 1984). Recommended for critically ill patients with delirium, obtundation, coma or shock
Tetanus	B/I	Single study showed benefit (Clin Ther 10:276, 1988)
Tuberculosis		
Pericarditis	A/I	Survival benefit: 40-80 mg prednisone/d with taper over weeks (JAMA 266:99, 1991)
Meningitis	B/I	Recommended when elevated intracranial pressure, focal neurologic deficits, altered consciousness; prednisone, 60 mg/d with taper at 1-2 wks over 4-6 weeks (Ped Infect Dis 10:179, 1991)
Debilitated patients	C/III	Severely debilitated patients show rapid symptomatic improvement; prednisone, 20-30 mg/d
Severe hypoxia	C/III	Improve severe hypoxemia: prednisone, 60-80 mg/d
Pleurisy	C/III	Data supporting recommendations categorized as C/III poor
Peritonitis	C/III	Supporting data are poor (NEJM 28:1091, 1969)
Herpes zoster		
Routine use (all pts)	E/I	Recommended only for patients >40 yrs to reduce post-herpetic neuralgia: prednisone, 50-60 mg/day x 1 wk with taper to none by week 3 (Lancet 2:126, 1987)
Old patients	C/III	

(continued)

170

Condition	Recommend*	Comment
Viral infections		
marrow suppression	C/III	Refers to marrow cytopenia or hypoplasia with parvovirus B19, EBV, HSV, VZV, CMV and HCV
EBV (infectious mono-		
nucleosis) routine use	D/II	Reduces fever and pharyngitis, but reluctance to use in
Airway obstruction	B/II	self-limited disease unless tonsil hypertrophy with
Hepatitis, myocarditis,		impending airway closure, prolonged course with high
encephalitis	C/III	fever or persistent morbidity: Prednisone, 80 mg/day x 2-3 days with taper to none after week 2 (JAMA 256: 1051, 1986)
Hantaan virus	E/I	JID 162:1213, 1990
Trichinosis	C/III	JAMA 230:537, 1974
CNS infections		
Bacterial meningitis	C/II	Efficacy shown in children with <u>H. influenzae</u> meningitis for reduction in hearing loss: Dexamethasone, 0.6 mg/kg/day x 4 days (NEJM 319:964, 1988) Data in adults with meningitis due to other organisms is sparce, but some recommend this for adults who are severely ill with mental status changes (Ann Intern Med 112:610, 1990)
Brain abscess	C-D/III	Recommended only when elevated intracranial pressure must be reduced (Neurosurgery 23:451, 1988)
Neurocysticercosis	C-D/III	Recommended for elevated intracranial pressure; this treatment may also reduce reaction to dying larvae caused by praziquantel (Rev Infect Dis 9:961, 1987)
Neuroborreliosis	D/III	No evidence of efficacy with facial nerve palsy (Laryngoscope 95:1341, 1985)
Cerebral malaria	E/I	(JID 150:325, 1988)
Airway infections		
P. carinii pneumonia	A/I	Three controlled trials show reduced risk of death and respiratory failure (NEJM 318:988, 1988; 323:1444, 1990; 323:1451, 1990). Recommended with pO_2 < 70 mm Hg or A-a gradient >35 mm Hg (NEJM 323: 1500, 1987)
Chronic bronchitis	C/III	Controlled trial showed no clear benefit (Ann Intern Med 106:196, 1987)
Acute epiglottitis	C/III	Consider when obstruction is likely (primarily children)

(continued)

Condition	Recommend*	Comment
Allergic broncho- pulmonary aspergillosis	B/II	Response is impressive: Prednisone, 45-60 mg/day (Arch Intern Med 146:1799, 1986). Inhaled steroids also effective (Allergy 43:24, 1988)
Heart Viral pericarditis	C/III	Symptomatic response impressive: Prednisone, 40-60 mg/day x 3-5 days, then taper over 3-4 wks. However, non-steroidals also effective, constrictive pericarditis is not prevented and concern that myocarditis may worsen
Viral myocarditis	C/III	Clinical trials variable. Steroids in coxsackievirus myocarditis in experimental animals cause increased myocardial necrosis and increased viral replication
Liver Acute viral hepatitis	E/I	Controlled trials show adverse outcome with prolongation of illness, more relapses and more chronic hepatitis (NEJM 294:681, 1976)
Chronic hepatitis HBV	E/I	Controlled trials show adverse outcome (Lancet 2:1136, 1989; NEJM 304:380, 1981; Ann Intern Med 109:89, 1988)
Chronic hepatitis HCV	E/III	(Ann Intern Med 112:921, 1990)
Aphthous ulcers	C/III	Anecdotal case reports indicate dramatic response in AIDS patients (Ann Intern Med 109:338, 1988)
Eye Endophthalmitis bacteria	C/III	Retrospective studies and experimental animal studies support efficacy (Inf Dis Clin N Amer 3:533, 1989)
Eye infections - viruses, protozoa, etc.	C/III	

*A-E: Categories for strength of recommendation
A = good evidence for use; B = moderate evidence for use; C = poor evidence for or against use; D = moderate evidence against use; E = good evidence against use

I-III: Categories for quality of evidence
I = at least one proper study; II = evidence from at least one clinical study with suboptimal design; III = evidence based on opinions of authorities

PATHOGENS ASSOCIATED WITH IMMUNODEFICIENCY STATUS

Condition	Usual conditions	Pathogens
Neutropenia (<500/ml)	Cancer chemotherapy; adverse drug reaction; leukemia	Bacteria: Aerobic GNB (coliforms and pseudomonads) Fungi: Aspergillus, Phycomycetes
Cell-mediated immunity	Organ transplantation: HIV infection; lymphoma (especially Hodgkin's disease); cortico-steroid therapy	Bacteria: Listeria, Salmonella, Nocardia, Mycobacteria (M. tuberculosis & M. avium), Legionella Viruses: CMV, H. simplex, Varicella-zoster Parasites: Pneumocystis carinii; Toxoplasma; Strongyloides stercoralis; Cryptosporidia Fungi: Candida, Phycomycetes (Mucor), Cryptococcus
Hypogammaglobulinemia or dysgamma-globulinemia	Multiple myeloma; congenital or acquired deficiency; chronic lymphocytic leukemia	Bacteria: S. pneumoniae, H. influenzae (type B) Parasites: Giardia Viruses: Enteroviruses
Complement deficiencies C2, 3	Congenital	Bacteria: S. pneumoniae, H. influenzae
C5		S. pneumoniae, S. aureus Enterobacteriaceae
C6-8		Neisseria meningitidis
Alternative pathway		S. pneumoniae, H. influenzae, Salmonella
Hyposplenism	Splenectomy; hemolytic anemia	S. pneumoniae, H. influenzae, DF-2

173

Guidelines for use of antimicrobial agents in neutropenic patients with unexplained fever (Adapted from: Working Committee, Infectious Diseases Society of America, Hughes W et al, J Infect Dis 161:381, 1990)

Regimens	Advantages	Disadvantages
Aminoglycoside (gent, tobra or amikacin) plus anti-pseudomonad betalactam (ticarcillin, piperacillin, azlocillin, mezlocillin, ticarcillin-clavulanate, cefoperazone or ceftazidime)	1. Potential synergy vs GNB 2. Activity vs anaerobes (except ceftazidime) 3. Minimal emergence of resistance 4. Preferred regimen when P. aeruginosa is suspected	1. Potential ototoxicity and nephrotoxicity (aminoglycoside) 2. Lack of activity vs some GPC (esp meth-resistant S. aureus and S. epidermidis 3. Need to monitor amino glycoside levels
Two betalactam drugs (third generation cephalosporin such as ceftazidime or cefoperazone plus a ureidopenicillin such as piperacillin or mezlocillin)	1. Reduced toxicity 2. Effective in clinical trials 3. Sometimes preferred in presence of renal failure or nephrotoxic drugs	1. Selection of resistant strains 2. Possible antagonism 3. Lack of activity vs some GPC
Single drug (ceftazidime, imipenem or cefoperazone)	1. Reduced toxicity 2. As effective as multiple drug regimens in most trials 3. Easily used in combination with other nephrotoxic drugs or in patients with renal failure	1. Reduced activity vs many GPC and some GNB 2. Must monitor closely for non-response, emergence of resistance and secondary infections 3. Ceftazidime has minimal activity vs anaerobes 4. Preferred for patients with brief and mild neutropenia (500-1000/μl)
Vancomycin plus aminoglycoside plus antipseudomonad betalactam (see agents above)	1. Broadest spectrum including GPC 2. Preferred regimen if meth-resistant S. aureus suspected: line infection, colonized, hospital-acquired infection	1. Some believe decision to treat GPC can await culture results 2. Potential ototoxicity (vancomycin + ceftazidime is another option) 3. Cost

174

Guide to initial management of febrile neutropenic patients: Reprinted from Hughes WT et al, J Infect Dis 161:381, 1990 (with permission)

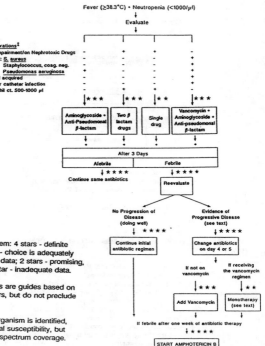

Note:

1. Star rating system: 4 stars - definite choice; 3 stars - choice is adequately supported with data; 2 stars - promising, not proven; 1 star - inadequate data.

2. ‡ Considerations are guides based on modifying factors, but do not preclude other options.

3. • If causative organism is identified, modify to optimal susceptibility, but maintain broad spectrum coverage.

Common infections by time after marrow
transplantation*

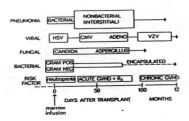

* Meyers JD: Infections in marrow transplant
recipients. In Mandell J, et al. Principles
and Practice of Infectious Diseases, Churchill
Livingstone, NY, 3rd edition, 1990, pp 2291.

TOXIC SHOCK SYNDROME: Case definition of Centers for Disease Control (MMWR 29:229,1980)

1. Fever: Temperature ≥ 38.9°C (102°F).
2. Rash: Diffuse macular erythroderma.
3. Desquamation: 1-2 wks afer onset, especially palms and soles.
4. Hypotension: Systolic < 90 mmHg for adults or < 5th percentile by age for children, or orthostatic syncope.
5. Involvement of three or more of the following organs
    GI: Vomiting or diarrhea at onset
    Muscular: Severe myalgia or creatine phosphokinase > 2x normal
    Mucous membrane: Vaginal, oropharyngeal or conjunctival hyperemia
    Renal: BUN or creatinine ≥ 2x normal or ≥ 5 WBC/HPF in absence of UTI
    Hepatic: Bilirubin or transaminase levels ≥ 2x normal
    Hematological: Platelets < 100,000/mm³
    CNS: Disoriented or altered consciousness without focal neurologic signs
    when fever and neurologic signs are absent
6. Negative results for the following (if obtained): Cultures of blood, throat
    and cerebrospinal fluid; negative serology for Rocky Mountain spotted
    fever, leptospirosis or measles.

ANAEROBIC BACTERIAL INFECTIONS

1. Activity of antibiotics versus Bacteroides fragilis (Data for 557 strains collected from 8 U.S. medical centers in 1986, Cuchural GJ Jr et al: Antimicrob Ag Chemother 34:479,1990)

Agent	Resistant	Agent	Resistant
Metronidazole	0	Piperacillin	16%
Chloramphenicol	0	Moxalactam	23%/17%
Imipenem	0.2%	Cefotetan	36%/22%
Ticarcillin-		Ceftizoxime	33%/20%
clavulanate	1.7%	Cefotaxime	53%/33%
Clindamycin	6.0%	Cefoperazone	66%/27%
Cefoxitin	11%/2%*	Ceftazidime	87%/74%

* Two figures provided indicating arbitrary breakpoints in susceptibility testing; first figure indicates % resistant at 16 mcg/ml, 2nd figure indicates % resistant at 32 mcg/ml.

2. In vitro susceptibility of various anaerobes (from Finegold SM and Wexler HM: Antimicrob Ag Chemother, 32:611,1988)

	Chloro	Clinda	Erythro	Metro	Pen	Tetra	Vanco
Microaerophilic and anaerobic GPC	3*	2-3	2-3	2	4	2	3
B. fragilis group	3	2-3	1-2	3	1	1-2	1
Bacteroides sp (other)	3	3	2-3	3	2-3	2	1
Fusobacteria	3	2-3	1	3	3-4	2-3	1
C. perfringens	3	3	3	3	3	2	3
Clostridia (other)	3	2	2-3	3	3	2	2-3
Actinomyces	3	3	3	1-2	4	2-3	2-3

* 1 = poor activity; 2 = moderate activity, 3= good activity; 4 = drug of choice.

3. Susceptibility of Anaerobic bacteria. National Committee for Clinical Laboratory Standards, Working Group on Anaerobic Susceptibility Testing (J Clin Micro 26:1253, 1988)

Essentially always active
Metronidazole (except some nonsporulating GPB)
Chloramphenicol
Imipenem
Betalactam-betalactamase inhibitor combinations

Unpredictable activity
Cephalosporins (other)
Penicillins (other - esp antistaphylococcal agents)
Trimethoprim-sulfamethoxazole
Vacomycin
Erythromycin

Usually active
Clindamycin
Cefoxitin
Cefotetan
Antipseudomonad penicillins
Moxalactam

Virtually never active
Aztreonam
Aminoglycoside
Quinolones

FEVER OF UNKNOWN ORIGIN

A.   Definition (Petersdorf RG & Beeson PB, Medicine 40:1,1961)

  1)   Illness ≥ 3 weeks.
  2)   Documented fever ≥ 101°F (38.3°C).
  3)   Negative diagnostic evaluation with 1 week in hospital.

B.   Causes (Adapted from: Larson E et al, Medicine 61:269,1982)*

Infections	32	Neoplastic diseases	33
Abdominal abscesses	11	Lymphoma	6
Mycobacteria	5	Hodgkin's	4
Endocarditis	0	Leukemia	5
HIV infection**	0	Lymphomatoid granulomatosis	2
Cytomegalovirus	4	Malignant histocytosis	4
Miscellaneous***	12	Pre-leukemia	1
Collagen disease	8	Solid tumor****	11
Still's disease	4	Miscellaneous	10
Polyarteritis nodosa	2	Hematoma	3
Rheumatic fever	1	Pulmonary emboli	1
Polymyalgia rheumatica	0	Familial Mediterranean	
Rheumatic fever	1	fever	1
Systemic lupus	0	Myxoma	1
Granulomatous disease	9	Periodic fever	0
Granulomatous hepatitis	4	Factitious fever	3
Sarcoidosis	2	Non-specific pericarditis	1
Giant cell arteritis	1	Undiagnosed	13
Crohn's disease	2		

*   This represents an updated version (105 cases; 1970-1980) of the classical
     report by Petersdorf and Beeson (100 cases, 1952-1957); more recent
     developments include AIDS and extensive use of scans.
**   The Seattle study predated AIDS, but HIV infection would now constitute an
     important diagnostic consideration.
*** Includes sinusitis, dental infections, osteomyelitis, amebiasis, candidiasis,
     urinary tract infection.
**** All were solid tumors in the abdomen including hepatoma (2) and
     hypernephroma (2).

LYME DISEASE: CASE DEFINITION OF THE CENTERS FOR DISEASE CONTROL (reprinted with permission from: Rahn DW and Malawista SE, Ann Intern Med 114:473, 1991 and MMWR 40:417, 1991)

Lyme Disease National Surveillance Case Definition

Lyme disease is a systemic, tick-borne disease with protean manifestations, including dermatologic, rheumatologic, neurologic, and cardiac abnormalities. The best clinical marker for the disease is the initial skin lesion, erythema migrans, that occurs in 60% to 80% of patients.

Case definition for the national surveillance of Lyme disease:

1. A person with erythema migrans; or
2. A person with at least one late manifestation and laboratory confirmation of infection.

General definitions:

1. Erythema migrans: For purposes of surveillance, erythema migrans is a skin lesion that typically begins as a red macule or papule and expands over a period of days or weeks to form a large round lesion, often with partial central clearing. To be considered erythema migrans, a solitary lesion must measure at least 5 cm. Secondary lesions may also occur. Annular erythematous lesions developing within several hours of a tick bite represent hypersensitivity reactions and do not qualify as erythema migrans. In most patients, the expanding erythema migrans lesion is accompanied by other acute symptoms, particularly fatigue, fever, headache, mildly stiff neck, arthralgias, and myalgias. These symptoms are typically intermittent. The diagnosis of erythema migrans must be made by a physician. Laboratory confirmation is recommended for patients with no known exposure.

2. Late manifestations: These manifestations include any of the following when an alternate explanation is not found:
   a. Musculoskeletal system: Recurrent, brief attacks (lasting weeks or months) of objective joint swelling in one or a few joints. Manifestations that are not considered to be criteria for diagnosis include chronic progressive arthritis that is not preceded by brief attacks and chronic symmetric polyarthritis. Additionally, arthralgias, myalgias, or fibromyalgia syndromes alone are not accepted as criteria for musculoskeletal involvement.

   b. Nervous system: Lymphocytic meningitis, cranial neuritis, particularly facial palsy (may be bilateral), radiculo-

neuropathy or, rarely, encephalomyelitis alone or in combination. Encephalomyelitis must be confirmed with evidence of antibody production against *Borrelia burgdorferi* in the cerebrospinal fluid, shown by a higher titer of antibody in the cerebrospinal fluid than in the serum. Headache, fatigue, paresthesias, or mildly stiff neck alone are not accepted as criteria for neurologic involvement.

   c. Cardiovascular system: Acute-onset, high-grade (second- or third-degree) atrioventricular conduction defects that resolve in days to weeks and are sometimes associated with myocarditis. Palpitations, bradycardia, bundle-branch block, or myocarditis alone are not accepted as criteria for cardiovascular involvement

3. Exposure: Exposure is defined as having been in wooded, brushy, or grassy areas (potential tick habitats) in an endemic county no more than 30 days before the onset of erythema migrans. A history of tick bite is not required.

4. Endemic county: A county in which at least two definite cases have been previously acquired or in which a tick vector has been shown to be infected with *B. burgdorferi*.

5. Laboratory confirmation: Laboratory confirmation of infection with *B. burgdorferi* is established when a laboratory isolates the spirochete from tissue or blood fluid, detects diagnostic levels of immunoglobulin M or immunoglobulin G antibodies to the spirochete in the serum or the cerebrospinal fluid or detects an important change in antibody levels in paired acute and convalescent serum samples. States may determine the criteria for laboratory confirmation and diagnostic levels of antibody. Syphilis and other known biologic causes of false-positive serologic test results should be excluded, although laboratory confirmation is based on serologic testing along.

---

* This epidemiologic case definition is intended for surveillance purposes only.

TREATMENT OF LYME DISEASE
Recommendations of Rahn DH and Malawista SE, Yale University School of Medicine,
Ann Intern Med 114:472, 1991 and Medical Letter consultants 34:17, 1992

Recommendations for Antibiotic Treatment*

Tick bite: Doxycycline 100 mg orally twice daily for 14 days is cost-effective in preventing
Lyme disease if the prevalence of *B. burgdorferi* in ticks exceeds 10%. Rates for I.
<u>dammini</u> ticks in New England and Mid-Atlantic states are 0.1-1% for larvae, 25% for
nymphs and 50% for adult ticks. Rates for *I. pacificus* in Western states are 1-3%
(NEJM 327:534, 1992).

Early Lyme disease+
    Doxycycline, 100 mg bid or tid for 10 to 30 days
    Amoxicillin, 250-500 mg three times daily for 10 to 30 days
    Erythromycin, 250 mg four times daily for 10 to 30 days
        (less effective than doxycycline or amoxicillin)
    Cefuroxime axetil, 500 mg bid x 10 to 30 days (Ann Intern Med 117:273, 1992)

Lyme carditis
    Ceftriaxone, 2 g daily intravenously for 14 to 21 days
    Penicillin G, 20 million units intravenously for 14 to 21 days
    Doxycycline, 100 mg orally twice daily for 14 to 30 days
    Amoxicillin, 500 mg orally three times daily for 14 to 30 days

Neurologic manifestations
    Facial nerve paralysis
        For an isolated finding, oral regimens for early disease,
            use for at least 21 to 30 days
            For a finding associated with other neurologic manifestations,
                intravenous therapy (see below)
    Lyme meningitis, radiculoneuropathy, peripheral neuropathy and encephalitis
        Ceftriaxone, 2 g daily by single dose for 14 to 21 days
        Penicillin G, 20 million units daily in divided doses for 14 to 21 days

Lyme arthritis
    Doxycycline, 100 mg orally twice daily for 30 days
    Amoxicillin and probenecid, 500 mg each orally four times daily for 30 days
    Penicillin G, 20 million units intravenously in divided doses daily for 14 to 21 days
    Ceftriaxone, 2 g intravenously daily for 14 days

In pregnant women
    For localized early Lyme disease, amoxicillin, 500 mg three times daily for 21 days
    For disseminated early Lyme disease or any manifestation of late disease, penicillin G,
        20 million units daily for 14 to 21 days
    For asymptomatic seropositivity, no treatment necessary

* These guidelines are to be modified by new findings and should always be applied with
close attention to the clinical course of individual patients. Most authorities use the
longest duration of treatment suggested.
+ Shorter courses are reserved for disease that is limited to a single skin lesion only.

Condition	Agent	Laboratory diagnosis	Treatment
Superficial erythematous lesions			
Abscess	S. aureus	Culture and Gram stain Anaerobes	Drainage
Acne rosacea	?	Appearance	Doxycycline* Metronidazole (0.75% topical) Accutane
Acne vulgaris	Propioni- bacterium acnes	Appearance	Tetracycline* Topical clindamycin
Cellulitis: Diffuse spreading infection of deep dermis	Gr A strep; S. aureus (Vibrio sp. & Aeromonas sp. with fresh or salt water exposure)	Culture advanced edge of inflammation (rarely positive), 3-mm dermal punch, ulcerated portal of entry, blood Serial DNase titer (gr A strep)	Penicillinase-resistant penicillin*, vancomycin, clindamycin, cephalosporin-1st gen, erythromycin
Erysipelas: Superficial infection with raised edge	Gr A strep	Culture: as above Serial DNase titer	Penicillin*, clindamycin, cephalosporin - 1st gen
Lymphangitis	Gr A strep	As above	As above
Folliculitis Infected hair follicle(s)	S. aureus (P. aeruginosa whirlpools, hot tubs, etc)	Culture and gram stain (usually unnecessary)	Local compresses or topical antibiotics. Fever, cellulitis or mid-face involvement - treat as furunculosis
Furunculosis carbuncle: Abscess that starts in hair follicle; carbuncle is deeper and more extensive	S. aureus	Culture and Gram stain	Drainage ± penicillinase-resistant penicillin*, clindamycin, vancomycin, cephalosporin - 1st gen, erythromycin, amoxicillin-clavulanate

(continued)

Condition	Agent	Laboratory diagnosis	Treatment
Recurrent furunculosis			Bathe with hexchlorophene May be controlled with chronic clindamycin, 150 mg qd x 3 mo.* Nasal carriers of staph - mupirocin to ant. nares or rifampin, 300 mg bid x 5 days
Paronychia: Infection of nail fold	<u>S. aureus</u> <u>Candida</u>	Culture and Gram stain	
Impetigo: Infection of epidermis	Gr A strep (<u>S. aureus</u>)	Culture and Gram stain	Penicillin V*, penicillin G benzathine, erythromycin or mupirocin; cloxacillin, cephalexin or amoxicillin + clavulanate
Whitlow: Infection of distal phalanx finger	<u>S. aureus</u> H. simplex	Culture and Gram stain; viral culture, Tzank prep or FA stain for H. simplex	Penicillinase- resistant penicillin*, clindamycin, cephalosporin - 1st gen.
Fungal infections: Keratinized tissue-skin, nails, hair (see pg 118)	<u>Candida</u>-red, moist, satellite lesions, esp skin folds	Scrapings for KOH prep, culture on Sabouraud medium	<u>Skin</u>: Topical anti-fungal agent: Miconazole, clothrimazole, econazole, naftifine or ciclopirox
	Dermatophytes- <u>Epidermophyton</u>, <u>Trichophyton</u>, <u>Microsporum</u>, "ring worm"	Scrapings for KOH prep and culture; Wood's light	<u>Skin</u>: Topical agents (as above) or oral ketoconazole <u>Nail</u>: Griseofulvin or ketoconazole <u>Scalp</u>: Selenium sulfide shampoo + griseofulvin
	Tinea versicolar- <u>Malassezia furfur</u>; red or hypopigmented macules		<u>Skin</u>: Topical agents (as above), oral ketoconazole or topical selenium sulfide
<u>Bites</u> Dog & cat	<u>P. multocida</u> Dysgonic fermenter type 2 (DF$_2$) <u>S. aureus</u>, anaerobes	Culture and Gram stain	Ampicillin + clavulanate (Augmentin)*, penicillin V ± cephalexin; tetracycline

(continued)

182

Condition	Agent	Laboratory diagnosis	Treatment
Human including clenched-fist injury	Oral flora (strep, anaerobes, etc) <u>S. aureus</u>, <u>Eikenella corrodens</u>	Culture and Gram stain	Amoxicillin-clavulanic acid (Augmentin)*, penicillin V ± cephalexin
Rat	<u>Strepto-bacillus moniliformis</u>	<u>S. moniliformis</u>: Giemsa stain of blood or pus; culture; serology	Penicillin*, tetracycline
	<u>Spirillum minus</u>	<u>S. minus</u>: Giemsa stain of blood or exudate	Penicillin*, tetracycline
<u>Cat scratch disease</u>	<u>Rochalimaea henselae</u> or <u>Afifpia felix</u>	Warthin-Starry stain of biopsy	Efficacy not established Sulfa-trimethoprim(?) Ciprofloxacin (?) Amoxicillin-clavulanate(?)
<u>Burns</u>			
	S. aureus, GNB <u>Candida albicans</u> <u>Aspergillus</u>, Herpes simplex, Gr A strep	Quantitative culture and stain of biopsy	Removal of eschar Topical sulfa (silver sulfadiazine or mafenide) Empiric antibiotics - Aminoglycoside + nafcillin, anti-pseudomonad, penicillin, ticarcillin clavulanate, vancomycin or cephalosporin
<u>Sinus tract</u> Osteomyelitis	<u>S. aureus</u>, <u>S. epid.</u>, GNB, anaerobes	Culture of sinus tract drainage does not reliably reflect agent(s) of osetomyelitis	Antibiotics optimally based on bone biopsy
Lymphadenitis	<u>S. aureus</u> Mycobacteria (scrofula)	Culture and Gram stain AFB smear and culture	Anti-staphylococcal agent TB-Antituberculous drugs M. scrofulaceum-excision
Actinomycosis	<u>A. israelii</u> <u>A. naeslundii</u> <u>A. odontolyticus</u> <u>Arachnia proprionica</u>	FA stain, anaerobic culture	Penicillin G*, amoxicillin, clindamycin, tetracycline

(continued)

Condition	Agent	Laboratory diagnosis	Treatment
Madura foot	Nocardia	AFB stain, culture for <u>Nocardia</u>	Sulfonamides
	Fungi - Petriellidium boydii, Madurella mycetomatis, Phialophora verrucosa	KOH, culture on Sabouraud medium	
<u>Nodules/ulcers</u>			
Sporotrichoid (cutaneous inoculation with lymphatic spread)	<u>Sporothrix schenckii</u> (thorns)	Histology (PAS, GMS), culture on Sabouraud medium	Oral KI
	<u>M. marinum</u> (tidal water, swimming pool or tropical fish tank)	Histology, AFB stain & culture (at 30-32°C)	Rifampin + ethambutol Minocycline TMP-SMX
	Nocardia	Histology, AFB stain, culture for <u>Nocardia</u>	Sulfonamide
Nodules/ulcers (from hemato-genous dissem-ination)	Blastomycosis Endemic area	Culture biopsy on Sabouraud medium	Ketoconazole, amphotericin B
	Cryptococcus Defective cell mediated immunity	Blood for cryptococcal antigen and culture; histopathology and culture of biopsy	Amphotericin B, fluconazole
	<u>Candida</u> - Defective cell-mediated immunity	Blood culture; histopathology and culture of biopsy	Amphotericin B
Diabetic foot ulcer and decubitus ulcer	Mixed aerobes-anaerobes <u>S. aureus</u> Gr A strep	Culture and Gram stain of wound edge or dermal punch biopsy	Local care - debridement, bedrest Antibiotics - for fever, extensive cellulitis, regional adenopathy or osteomyelitis Agents - parenteral agents as for intra-abdominal sepsis Oral regimen - ciprofloxacin + metronidazole or clindamycin

* Preferred regimen

Deep and Serious Soft Tissue Infections
(from Bartlett JG, Cecil Textbook of Medicine, W.B. Saunders Co., 1992, pg 1679)

	Gas-Forming Cellulitis	Synergistic Necrotizing Cellulitis	Gas Gangrene	"Streptococcal" Myonecrosis	Necrotizing Fasciitis	Infected Vascular Gangrene	Streptococcal
Predisposing conditions	Traumatic	Diabetes, prior local lesions, perirectal lesions	Traumatic or surgical wound	Trauma, surgery	Diabetes, trauma, surgery, perineal infection	Arterial insufficiency	Traumatic or surgical wound
Incubation period	> 3 days	3-14 days	1-4 days	3-4 days	1-4 days	> 5 days	6 hours-2 days
Etiologic organism(s)	Clostridia, others	Mixed aerobic-anaerobic flora	Clostridia, esp. C. perfringens	Anaerobic streptococci	Mixed aerobic anaerobic flora	Mixed aerobic-anaerobic flora	S. pyogenes
Systemic toxicity	Minimal	Moderate to severe	Severe	Minimal until late in course	Moderate to severe	Minimal	Severe
Course	Gradual	Acute	Acute	Subacute	Acute to subacute	Subacute	Acute
Wound findings Local pain	Minimal	Moderate to severe	Severe	Late only	Minimal to moderate	Variable	Severe
Skin appearance	Swollen, minimal discoloration	Erythematous or gangrene	Tense and blanched, yellow-bronze, necrosis with hemorrhagic bullae	Erythema or yellow-bronze	Blanched, erythema, necrosis with hemorrhagic bullae	Erythema or necrosis	Erythema, necrosis
Gas	Abundant	Variable	Usually present	Variable	Variable	Variable	No
Muscle involvement	No	Variable	Myonecrosis	Myonecrosis	No	Myonecrosis limited to area of vascular insufficiency	No
Discharge	Thin, dark, sweetish or foul odor	Dark pus or "dishwater," putrid	Serosanguineous, sweet or foul odor	Seropurulent	Seropurulent or "dishwater," putrid	Minimal	None or serosanguineous
Gram stain	PMNs, Gram-positive bacilli	PMNs, mixed flora	Sparse PMNs, Gram-positive bacilli	PMNs, Gram-positive cocci	PMNs, mixed flora	PMNs, mixed flora	PMNs, Gram-positive cocci in chains
Surgical therapy	Debridement	Wide filleting incisions	Extensive excision, amputation	Excision of necrotic muscle	Wide filleting incisions	Amputation	Debridement of necrotic tissue

185

BONE AND JOINT INFECTIONS

I. Osteomyelitis

A. Classification

	Hematogenous	Contiguous infection	Vascular insufficiency
Age	1-20 yrs	> 50 yrs	> 50 yrs
Bones	Long bones	Femur, tibia	Feet
	Vertebrae	Skull, mandible	
Associated conditions	Trauma	Surgery	Diabetes
	Bacteremia	Soft tissue	Neuropathy
	(any source)	infection	Vascular disease
Bacteriology	S. aureus	Mixed	Mixed
	Gram-neg rods	S. aureus	S. aureus
		Gram-neg rods	Streptococci
		Anaerobes	Gram-neg rods

B. Special conditions

	Bones	Bacteriology
Sickle cell disease	Multiple	Salmonella
IV drug abuse	Clavicle	S. aureus
	Vertebrae	Pseudomonas
Penetrating injury	Foot	Pseudomonas
Hemodialysis	Ribs	S. aureus
	Thoracic vertebrae	S. aureus
Chronic		
Brodie's abscess	Distal tibia	S. aureus
Tuberculosis	Spine (Potts')	M. tuberculosis
	Hip, knee	
Prosthetic joint	Site of prosthesis	S. aureus
		S. epidermidis

C. Treatment

<u>Acute</u>: Antibiotics x 4-6 weeks (S. aureus - nafcillin or oxacillin ± rifampin) + drainage of purulent collections.

<u>Chronic</u>: Antibiotics, intravenous x 4-6 weeks, then oral x 2 mo. (S. aureus - nafcillin IV ± rifampin <u>or</u> cloxacillin, 5 gm/day po + probenecid, 2 gm/day) + surgical debridement (Black J et al, J Infect Dis 155:968,1987).

<u>Empiric treatment</u>:

1. Settings in which <u>S</u>. aureus is anticipated pathogen

    <u>Preferred</u>: Nafcillin or oxacillin with or without an aminoglycoside, vancomycin with or without aminoglycoside, clindamycin with or without aminoglycoside

2. Patient with hemoglobinopathy

    <u>Preferred</u>: Nafcillin (or oxacillin) <u>plus</u> ampicillin

    <u>Alternatives</u>: Nafcillin (or oxacillin) plus cefotaxime (or ceftriaxone) <u>or</u> nafcillin (or oxacillin) plus chloramphenicol <u>or</u> cefazolin (or cephalothin or cephapirin) plus chloramphenicol

3. Osteomyelitis with vascular insufficiency, decubitus ulcer, diabetic foot ulcer, etc.
   Preferred: Aminoglycoside plus clindamycin, cefoxitin, imipenem, betalactam-betalactamase inhibitor or anti-pseudomonad penicillin
   Alternatives: Aztreonam plus clindamycin; beta-betalactamase inhibitor (alone); imipenem (alone); quinolone plus metronidazole or quinolone plus clindamycin
   Oral regimens: Quinolone with or without metronidazole or clindamycin; cefixime plus clindamycin; amoxicillin-clavulanate

II. Septic arthritis

A. Acute monarticular arthritis

1. Differential diagnosis: Septic arthritis, rheumatoid arthritis, gout and chondrocalcinosis (pseudogout)

2. Septic arthritis in adults

a. Agent	Treatment (alternatives)	Comment
S. aureus	Penicillinase resistant penicillin (cephalosporin, vancomycin, clindamycin) x 3 weeks	Accounts for 50-80% of non-gonococcal arthritis cases Cephalosporin-1st generation preferred
N. gonorrhoeae	Ceftriaxone 1 gm IV daily x 24-48 hrs, then oral agent (cefuroxime axetil, ciprofloxacin or amoxicillin + clavulanic acid or cefixime) to complete ≥ 7 day course	Most common cause of monarticular arthritis in young sexually active adults Skin lesions rarely present and blood cultures usually neg with gonococcal monarticular arthritis; joint fluid often culture positive
Streptococci	Penicillin (cephalosporin-1st gen, vancomycin, clindamycin) x 2 wks	Accounts for 10-20% of non-gonococcal septic arthritis cases
Gram-negative bacilli	Based on in vitro sensitivity tests Treat x 3 wks	Accounts for 10-20% of non-gonococcal septic arthritis cases Most commonly in chronically debilitated host, immuno-suppressed, prior joint disease Heroin addicts prone to sacroiliac or sternoclavicular septic arthritis due to pseudomonas aeruginosa

b. Empiric treatment (negative joint fluid gram stain and pending culture)

   (1) Sexually active adolesents and adults ages 15-40 yrs: Treat for disseminated gonococcal infection with ceftriaxone followed by oral agent to complete 1 wk course of treatment (see pg 215). Some authorities add nafcillin or oxacillin for S. aureus.

(2) Older adults (> 40 yrs)

Preferred: Penicillinase-resistant penicillin (nafcillin with or without an aminoglycoside or penicillinase-resistant penicillin with or without a third generation cephalosporin.

Alternative: Cephalosporin (1st generation) with or without an aminoglycoside or vancomycin with or without an aminoglycoside or imipenem with or without an aminoglycoside.

3. Prosthetic joint:

a. Bacteriology: S. aureus (20-30%), S. epidermidis (20-30%), streptococci (15-25%), gram-negative bacilli (15-25%), anaerobes (5-10%).

b. Management: Surgical drainage, antimicrobials ≥ 6 wks, retention of prosthesis: 20-30% success
Removal of prosthesis, bactericidal antibiotics x 6 wks, then reimplantation: 90-95% success
Removal of prosthesis and reimplantation of prosthesis with antibiotic impregnated cement plus course of bactericidal antibiotics: 70-80% success

c. Empiric treatment: Vancomycin plus aminoglycoside, 3rd generation cephalosporin or imipenem

B. Chronic Monarticular Arthritis

1. Bacteria: Brucella, Nocardia

2. Mycobacteria: M. tuberculosis, M. kansasii, M. marinum. M. avium-intracellulare, M. fortuitum (See pp 133-134).

3. Fungi: Sporothrix schenckii, Coccidioides immitis, Blastomyces dermatitidis, Pseudoallescheria boydii (See pp 111-117).

C. Polyarticular Arthritis

1. Bacteria: Neisseria gonorrhoeae (usually accompanied by skin lesions, positive cultures of blood and/or genital tract, negative joint cultures); N. meningitidis; Borrelia burgdorferi (Lyme disease, see pp 171-172); pyogenic (10% of cases of septic arthritis have two or more joints involved).

2. Viral: Hepatitis B (positive serum HBsAg, seen in pre-icteric phase, ascribed to immune-complexes, hands most frequently involved); rubella (usually small joints of hand, women >men, simultaneous rash, also seen with rubella vaccine in up to 40% of susceptible postpubertal women); parvovirus B19 (hand/wrists and/or knees; adults > children; women > men); mumps (0.5% of mumps cases, large and small joints, accompanies parotitis, men > women).

3. Miscellaneous: Acute rheumatic fever (Jones' criteria including evidence of preceding streptococcal infection); Reiter's syndrome (conjunctivitis and urethritis, associated infections - Shigella, Salmonella, Campylobacter, Yersinia).

OCULAR AND PERIOCULAR INFECTIONS

Condition	Microbiology	Treatment	Comment
Conjunctivitis	S. pneumoniae	Topical sulfaceta-mide, bacitracin, erythromycin	Hyperemia ± discharge photophobia, pain vision intact
	N. gonorrhoeae	Ceftriaxone, 250 mg x 1	Most are self-limited Pharyngoconjunctival
	C. trachomatis	Erythromycin x 3 wks	fever - Adenovirus 3 & 7 Epidemic keratoconjunc-
	Adenovirus	None	tivitis - Adenovirus 8
	Allergic or immune-mediated	Topical prednisone	Lab - conjunctival scraping: bacteria -
	Unknown (empiric)	Topical sulfaceta-mide or neomycin-bacitracin- poly-myxin or bacitracin-polymyxin	PMNs, viral - mononuclear; herpetic - multinucleated cells; chlamydia-mixed; allergic-eosinophils
Keratitis	S. aureus; S. pneumoniae; P. aeruginosa; Moraxella; Serratia	Usually hospitalize for treatment to prevent perfora-tion Antibiotics-systemic, sub-conjunctival and/or topical ± corticosteroids	Pain; no discharge; decreased vision Lab-conjunctival scrapings for stain (Gram, Giemsa, PAS & methenamine silver) + culture for bacteria and fungi Systemic antibiotics for deep corneal ulcers with bacterial infection
	Herpes simplex	Trifluridine/vidarabine and/or corticosteroids	Supportive care with cytoplegics, use of corticosteroids
	Herpes zoster	Acyclovir	controversial
	Fungal-Fusarium solani, Aspergillus, Candida	Topical natamycin, miconazole or flucytosine ± systemic anti-fungal	For topical antibiotics use solutions
	Acanthamoeba	Topical propamadine isethionate, dibromopropamadine isethionate + neomycin; usually requires corneal transplant	
Endophthalmitis	Bacteria Post-ocular surgery - S. aureus, Pseudomonas, S. epidermidis, P. acnes	IV antibiotics ± intravitreal antibiotics, corticosteroids, vitrectomy	Lab-Aspiration of aqueous and vitreous cavity for stain (Gram, Giemsa, PAS, methenamine silver) and culture for bacteria and fungi (continued)

189

Condition	Microbiology	Treatment	Comment
Endophthalmitis *(continued)*	Penetrating trauma - <u>Bacillus</u> sp.		
	Hematogenous - <u>S. pneumoniae</u>, <u>N. meningitidis</u> (others)		
	<u>Fungal</u>		
	Post-ocular surgery <u>Neurospora</u>, <u>Candida</u>, <u>Scedosporium</u>, <u>Paecilomyces</u>	IV amphotericin + topical natamycin ± corticosteroids vitrectomy	
	Hematogenous - <u>Candida</u>, <u>Aspergillus</u>	IV amphotericin B	
	Histoplasmosis	Systemic corticosteroids	
	<u>Parasitic</u>		
	Toxoplasmosis	Systemic + local corticosteroids ± pyrimethamine and sulfadiazine	
	Toxocara	Systemic or intra-ocular corticosteroids	
	<u>Virus</u>: Herpes simplex, H. zoster	Topical atropine + corticosteroids, Acyclovir (?)	Recurrence rate of H. simplex: 30-40%
Periorbital **Lid**			
Blepharitis	<u>S. aureus</u> - Seborrhea	Topical bacitracin or erythromycin ± topical corticosteroid	
Hordeolum	<u>S. aureus</u>	Topical bacitracin or erythromycin + warm compresses	
Chalazion	Chronic granuloma	Observation or curettage	
Lacrimal apparatus			
Canaliculitis	Anaerobes	Topical penicillin + antibiotic irrigation	
Dacryocystitis	Acute - <u>S. aureus</u>	Systemic antistaphylococcal agent; then digital message + antibiotic drops	
	Chronic - <u>S. pneumoniae</u> <u>S. aureus</u>, <u>Pseudomonas</u>, mixed	Systemic antibiotics; digital message	

(continued)

Condition	Microbiology	Treatment	Comment
Orbital	S. aureus (S. pneumoniae, S. pyogenes) Fungi - Phycomycosis, Aspergillus, Bipolaris, Curvularia, Drechslera	IV antibiotics- Cephalosporin, Cefuroxime or 3rd gen. Amphotericin B+ surgery	Over 80% have associated sinusitis Treat sinusitis

INFECTIONS OF THE CENTRAL NERVOUS SYSTEM

I. Cerebrospinal Fluid

A. <u>Normal findings</u>
   1. Opening pressure: 5-15 mm Hg or 65-195 mm H_2O

   2. Leukocyte count: <10 mononuclear cells/mm^3 (5-10/ml suspect);
      1 PMN (5%)

      Bloody tap: Usually 1 WBC/700 RBC with normal peripheral RBC
         and WBC counts; if abnormal: true CSF WBC = WBC (CSF) - WBC
         (blood) x RBC (CSF)/RBC (blood)
      Note: WBCs begin to disintegrate after 90 minutes

   3. Protein: 15-45 mg/dl (higher in elderly)
      Formula: 23.8 x 0.39 x age $\pm$ 15 mg/100 ml or (more simply) less
         than patient's age (> 35 yrs)
      Traumatic tap: 1 mg/1000 RBCs

   4. Glucose: 40-80 mg% or CSF/blood glucose ratio > 0.6
      (with high serum glucose usual ratio is 0.3)

B. <u>Abnormal CSF with non-infectious causes</u>

   1. Traumatic tap: Increased protein; RBCs; WBC count and differential
      proportionate to RBCs in peripheral blood; clear and colorless
      supernatant of centrifuged CSF.

   2. Chemical meningitis (injection of anesthetics, chemotherapeutic
      agents, air, radiographic dyes): Increased protein, lymphocytes
      (occasionally PMNs).

   3. Cerebral contusion, subarachnoid hemorrhage, intracerebral bleed:
      RBCs, increased protein (1 mg/1000 RBCs), disproportionately
      increased PMNs (peak at 72-96 hrs); decreased glucose in 15-20%).

   4. Vasculitis (SLE, etc): Increased protein (50-100 mg/dl), increased
      WBCs (usually mononuclear cells, occasionally PMNs); normal glucose.

   5. Postictal (repeated generalized seizures): RBCs (0-500/mm^3), WBCs
      (10-100/mm^3 with variable % PMNs with peak at 1 day), protein
      normal or slight increase.

   6. Tumors (esp. glioblastomas, leukemia, lymphoma, breast cancer,
      pancreatic cancer): Low glucose, increased protein, moderate PMNs.

   7. Neurosurgery: Blood; increased protein; WBCs (disproportionate to
      RBCs with predominance of mononuclear cells) up to 2 weeks post-op.

   8. Sarcoidosis: Increased protein; WBCs (up to 100/mm^3 predominately
      mononuclear cells); low glucose in 10%.

(continued)

192

C. **Doses of Drugs for CNS Infections***

1. Aminoglycosides and vancomycin

Agent	Systemic	Intrathecal/intraventricular
Gentamicin	1.7-2.0 mg/kg q8h (see pg 33, 34)	4-8 mg q24h
Tobramycin	1.7-2.0 mg/kg q8h (see pg 33, 34)	4-8 mg q24h
Amikacin	5.0-7.5 mg/kg q8h (see pg 33, 34)	10-20 mg q24h
Vancomycin	1 gm q12h	5-20 mg q24h

2. Cephalosporins

   Cefuroxime: 9 gm/day in 3 doses
   Cefotaxime: 12 gm/day in 6 doses**
   Ceftizoxime: 9 gm/day in 3 doses**
   Ceftriaxone: 4-6 gm/day in 2 doses**
   Ceftazidime: 6-12 gm/day in 3 doses**

3. Chloramphenicol: 4-6 gm/day in 4 doses**

4. Penicillins

   Ampicillin: 12 gm/day in 6 doses**

   Antipseudomonad penicillins
      Ticarcillin: 18-24 gm/day in 6 doses (40-60 mg/kg q 4 h)
      Mezlocillin: 18-24 gm/day in 6 doses (40-60 mg/kg q 4 h)
      Azlocillin: 18-24 gm/day in 6 doses (40-60 mg/kg q 4 h)
      Pipericillin: 18-24 gm/day in 6 doses (40-60 mg/kg q 4 h)

   Antistaphylococcal penicillins
      Nafcillin: 9-12 gm/day in 6 doses
      Oxacillin: 9-12 gm/day in 6 doses

   Penicillin G: 20-24 million units/day in 6 doses**

5. Trimethoprim-sulfamethoxazole: 15-20 mg/kg/day (trimethoprim) in 4 doses

   Metronidazole: 2 gm/day in 2-4 doses
   Vancomycin: 2 gm/day in 2 doses**

---

*   Assume adult patient with normal renal function.
** Recommendation of Tunkel AR et al, Ann Intern Med 112:610, 1990.

II. MENINGITIS (Medical Letter 34:49, 1992)

A. Likely pathogens and treatment

Setting	Likely agent	Empiric treatment*		Comment
		Preferred	Alternative	
Adult Immunocompetent, community-acquired	S. pneumoniae N. meningitidis	Cefotaxime Ceftriaxone	Penicillin G Chloramphenicol Cefuroxime Ceftazidime Ampicillin	Chloramphenicol is not effective against some GNB and some S. pneumoniae. GNB are rare except in newborns, adults >60 yrs, post-neurosurgery or immunosuppressed patients. In children, early use of decadron decreased incidence of hearing loss with H. influenzae meningitis (NEJM 324: 525, 1991); some recommend this for adults with pyogenic meningitis and mental status changes (JID 165:1, 1992)
Penicillin allergy	Same	Chloramphenicol	As above	Cephalosporins can usually be used with penicillin allergy unless reaction was IgE mediated. Vancomycin may not reach effective CSF levels: combine with rifampin for resistant S. pneumoniae
Immunosuppressed Defective humoral immunity, asplenia, complement defect	S. pneumoniae N. meningitidis	As above	As above	
Defective cell-mediated immunity	Listeria Cryptococcus	Ampicillin ± aminoglycoside	Trimethoprim-sulfamethoxazole	Cephalosporins not active vs Listeria. Negative cryptococcal antigen assay of blood and CSF virtually excludes this diagnosis

(continued)

194

Setting	Likely agent	Empiric treatment*		Comment
		Preferred	Alternative	
Post-neurosurgical procedure	Enterobacteriacae Pseudomonas sp. Staph. aureus	Aminoglycoside + antipseudomonad penicillin (or ceftazidime) + antistaph penicillin (or vancomycin)	Chloramphenicol	In vitro sensitivity tests required, bactericidal activity preferred. Infections that are refractory or involve resistant GNB may require intrathecal or intraventricular aminoglycosides
Cranial or spinal trauma Early (0-3 days)	S. pneumoniae	Penicillin or ampicillin	Chloramphenicol	Occasional cases with H. influenzae or Strep pyogenes
Late (over 3 days)	Enterobacteriacae Pseudomonas S. aureus S. pneumoniae	Treat as recommended for postsurgical complication		
Ventricular shunt	S. epidermidis	Vancomycin ± rifampin	Anti-staphylococcal penicillin	In vitro sensitivity tests required. Necessity to remove shunt is highly variable; most advocate antibiotics via shunt

* Antibiotic recommendations assuming clinical (± initial CSF analysis) evidence supporting this diagnosis with no direct clues to the etiologic agent.

B. Treatment by organism (See Tunkel A et al. Ann Intern Med 112:610,1990)

Organism	Preferred drug	Alternative	Comment
Strep pneumoniae	Penicillin G or ampicillin Cefotaxime Ceftriaxone	Chloramphenicol Cefuroxime Ceftizoxime	Test susceptibility to penicillin. Resistant strains: chloramphenicol or vancomycin + rifampin. Treat ≥ 10 days
Neisseria meningitidis	Penicillin G or ampicillin	(As above)	Intimate contacts should receive rifampin. Treat ≥ 7 days

(continued)

Organism	Preferred drug	Alternative	Comment
Haemophilus influenzae	Ampicillin (Ampicillin-sensitive strains)	Chloramphenicol Cefotaxime Ceftizoxime Ceftriaxone Ceftazidime	If children < 4 yrs in household, contacts should receive rifampin prophylaxis (type B only) Treat ≥ 10 days Cefuroxime found inferior to ceftriaxone (NEJM 322:141,1990)
Listeria monocytogenes	Ampicillin ± gentamicin	Trimethoprim-sulfamethoxazole	Cephalosporins are not effective Treat 14-21 days
E. coli and other coliforms	Cefotaxime Ceftizoxime Ceftriaxone Ceftazidime	Aminoglycoside ± antipseudomonad penicillin or ampicillin Sulfa-trimethoprim Aztreonam* Quinolone*	In vitro sensitivity tests required; MBC data preferred Chloramphenicol lacks bactericidal activity vs GNB - not recommended Aminoglycoside is given systemically ± intrathecally Treat ≥ 21 days Ceftazidime should be reserved for suspected or established P. aeruginosa
Pseudomonas aeruginosa	Aminoglycoside + ceftazidime	Aminoglycoside + antipseudomonad penicillin (ticarcillin, mezlocillin, piperacillin, Aminoglycoside + aztreonam,* imipenem,* quinolones*	Sulfa-trimethoprim-Acinetobacter, Ps. cepacia and Flavobacterium Aminoglycoside is given systemically ± intrathecally
Staph aureus	Antistaphylococcal penicillin ± rifampin	Vancomycin + rifampin Trimethoprim-sulfa + rifampin or ciprofloxacin	Vancomycin + rifampin for methicillin-resistant S. aureus
Staph epidermidis	Vancomycin + rifampin	Teicoplanin	

* Effectiveness in meningitis is not known

196

C. **Differential diagnosis of chronic meningitis*** (Adapted from Harris AA, Levin S: Infect Dis Clin Prat 1:158, 1992)

Infectious disease		Neoplastic	Miscellaneous
<u>Bacteria</u>	<u>Fungi</u>	Leukemia	Systemic lupus**
M. tuberculosis	<u>Cryptococcus</u>	Lymphoma	Wegener's granulomatosis**
Atypical mycobacteria	<u>Coccidioides</u>**	Metastatic	CNS vasculitis
<u>Treponema pallidum</u>**	<u>Histoplasia</u>**	Breast	Granulomatous vasculitis
<u>Borellia burgdorferi</u>**	<u>Blastomyces</u>	Lung	Sarcoidosis
<u>Leptospira</u>	<u>Sporotrichum</u>	Thyroid	Behçet's disease
<u>Brucella</u>**	Pseudoallescheria	Renal	Vogt-Koyanagi's and
<u>Listeria</u>	Alternaria	Melanoma	Harada's syndromes
<u>Actinomyces/Arachnia</u>	Fusaria	Primary CNS	Benign lymphacytic
<u>Nocardia</u>	<u>Aspergillus</u>	Astrocytoma	meningitis
<u>Parasites</u>	<u>Zygomycetes</u>	Glioblastoma	
<u>Toxoplasma gondii</u>	<u>Cladosporium</u>	Ependymoma	
<u>Cysticercus</u>	<u>Viruses</u>	Pinealoma	
<u>Angiostrongylus</u>	HIV**	Medulloblastoma	
Spinigerum	Echovirus		
<u>Schistosoma</u>			

* Defined as illness present for ≥ 4 wks with or without therapy; CSF analysis usually shows lymphocytic pleocytosis. Analysis of 83 previously healthy persons in New Zealand showed 40% had tuberculosis, 7% had cryptococcosis, 8% had malignancy and 34% were enigmatic (Q J Med 63:283, 1987)

** Evaluation: Culture, serum serology,** CT scan or MRI (brain abscess, cysticercosis, toxoplasmosis), cytology CSF (lymphoma, metastatic ca, eosinophilic (parasitic, cocardioidomycosis), CSF serology or antigen (cryptococcosis, coccidioidomycosis, syphilis, histoplasmosis), blind meningeal biopsy (rarely positive), empiric treatment (TB, then penicillin, then amphotericin B., then ? cortico-steroids)

D. **Aseptic Meningitis: Infectious and Non-infectious Causes*** (from American Academy of Pediatrics, Pediatrics 78 (Supplement):970, 1986)

<u>Infectious Agents and Diseases</u>
Bacteria: Partially treated meningitis, <u>Mycobacterium</u> <u>tuberculosis</u>, parameningeal focus (brain abscess, epidural abscess), acute or subacute bacterial endocarditis
Viruses: Enteroviruses, mumps, lymphocytic choriomeningitis, Epstein-Barr, arboviruses (Eastern equine, Western equine, St. Louis), cytomegalovirus, varicella-zoster, herpes simplex, human immuno-deficiency virus
Rickettsiae: Rocky Mountain spotted fever
Spirochetes: Syphilis, leptospirosis, Lyme disease
Mycoplasma: <u>M</u>. <u>pneumoniae</u>, <u>M</u>. <u>hominis</u> (neonates)
Fungi: <u>Candida</u> <u>albicans</u>, <u>Coccidioides</u> <u>immitis</u>, <u>Cryptococcus</u> <u>neoformans</u>
Protozoa: <u>Toxoplasma</u> <u>gondii</u>, malaria, amebas, visceral larval migrans (<u>Taenia</u> <u>canis</u>)
Nematode: Rat lung worm larvae (eosinophilic meningitis)
Cestodes: Cysticercosis
<u>Non-infectious Diseases</u>
Malignancy: Primary medulloblastoma, metastatic leukemia, Hodgkin's disease
Collagen-vascular disease: Lupus erythematosus
Trauma: Subarachnoid bleed, traumatic lumbar puncture, neurosurgery
Granulomatous disease: Sarcoidosis
Direct toxin: Intrathecal injections of contrast medium, spinal anesthesia

197

Poison: Lead, mercury
Autoimmune disease: Guillain-Barré syndrome
Unknown: Multiple sclerosis, Mollaret's meningitis, Behçet's syndrome,
Vogt-Koyanagi's syndrome, Harada's syndrome, Kawasaki disease

* Aseptic meningitis is defined as meningitis in the absence of evidence of
a bacterial pathogen detectable in CSF by usual laboratory techniques.

E. **Empiric treatment meningitis** (assumes no LP or negative LP for likely pathogens)
(Medical Letter 34:49, 1992)

Age 3 mo-18 yrs: Cefotaxime or ceftriaxone
18-50 yrs: Cefotaxime or ceftriazone; alternatives
are ampicillin or pencillin G
> 50 yrs: Ampicillin plus cefotaxime or ceftriaxone

III. Brain abscess

Associated condition	Likely pathogens	Treatment
Sinusitis	Anaerobic, micro-aerophilic and aerobic streptococci, <u>Bacteroides</u> sp.	Metronidazole + penicillin or chloramphenicol + penicillin
Otitis	<u>Bacteroides fragilis</u>, <u>Bacteroides</u> sp., streptococci, <u>Enterobacteriaceae</u>	Metronidazole + penicillin or chloramphenicol + penicillin
Trauma, post-neurosurgery	<u>Staph. aureus</u>	Penicillinase-resistant penicillin Vancomycin ± rifampin
	<u>Enterobacteriaceae</u>	Cefotaxime, ceftriaxone, ceftizoxime, ceftazidime Aminoglycoside + cephalosporin
	<u>Pseudomonas aeruginosa</u>	Aminoglycoside + ceftazidime or an anti-pseudomonad penicillin
Endocarditis	<u>Staph. aureus</u>	Penicillinase-resistant penicillin or vancomycin
	<u>Streptococcus</u> sp.	Penicillin or penicillin + aminoglycoside
Cyanotic heart disease	<u>Streptococcus</u> sp.	Penicillin or metronidazole + penicillin

UPPER RESPIRATORY TRACT INFECTIONS

Condition	Usual pathogens	Preferred treatment	Alternatives	Comment
Ear & Mastoids				
Acute otitis media	<u>S. pneumoniae</u> <u>H. influenzae</u> <u>M. catarrhalis</u>	Amoxicillin	Trimethoprim-sulfamethoxazole Amoxicillin + clavulanate Erythromycin + sulfoxazole Cefuroxime axetil Cefixime, Loracarbef Cefaclor, Cefprozil Cefpodoxime Tetracycline Parenteral: Cephalosporin-3rd gen	Tympanocentesis rarely indicated Less frequent pathogens: <u>S. aureus</u>, <u>Strep. progenes</u>. Oral or nasal decongestants ± antihistamine
Chronic suppurative otitis media	<u>Pseudomonas</u> <u>Staph. aureus</u>	Neomycin/polymyxin/ hydrocortisone otic drops	Chloramphenicol otic drops	Persistent effusion: myringotomy
Malignant otitis externa	<u>P. aeruginosa</u>	Tobramycin or amikacin + ticarcillin, mezlocillin or piperacillin Ciprofloxacin ± rifampin	Tobramycin or amikacin + cefoperazone, ceftazidime, aztreonam, imipenem, or ciprofloxacin	Surgical drainage and/or debridement sometimes required Treat 4-8 weeks Oral regimen - See Rubin J. Arch Otolaryngol Head Neck Surg 115:1063,1989
Acute diffuse otitis externa ("swimmer's ear")	<u>P. aeruginosa</u> Coliforms <u>Staph. aureus</u>	Topical neomycin + polymyxin otic drops	Boric or acetic acid (2%) drops Topical chloramphenicol	Initially cleanse with 3% saline or 70-95% alcohol + acetic acid Systemic antibiotics for significant tissue infection
Otomycosis	<u>Aspergillus niger</u>	Boric or acetic acid drops	M-cresyl acetic otic drops	

(continued)

Condition	Usual pathogens	Preferred treatment	Alternatives	Comment
Acute mastoiditis	S. pneumoniae H. influenzae	Cefuroxime, trimethoprim-sulfamethoxazole, cephalosporin-3rd gen	Amoxicillin or ampicillin Amoxicillin + clavulanate	Surgery required for abscess in mastoid bone S. aureus is occasional pathogent, esp. in subacute cases
Chronic mastoiditis	Anaerobes Pseudomonas sp. Coliforms Staph. aureus	None		Surgery often required Pre-op: Tobramycin + ticarcillin or piperacillin
Sinusitis				
Acute sinusitis	H. influenzae S. pneumoniae M. catarrhalis	Amoxicillin	Trimethoprim-sulfamethoxazole Cefaclor, cefuroxime axetil, cefpodoxime Loracarbef, cefprozil Amoxicillin + clavulanate	Nasal decongestant Sinus lavage for refractory cases
Chronic sinusitis	Anaerobes S. aureus	Penicillin or amoxicillin	Amoxicillin + clavulanate Clindamycin	Usually reserve antibiotic treatment for acute flares Surgery may be required
Nosocomial sinusitis	Pseudomonas Coliforms	Aminoglycoside + anti-pseudomonad penicillin or aminoglycoside + cephalosporin-3rd gen (ceftazidime)	Imipenem, cephalosporin - 3rd gen	Complication of nasal intubation
Pharynx				
Pharyngitis	Strep. pyogenes (Corynebacterium hemolyticum, C. diphtheriae, N. gonorrhoeae, Mycoplasma, C. pneumoniae, viruses including EBV)	Penicillin po (strep only) x 10 days or benzathine penicillin IM x 1 Cefpodoxime Cefuroxime axetil	Erythromycin x 10 days Cephalosporin x 10 day Clarithromycin x 10 days Azithromycin x 5 days	If compliance questionable use benzathine pen Gx1 IM Penicillin sometimes preferred due to established efficacy in preventing rheumatic fever although

(continued)

Condition	Usual pathogens	Preferred treatment	Alternatives	Comment
Pharyngitis (continued)				some report higher strep eradication rates with some cephalosporins Erythromycin: About 5% of Gr A strep are resistant
Gonococcal pharyngitis	N. gonorrhoeae	Ceftriaxone (250 mg x 1)	Ciprofloxacin (500 mg x 1)	
Peritonsillar or tonsillar abscess	Strep. pyogenes Peptostreptococci	Penicillin G	Clindamycin	Most cases are asymptomatic Drainage necessary
Membranous pharyngitis	C. diphtheriae Epstein-Barr virus Vincent's angina (anaerobes)	Penicillin or erythromycin (diphtheria) Penicillin/clindamycin (anaerobes)		Diphtheria: Antitoxin
Epiglottitis	H. influenzae	Cefotaxime, ceftizoxime, ceftriaxone, ceftazidime	Cefuroxime Chloramphenicol + ampicillin	Ensure patent airway (usually with endotracheal tube) Rifampin prophylaxis for household contacts < 4 yrs (x 4 days)
Laryngitis	Viruses (M. catarrhalis)			For M. catarrhalis: trimethoprim-sulfa, erythromycin, amoxicillin-clavulanate or cefaclor
Perimandibular Actinomycosis	A. israelii	Penicillin G or V	Clindamycin	Treat for 3-6 months: Tetracycline, erythromycin
Parotitis	S. aureus (anaerobes)	Penicillinase-resistant penicillin	Cephalosporin-1st gen Clindamycin, vancomycin	Surgical drainage usually required
Space infections	Anaerobes	Penicillin Clindamycin	Cefoxitin, penicillin + metronidazole	Surgical drainage required (continued)

Condition	Usual pathogens	Preferred treatment	Alternatives	Comment
Cervical				
Cervical adenitis				
Acute	S. aureus Strep. pyogenes Anaerobes Viral Toxoplasmosis	Penicillin (S. pyogenes, anaerobes) Penicillinase-resistant penicillin (S. aureus)	Erythromycin Clindamycin Amoxicillin + clavulanate (Bacterial infections) Oral cephalosporin (not cefixime)	
Chronic	Mycobacteria, cat scratch disease, HIV infection	TB: INH, rifampin + pyrazinamide M. scrofulaceum: excision		Non-infectious causes include tumors, lymphoma, sarcoid
Dental				
Periapical abscess Gum boil Gingivitis Pyorrhea	Anaerobes Streptococci	Penicillin Clindamycin	Metronidazole + penicillin	Metronidazole often preferred for periodontal disease, i.e., gingivitis, periodontitis
Stomatitis				
Thrush	C. albicans	Oral nystatin (swish and swallow) or clotrimazole troches	Ketoconazole po Fluconazole po	
Vincent's angina	Anaerobes	Penicillin Clindamycin	Metronidazole, tetracycline	
Aphthous stomatitis	No pathogen identified	Topical corticosteroid (Topicort gel)	Systemic corticosteroids (Prednisone, 40 mg/day, then rapid taper) Silver nitrate	
Herpetiform ulcers	H. simplex	Acyclovir		Usually reserved for immunocompromised hosts

Cost of Oral Drugs Commonly Advocated for Upper Respiratory Infections

	Wholesale price for 10 day supply*
Penicillins	
Penicillin G: 400,000 units po qid	$ 2.80**
Penicillin V: 500 mg po qid	$ 3.20** ($ 9.60)
Ampicillin: 500 mg po qid	$ 5.40** ($ 8.22)
Amoxicillin: 250 mg po tid	$ 2.40** ($ 6.30)
Amoxicillin + clavulanate 250 mg po tid	$51.00 --
Dicloxacillin: 500 mg po qid	$18.50** ($30.00)
Cephalosporins	
Cefaclor: 250 mg po qid	$73.20 --
Cephalexin: 250 mg po qid	$ 6.00** ($46.00)
Cephradine: 250 mg po qid	$11.36** ($32.80)
Cefuroxime axetil: 250 mg po bid	$55.80 --
Cefprozil: 250 mg po bid	$52.60
Clindamycin: 300 mg po tid	$64.11 --
Trimethoprim-sulfamethoxazole: 1 DS bid	$ 1.35** ($19.80)
Metronidazole: 500 mg po bid	$ 1.50** ($41.80)
Erythromycin: 500 mg po qid	$ 8.60** ($ 9.60)
Tetracycline: 500 mg po qid	$ 2.07** ($ 4.50)
Doxycycline: 100 mg po bid	$ 2.13** ($63.00)
Azithromycin: 6 250 mg tabs	$48.72
Clarithromycin: 250 mg bid	$50.00

* Approximate wholesale prices according to Medi-Span, Hospital Formulary
  Pricing Guide, Indianapolis, May, 1992. (Prices to patient will be
  higher.)

** Price provided is for generic product; price in parentheses is for a
   representative brand product when both brand and generic products are
   available.

PULMONARY INFECTIONS

A. Specimens and Tests for Detection of Lower Respiratory Pathogens. (Reprinted with permission from: Bartlett JG et al: Cumitech 7A, Sept 1987, pg 3)

Organism	Specimen	Test			
		Microscopy	Culture	Serology	Other
Bacteria					
Aerobic and facultatively anaerobic	Expectorated sputum, blood, TTA, empyema fluid, lung biopsy	Gram stain	X		
Anaerobic	TTA, empyema fluid	Gram stain	X		
Legionella sp.	Sputum, lung biopsy, pleural fluid, TTA, serum	FA	X	IFA, EIA	Urinary antigen[b]
Nocardia sp.	Expectorated sputum, TTA, bronchial washing, BAL fluid, tissue, abscess	Gram and/or modified carbol fuchsin stain	X		
Chlamydia sp.	Nasopharyngeal swab, lung aspirate or biopsy, serum		X[a]	CF for *C. psittaci*	PCR for *C. pneumoniae*[b] (experimental)
Mycoplasma sp.	Expectorated sputum, nasopharyngeal swab, serum		X[a]	CF, EIA or MI; cold agglutinins	
Mycobacteria	Expectorated or induced sputum, TTA, bronchial washing, BAL fluid,	Fluorochrome stain or carbol fuchsin	X		PPD
Fungi					
Deep-seated					
Blastomyces sp.	Expectorated or induced sputum, TTA, bronchial washing or biopsy, BAL fluid, tissue, serum	KOH with phase contrast; GMS stain	X	CF, ID	
Coccidioides sp.			X	CF, ID, LA	
Histoplasma sp.			X	CF, ID	Antigen assay BAL[b]
Opportunistic					
Aspergillus sp.	Lung biopsy	H&E, GMS stain	X	ID	CT scan[b]
Candida sp.	Lung biopsy	H&E, GMS stain	X		
Cryptococcus sp.	Expectorated sputum, serum, transbronch bx or BAL	H&E, GMS stain Calcofluor white	X	LA	Serum or BAL antigen assay[b]
Zygomycetes	Expectorated sputum, tissue	H&E, GMS stain	X		
Viruses: Influenza Paraflu, RSV, CMV	Nasal washings, nasopharyngeal aspirate or swab, BAL fluid, lung biopsy, serum	FA: influenza and RSV	X	CF, EIA, LA, FA	CMV: shell viral culture, FA stain of BAL or bx[b]
Pneumocystis sp.	Induced sputum or bronchial brushings, washings, BAL fluid	Toluidine blue, Giemsa, or GMS stain			

Abbreviations: CF, complement fixation; MI, metabolic inhibition; PPD, purified protein derivative; ID, immunodiffusion; LA, latex agglutination; H & E, hematoxylin and eosin; CIE, counterimmunoelectrophoresis; EIA, enzyme immunoassay; FA, fluorescent antibody stain; IFA, indirect fluorescent antibody.

a Few clinical microbiology labs offer these cultures and those that do infrequently recover the indicated organisms.

b Added by author.

B. PREFERRED ANTIBIOTICS FOR PNEUMONITIS

Agent	Preferred antimicrobial	Alternatives	Comment
Bacteria			
S. pneumoniae	Penicillin G or V	Ampicillin/amoxicillin Cephalosporins (1st gen) Erythromycin Clindamycin Chloramphenicol Ofloxacin	Quinolones (ciprofloxacin) and some 3rd gen cephalosporins (ceftriaxone) are relatively inactive Penicillin resistance (high level): 2.6% in U.S. (1990-1991), 20-40% in Spain, S. Africa, Mexico, Alaska and East Europe.
Enterobacteriaceae (coliforms)	Cephalosporin (3rd gen) ± aminoglycoside	Aminoglycoside Aztreonam Antipseudomonad penicillin, Imipenem or betalactam-betalactamase inhibitor Fluoroquinolone	In vitro sensitivity tests required Aminoglycoside + second agent may be required for multiply resistant GNB
Pseudomonas aeruginosa	Aminoglycoside + anti-pseudomonad penicillin, or ceftazidime	Ciprofloxacin ± aminoglycoside Imipenem + aminoglycoside Aztreonam + aminoglycoside	In vitro sensitivity tests required Aminoglycoside combinations required for serious infections
Moraxella catarrhalis (Branhamella catarrhalis)	Trimethoprim-sulfa Erythromycin	Tetracycline Amoxicillin + clavulanate Cephalosporins Fluoroquinolones	70-80% of strains produce betalactamase
S. aureus			
Methicillin-sensitive	Penicillinase-resistant penicillin (nafcillin, oxacillin) ± gentamcin or rifampin	Cephalosporin - 1st gen Vancomycin Clindamycin	May add aminoglycoside or rifampin for serious or refractory infections
Methicillin-resistant	Vancomycin ± gentamicin or rifampin	Teicoplanin, fluoroquinolone Sulfa-trimethoprim	

(continued)

205

Agent	Preferred antimicrobial	Alternatives	Comment
H. influenzae	Ampicillin/amoxicillin (susceptible strains) Cephalosporin (3rd gen)	Cefuroxime Sulfa-trimethoprim Tetracycline Chloramphenicol Betalactam-beta-lactamase inhibitor Fluoroquinolones	15-30% of strains are ampicillin resistant
Anaerobes	Clindamycin	Penicillin Metronidazole + penicillin Betalactam-beta-lactamase inhibitor Cefoxitin	Penicillins other than anti-staphylococcal agents are equally effective compared to penicillin G Cephalosporins (esp cefoxitin) are probably effective, but published experience is limited Metronidazole should not be used alone
Mycoplasma pneumoniae	Tetracycline Erythromycin		Treat for 1-2 weeks
Chlamydia pneumoniae (TWAR agent)	Tetracycline or erythromycin		Treat for 10-14 days
Chlamydia psittaci	Tetracycline	Erythromycin	Treat at least 10-14 days
Legionella	Erythromycin ± rifampin	Sulfa-trimethoprim + rifampin Doxycycline + rifampin Ciprofloxacin + rifampin Azithromycin or clarithromycin + rifampin	Treat for 3 weeks. Erythromycin is the only agent with established merit in clinical trials
Nocardia	Sulfonamide	Doxycycline Sulfa-trimethoprim Sulfa + minocycline or amikacin	Usual sulfa is sulfadiazine Treat 3-6 months

Agent	Preferred antimicrobial	Alternatives	Comment
Coxiella burnetii (Q fever)	Tetracycline	Chloramphenicol	

Mycobacteria: See section on Mycobacterial Infection:

Fungi: See section on Fungal Infections

Viruses: See section on Viral Infections

Parasites: See section on PCP Treatment

Pneumonia with no identified pathogen according to expectorated sputum stain and culture: community-acquired cases in immunocompetent adults

Agent	Preferred antimicrobial	Alternatives	Comment
Mycoplasma pneumoniae Chlamydia trachomatis Legionella sp. Anaerobes Viral (esp influenza) S. pneumoniae H. influenzae (S. aureus, GNB, Moraxella)	Outpatient: Erythromycin Hospital patient: Erythromycin + cefuroxime or 3rd generation cephalosporin	Outpatient: Cephalosporin, betalactam-betalactamase inhibitor, clarithromycin azithromycin, ofloxacin, tetracycline, sulfa-trimethoprim. Hospitalized patient: cefuroxime, cephalosprin-3rd gen; erythromycin ± sulfa-trimethoprim	Some cases are due to failure to detect fastidious bacteria such as S. pneumoniae and H. influenzae or lack of an adequate specimen Other possible agents: C. psittaci, C. psittaci Coxiella (Q fever), Nocardia, Actinomyces
Pneumonia, nosocomial Gram-negative bacilli (esp P. aeruginosa, Klebsiella sp. and Enterobacter), S. aureus and anaerobes	Aminoglycoside + ceftazidime or antipseudomonad penicillin ± vancomycin	Aminoglycoside + 3rd gen cephalosporin, imipenem aztreonam or betalactam-betalactamase inhibitor ± vancomycin. Antipseudomonad penicillin + 3rd gen cephalosporin. Monotherapy: Imipenem, betalactam-betalactamase inhibitor or ceftazidime.	GNB and S. aureus causing pneumonitis or tracheo-bronchitis (intubation, tracheostomy) should be easily detected with gram stain and culture of respiratory sections Sporadic and nosocomial outbreaks may be due to Legionella sp. and C pneumoniae has been implicated in 5-10% of cases; consider erythromycin in enigmatic cases

(continued)

C. Lung abscess

Agent	Preferred antimicrobial	Alternatives	Comment
Anaerobic bacteria	Clindamycin	Metronidazole + penicillin Penicillin/amoxicillin	Many antibiotics would probably work; suggestions are based on published reports with successful results in large numbers of patients

D. Bronchitis

Without chronic lung disease, intubation or tracheostomy

Agent	Preferred antimicrobial	Alternatives	Comment
Viral	None		Some cases due to Mycoplasma pneumoniae or Chlamydia pneumoniae: Tetracycline or erythromycin

Chronic bronchitis: exacerbation

Agent	Preferred antimicrobial	Alternatives	Comment
S. pneumoniae	Amoxicillin	Cefaclor, cefuroxime, cefpodoxime	
H. influenzae	Tetracycline	Cefixime, cefprozil, Loracarbef	
	Sulfa-trimethoprim	Amoxicillin + clavulanate	
		Ciprofloxacin	

Tracheobronchitis: intubation or tracheostomy - see nosocomial pneumonia

ENDOCARDITIS

I. **ANTICIPATED AGENTS**

    A. Non-addicts, native value

        Streptococcus sp: 55-65%

            Viridans strep (_S. sanguis, S. mutans, S. milleri, S. mitor_, etc): 35-40%

            Other (Microaerophilic, anaerobic and non-enterococcal gr D-

                S. bovis): 10-15%

        <u>Enterococcus faecalis</u>: 10-15%

        <u>Staphylococcal aureus</u>: 15-20%

        HACEK (<u>Hemophilus</u> sp., <u>Actinobacillus actinomycetemcomitans</u>,

            <u>Cardiobacterium hominis</u>, <u>Eikenella corrodens</u>, <u>Kingella kingii</u>): 5-10%

    B. Prosthetic valve

        <u>S</u>. <u>epidermidis</u> > 50% occurring within 2 months post-op

        Others: <u>S</u>. <u>aureus</u>, GNB, diphtheroids and <u>Candida</u>

    C. Narcotic addicts

        <u>S</u>. <u>aureus</u>: 50%

        Streptococci: 20%

        GNB, especially <u>Ps</u>. <u>aeruginosa</u>: 20%

        Fungi, especially <u>Candida</u> sp: 10%

II. **TREATMENT OF ENDOCARDITIS**

    A. **Medical Management (Committee on Rheumatic Fever, Endocarditis and Kawasaki Disease of the American Heart Association's Council on Cardiovascular Disease in the Young: Antimicrobial Treatment of Infective Endocarditis due to Viridans, Streptococci,Enterococci and Staphylococci. JAMA 261:1471, 1989)**

        1. <u>Streptococci</u>

            a) Penicillin-sensitive streptococci (minimum inhibitory concentration < 0.1 μg/mL)

                (1) <u>Penicillin only</u>: Aqueous penicillin G, 10-20 million units/day IV x 4 weeks. (Preferred regimen for patients with a relative contraindication to streptomycin including age > 65 years, renal impairment or prior 8th cranial nerve damage.)

                (2) <u>Penicillin + streptomycin x 4 weeks</u>: Procaine penicillin G, 1.2 million units IM q 6 h <u>or</u> aqueous penicillin G, 10-20 million units/day x 4 weeks <u>plus</u> streptomycin, 7.5 mg/kg IM (up to 500 mg) q 12 h or gentamicin, 1 mg/kg IM or IV (up to 80 mg) q 8 h for first 2 weeks. (The disadvantage of the procaine penicillin + streptomycin is the necessity of 140 IM injections.)

                (3) <u>Two week course</u>: Procaine penicillin G, 1.2 million units q 6 h IM <u>or</u> aqueous penicillin G, 10-20 million units <u>plus</u> streptomycin, 7.5 mg/kg IM (up to 500 mg) q 12 h. (Advocated as most cost-effective regimen by Mayo Clinic group for uncomplicated cases with relapse rates of < 1%.)

(4) <u>Penicillin allergy</u>: Vancomycin, 30 mg/kg/day IV x 4 weeks in 2-4 doses not to exceed 2 gm/day unless serum levels are monitored.

(5) <u>Penicillin allergy, cephalosporins</u>: Cephalothin, 2 gm q 4h x 4 wks or cefazolin, 1 gm IM or IV q 8 h x 4 wks. (Avoid in patients with immediate hypersensitivity to penicillin.)

Note

- Aqueous penicillin G should be given in 6 equally divided daily doses or by continuous infusion; disadvantage of procaine penicillin is the large number of IM injections.

- Streptococcus bovis and tolerant streptococci with MIC < 0.1 μg/mL may receive any of these regimens.

- Nutritionally deficient streptococci with MIC < 0.1 ug/mL should receive regimen #2 with IV penicillin; if susceptibility cannot be reliably determined treat for MIC > 0.1 mg/mL and < 0.5 μg/mL.

- Prosthetic valve endocarditis: Regimen #2 with IV penicillin for 6 weeks and aminoglycoside (streptomycin or gentamicin) for at least 2 weeks.

- Streptococci with MICs > 1000 mg/mL to streptomycin should be treated with gentamicin in aminoglycoside containing regimens. Gentamicin and streptomycin are considered equally effective for strains sensitive to both. An advantage of gentamicin is the ability to administer IV as well as IM.

- Cephalosporin regimens: Other cephalosporins may be effective, but clinical experience for agents other than cephalothin and cefazolin is limited.

- Two week treatment regimen is <u>not</u> recommended for complicated cases, e.g., shock, extracardiac foci of infection or intra-cardiac abscess.

- Desired peak serum levels if obtained: Streptomycin - 20 μg/mL, gentamicin - 3 μg/mL, vancomycin - 20-35 μg/mL (qid), or 30-45 μg/mL (bid).

b) Viridans streptococci and <u>Streptococcus bovis</u> relatively resistant to penicillin G (minimum inhibitory concentration > 0.1 μg/mL and < 0.5 μg/mL).

(1) Aqueous penicillin G, 20 million units/day IV x 4 weeks <u>plus</u> streptomycin, 7.5 mg/kg IM (up to 500 mg) q 12 h or gentamicin, 1.0 mg/kg (up to 80 mg) q 8 h x 2 wks.

       (2) <u>Penicillin allergy</u>: Vancomycin, 30 mg/kg/day x 4 wks
           in 2-4 daily doses.

       (3) <u>Penicillin allergy, cephalosporins</u>: Cephalothin, 2 gm IV
           q 4 h or cefazolin, 1 gm IM or IV q 8 h x 4 wks.

  c)   Penicillin-resistant streptococci including enterococci and
      strains with minimum inhibitory concentrations of > 0.5 μg/ml.

       (1) <u>Penicillin + aminoglycoside</u>:

Aq pen G 20-30		Strep, 7.5 mg/kg IM q12h
units/day IV <u>or</u>	<u>plus</u>	<u>or</u>
Ampicillin, 12 mg/		Gent, 1 mg/kg IM or IV
day IV		

       (2) <u>Penicillin allergy</u>: <u>Vancomycin + aminoglycoside</u>

Vanco, 30 mg/kg/		Streptomycin, 7.5 mg/kg IM q12h
day IV in 2-4	<u>plus</u>	<u>or</u>
doses		Gent, 1 mg/kg IM or IV q8h

<u>Note</u>

- Choice of aminoglycoside is usually determined by <u>in</u> <u>vitro</u> sensitivity testing. Gentamicin and streptomycin are considered equally effective for treatment of strains susceptible at 2000 μg/mL; high level resistance is more likely with streptomycin so that gentamicin is preferred when <u>in</u> <u>vitro</u> testing cannot be done. Other aminoglycosides should not be used.

- Occasional strains produce beta-lactamase and should be treated with vancomycin.

- Patients with symptoms for over 3 months before treatment and those with prosthetic valve endocarditis should receive combined treatment for 6 wks.

- Serum levels of aminoglycosides should be monitored. Desirable peak levels are: Streptomycin - 20 μg/mL and gentamicin - 3 μg/mL.

2.   <u>Staphylococcus aureus</u> or <u>S.</u> epidermidis

  a.   No prosthetic device - methicillin-sensitive

       (1) Nafcillin or oxacillin, 2 gm IV q 4 h x 4-6 wks $\pm$
           gentamicin, 1 mg/kg IV or IM q 8 h x 3-5 days.

       (2) <u>Penicillin allergy, cephalosporin</u>: Cephalothin, 2 gm IV q 4 h <u>or</u>
           cefazolin, 2 gm IV q 8 h x 4-6 wks $\pm$ gentamicin, 1 mg/kg
           IV or IM q 8 h x 3-5 days (should not be used with
           immediate type penicillin hypersensitivity).

(3) <u>Penicillin allergy</u>: Vancomycin, 30 mg/kg/day in 2-4 doses (not to exceed 2 gm/day unless serum levels monitored) x 4-6 wks.

(4) <u>Methicillin-resistant strain</u>: Vancomycin, 30 mg/kg/day in 2-4 doses (not to exceed 2 gm/day unless serum levels monitored) x 4-6 wks.

B. Prosthetic valve or prosthetic material

1. Methicillin-sensitive strains: Nafcillin, 2 gm IV q 4 h x $\geq$ 6 wks <u>plus</u> rifampin, 300 mg po q 8 h x $\geq$ 6 wks <u>plus</u> gentamicin, 1 mg/kg IV or IM (not to exceed 80 mg) x 2 wks.

2. Methicillin-resistant strains: Vancomycin, 30 mg/kg/day in 2-4 doses (not to exceed 2 gm/day unless serum levels monitored) x $\geq$ 6 wks <u>plus</u> rifampin, 300 mg po q 8 h x $\geq$ 6 wks <u>plus</u> gentamicin, 1 mg/kg IV or IM (not to exceed 80 mg) x 2 wks.

<u>Note</u>

- Methicillin-resistant staphylococci should be considered resistant to cephalosporins.

- Tolerance has no important effect on antibiotic selection.

- The occasional strains of staphylococci that are sensitive to penicillin G at $\leq$ 0.1 μg/mL may be treated with regimens advocated for penicillin-sensitive streptococci.

- For native valve endocarditis, the addition of gentamicin to nafcillin or oxacillin causes a more rapid clearing of bacteremia, but has no impact on cure rates; use of gentamicin (or rifampin) with either methicillin-sensitive or methicillin-resistant strains is arbitrary. With vancomycin regimens, there is evidence for synergistic nephrotoxic effects and no enhanced efficacy; addition of aminoglycosides should be restricted to cases involving aminoglycoside-sensitive strains and duration limited to 3-5 days.

- Coagulase-negative strains infecting prosthetic valves should be considered methicillin-resistant unless sensitivity is conclusively demonstrated.

- Aminoglycoside selection for coagulase- negative strains should be selected on the basis of <u>in vitro</u> sensitivity tests; if not active, these agents should be omitted.

C. Empiric treatment for acute endocarditis (Recommendations of AMA's Drug Evaluations, AMA, Chicago, II/INF - 2:10, 1991)

    1. <u>Native valve</u>
        a) Nafcillin or oxacillin: 2 gm IV q 4h <u>plus</u> Gentamicin (normal renal function): 1 mg/kg IV q 8h (adjust to keep peak serum level of about 3 mcg/ml) <u>plus</u> Aqueous penicillin G: 20 million units/day IV <u>or</u> ampicillin: 12 gm/day IV

        b) Vancomycin: 30 mg/kg/day IV (up to 2 gm/day) Gentamicin (above doses)

    2. <u>Prosthetic valve</u>
        a) Vancomycin (above doses) <u>plus</u> Gentamicin (above doses) <u>plus</u> Ampicillin (above doses)

        b) Vancomycin (above doses) <u>plus</u> Gentamicin (above doses) <u>plus</u> Cephalosporin - 3rd generation: cefotaxime - 12 gm/day, ceftizoxime - 12 gm/day <u>or</u> ceftriaxone - 4 gm/day

III. Indications for Cardiac Surgery in Patients with Endocarditis (Alsip SG, et al: Amer J Med 78(suppl 6B):138,1985)

    1. <u>Indications for urgent cardiac surgery</u>

        Hemodynamic compromise
            Severe heart failure (esp with aortic insufficiency)
            Vascular obstruction
        Uncontrolled infection
            Fungal endocarditis
            Persistent bacteremia (or persistent signs of sepsis)
            Lack of effective antimicrobial agents
        Unstable prosthetic valve

    2. <u>Relative indications for cardiac surgery</u>

        a. Native valve
            Bacterial agent other than susceptible streptococci (such as <u>S</u>. aureus or gram-neg bacilli)
            Relapse (esp if non-streptococcal agent)
            Evidence of intracardiac extension
                Rupture of sinus of Valsalva or ventricular septum
                Ruptured chordae tendineae or papillary muscle
                Heart block (new conduction disturbance)
                Abscess shown by echo or catheterization
            Two or more emboli
            Vegetations demonstrated by echo (especially large vegetation or aortic valve vegetations)
            Mitral valve preclosure by echo (correlates with severe acute aortic insufficiency)

    b.   Prosthetic valve
        Early post-operative endocarditis (< 8 wks)
        Nonstreptococcal late endocarditis
        Periprosthetic leak
        Two or more emboli
        Relapse
        Evidence of intracardiac extension (see above)
        Miscellaneous: Heart failure, aortic valve involvement, new
            or increased regurgitant murmur or mechanical valve versus
            bioprosthesis

3.   <u>Point system</u>: Urgent surgery should be strongly considered with 5
    accumulated points (Cobbs CG and Gnann JW: Indications for surgery in
    infective endocarditis. <u>In</u> Sande MA, Kaye D (Eds), Contemporary Issues
    in Infectious Disease. Churchill Livingstone, New York, 1984,
    pp 201-212).

	Native valve	Prosthetic valve
Heart failure		
Severe	5	5
Moderate	3	5
Mild	1	2
Fungal etiology	5	5
Persistent bacteremia	5	5
Organism other than susceptible strep	1	2
Relapse	2	3
One major embolus	2	2
Two or more systemic emboli	4	4
Vegetations by echocardiography	1	1
Ruptured chordae tendinae or papillary mm	3	-
Ruptured sinus of Valsalva	4	4
Ruptured ventricular septum	4	4
Heart block	3	3
Early mitral valve closure by echo	2	-
Unstable prosthesis	-	5
Early prosthetic valve endocarditis	-	2
Periprosthetic leak	-	2

INTRA-ABDOMINAL SEPSIS: ANTIBIOTIC SELECTION

I. **Peritonitis**

    A. <u>Polymicrobial infection</u>

        1. Combination treatment*

            An aminoglycoside vs. coliforms**

            a. Gentamicin, 2.0 mg/kg, then 1.7 mg/kg IV q 8 h (usually preferred) <u>or</u>

            b. Tobramycin, 2.0 mg/kg, then 1.7 mg/kg IV q 8 h <u>or</u>

            c. Amikacin, 7.5 mg/kg, then 5.0 mg/kg IV q 8 h <u>or</u>

            Plus an agent vs. anaerobes

            a. Clindamycin, 600 mg IV q 8 h <u>or</u>

            b. Cefoxitin, 2 gm IV q 6 h <u>or</u>

            c. Metronidazole, 500 mg IV q 8 h

---

    *   Some authorities add an agent for the enterococcus: Ampicillin, 1-2 gm IV q 6 h.

    ** Aztreonam, 1-1.5 gm IV q6-8h, may be used in place of aminoglycoside in combination with metronidazole or clindamycin.

        2. Single drug treatment

            a. Cefoxitin, 2 gm IV q 6 h (not advocated as single agent if infection was acquired during hospitalization or if there has been antibiotic administration during prior 2 weeks). Alternatives to cefoxitin are: cefotetan, 1 gm IV q 12 h or cefmetazole, 2 gm q6-12h.

            b. Imipenem, 500 mg IV q 6-8 h (See Solomkin J et al. Ann Surg 212:581,1990).

            c. Ticarcillin, 3 gm + clavulanic acid, 100 mg (Timentin) IV q 4-6 h

            d. Ampicillin, 2 gm + sulbactam, 1 gm (Unasyn) IV q 6 h

    B. <u>Monomicrobial infections</u>

        1. Spontaneous peritonitis or "primary peritonitis"

            a. Gentamicin or tobramycin, 2 mg/kg IV, then 1.7 mg/kg q 8 h <u>plus</u> a betalactam: Cefoxitin, 2 gm IV q 6 h; cefotaxime, 1.5-2 gm IV q 6 h; ampicillin, 2 gm IV q 6 h; or piperacillin, 4-5 gm IV q 6 h

            b. Cefotaxime, 1.5-2 gm IV q 6 h $\pm$ ampicillin, 2 gm IV q 6 h

2. Peritonitis associated with peritoneal dialysis

    a. Vancomycin, 1 gm IV (single dose)

    b. Antibiotics added to dialysate based on <u>in vitro</u> sensitivity:
Nafcillin, 10 mg/L; ampicillin, 20 mg/L; ticarcillin, 100
100 mg/L; penicillin G, 1,000-2,000 units/L; cephalothin,
20 mg/L; gentamicin or tobramycin, 5 mg/L; amikacin,
25 mg/L; clindamycin, 10 mg/L

3. Candida peritonitis (diagnostic criteria and indications to
treat in absence of peritoneal dialysis are nebulous)

    a. Amphotericin B, 200-1000 mg (total dose) 1 mg IV over 6 hrs,
then increase by 5-10 mg/day to maintenance dose of 20-30
mg/day

    b. Peritoneal dialysis: Systemic amphotericin B (above regimen)
plus addition to dialysate, 2-5 μg/ml

4. Tuberculous
INH, 300 mg/day po, <u>plus</u> rifampin, 600 mg/day po, <u>plus</u>
pyrazinamide, 15-30 mg/kg/day po x 2 months, then INH <u>plus</u>
rifampin x 7-22 months

II. Localized Infections

A. <u>Intra-abdominal abscess(es)</u> (not further defined): Use regimens
recommended for polymicrobial infections with peritonitis.

B. <u>Liver abscess</u>

1. Amebic

    a. Preferred: Metronidazole, 750 mg po or IV tid x 10 days plus
diloxanide furate, 500 mg po tid x 10 day or paromomycin, 500 mg
po bid x 7 days.

    b. Alternative: Emetine, 1 mg/kg/day IM x 5 days (or dehydro-
emetine, 1-1.5 mg/kg day x 5 days) <u>followed by</u> chloroquine,
500 mg po bid x 2 days, then 250 mg po bid x 3 weeks <u>plus</u>
iodoquinol, 650 mg po tid x 20 days

2. Pyogenic

    a. Gentamicin <u>or</u> tobramycin, 2.0 mg/kg IV, then 1.7 mg/kg IV
q 8 h <u>plus</u> metronidazole, 500 mg IV q 8 h; clindamycin,
600 mg IV q 8 h, or cefoxitin, 2 gm IV q 6 h <u>plus</u> ampicillin,
2 gm IV q 6 h or penicillin G, 2 million units IV q 6 h

    b. Gentamicin or tobramycin (above doses) <u>plus</u> clindamycin (above
doses), cefoxitin (above doses) <u>or</u> piperacillin 4-5 gm IV q 6 h

C. Biliary tract infections

1. Cholecystitis

   a. Combination treatment: Gentamicin or tobramycin, 2.0 mg/kg IV, then 1.7 mg/kg IV q 8 h plus ampicillin, 2 gm IV q 6 h, piperacillin, 2-5 gm IV q 6 h, or cefoperazone, 1-2 gm IV q 12 h*

   b. Single agent: Cefoperazone, 1-2 gm IV q 12 h*. Ampicillin + sulbactam, 1-2 gm IV q 6 h; ticarcillin-clavulanate, 2-3 gm IV q 6 h; for mild infections the usual recommendation is cefazolin, 1-2 gm IM or IV q 8 h, or ampicillin 1-2 gm IV q 6 h.

   ---

   * Other cephalosporins (2nd and 3rd generation) are probably equally effective. Some authorities add ampicillin (1-2 gm IV q 6 h) to cephalosporin containing regimens.

2. Ascending cholangitis, empyema of the gallbladder, or emphysematous cholecystitis: Treat with regimens advocated for peritonitis or intra-abdominal abscess.

D. Appendicitis (adult doses) (Role of antibiotics in nonperforative appendicitis is unclear.)

1. Combination treatment: Gentamicin or tobramycin, 2.0 mg/kg IV, then 1.7 mg/kg q 8 h plus clindamycin, 600 mg IV q 8 h, cefoxitin, 2 gm IV q 6 h or metronidazole, 500 mg IV q 6 h

2. Single agent: Cefoxitin, 2 gm IV q 6 h

E. Diverticulitis (Role of antibiotics in uncomplicated diverticulitis is unclear.)

1. Ambulatory patient

   a. Ampicillin, 500 mg po qid
   b. Tetracycline, 500 mg po qid
   c. Amoxicillin plus clavulanic acid (Augmentin), 500 mg po qid
   d. Cephalexin, 500 mg po qid plus metronidazole, 500 mg po qid

2. Hospitalized patients: Use regimens advocated for peritonitis or intra-abdominal abscess.

217

HEPATITIS

A. Types, clinical features and prognosis (MMWR 34:313,1985; MMWR 37:341, 1988; MMWR 39:1, 1990 and MMWR 40:RR (2:1, 1991)

Type	Source	Incubation period	Diagnosis of acute viral hepatitis*	Prognosis
A (HAV)	Person-to-person fecal-oral Contaminated food & water (epidemic) Seroprevalence: Anti-HAV in adults U.S.: 40-50%	15-50 days Avg: 28 days	IgM-anti-HAV	Self limited: > 99% Fulminant & fatal: 0.6% No carrier state or chronic infection Severity increases with age
B (HBV)	Sexual contact or contaminated needles from HBsAg carrier source (transmission via blood transfusions is rare due to HBsAg screening) Efficacy of transmission increased if source is HBeAg positive Seroprevalence (any marker, U.S.) (see pg 83) General population: 3-14% blacks: 14%; whites: 3% IV drug abuse: 60-80% Gay men: 35-80% Hemodialysis patients: 20-80% Health care workers (unvaccinated, frequent blood exp): 15-30% (unvaccinated, no frequent blood exp): 3-10%	45-160 days Avg: 120 days	HBsAg and/or IgM anti-HBc	Fulminant & fatal: 1.4% Carrier state, (defined as HBsAg-pos, twice separated by 6 months or HBsAg pos and IgM anti-HBc neg): 6-10% of adults; 25-50% of children < 5 yrs (this means 6-10% of adults with any marker will be HBsAg pos) Chronic carriers: 25% develop chronic active hepatitis that progresses to cirrhosis in 15-30%, fatal cirrhosis in 1%/yr and/or fatal hepatocellular carcinoma in 0.25%/yr Perinatal with HBsAg-pos and HBeAg-pos mother: 70-90% acquire perinatal HBV infection and 85-90% of these will become chronic carriers; > 25% of these carriers will develop cirrhosis or hepatocellular carcinoma Risk of transmission with needlestick from HBsAg-pos source: 6-30%

(continued)

218

Type	Source	Incubation period	Diagnosis of acute viral hepatitis*	Prognosis
C (HCV) (parenterally transmitted non-A,non-B) also causes sporadic NANB hepatitis	Contaminated transfused blood: 10%; IVDA-40%; heterosexual contact-10%; unknown-40% Seroprevalence rates (U.S.) Blood donors: 0.5-0.6% General population: 2% Hemophiliacs: 60-90% IV drug abuse: 60-90% Dialysis patients: 15-20% Gay men: 8%; Cryptogenic cirrhosis: 50-70% Chronic NANB hepatitis: 90-96%	14-84 days	Neg IgM anti-HAV, neg HBsAg and/or IgM anti-HBc; anti-HCV now available, but requires mean of 6 mo. to seroconvert with acute hepatitis; only about 30% of positive serologic tests in blood donors are true positives False positives with hyper-globulinemia including 5-6% with autoimmune chronic active hepatitis "2nd gen" tests such as RIBA-2 and PCR for HCV RNA (increased sensitivity, increased specificity and more rapid seroconversion) Preferred diagnostic tests are	Fulminant & fatal: rare Chronic hepatitis: 50%; cirrhosis: 10% (20% of those with chronic hepatitis); relationship to hepatocellular carcinoma is probable
Delta	Defective virus that requires presence of active HBV, e.g., co-infection with HBV or superinfection in HBsAg carrier; main source is blood (IV drug abuse, hemophilia) Seroprevalence in HBsAg carriers: IV drug abusers: 10-40% Hemophiliacs: 50-80% Hemodialysis patients: 20%	Superinfection: 30-60 days Co-infection: same as HBV	HBsAg + anti-HDV, but in delta hepatitis anti-HDV appears late and is short lived Co-infection: IgM anti-HBc + anti-HDV Superinfection: persistent HBs + anti-HDV in high titer (> 1:100)	Acute co-infection with HBV: 1-10% acute fatality; < 5% chronic hepatitis Acute superinfection: 5-20% acute fatility >75% develop chronic hepatitis with 70-80% developing cirrhosis Epidemics in underdeveloped countries: fulminant fatal hepatitis in 10-20% of children Chronic delta hepatitis: Worsens prognosis of chronic HBV infection

(continued)

219

Type	Source	Incubation period	Diagnosis of acute viral hepatitis*	Prognosis
Delta	Endemic areas (Mediterranean Basin, Middle East, Amazon Basin): 20-40% Medical care workers and gay men: low			
E (HEV) (enterally transmitted non-A,non-B or epidemic (NANB)	Epidemic fecal-oral (Burma, Borneo, Somalia, Pakistan, China, Soviet Union, throughout Africa)	20-60 days (mean 40 days)	As above but neg anti-HCV at 1 yr No chronic infection	Mortality < 2% except for pregnant women with mortality of 10-20% Usually mild disease predominately in adults > 15 yrs; chronic liver disease has not been reported

* Symptoms or signs of viral hepatitis, serum aminotransferase > 2.5 x upper limit of normal, and absence of other causes of liver injury.

Centers for Disease Control Hepatitis Hotline: Automated telephone information system concerning modes of transmission, prevention, serologic diagnosis, statistics and infection control (404) 332-4555.

B. Hepatitis nomenclature (MMWR 39:6,1990)

	Abbreviation	Term	Definition/Comments
Hepatitis A	HAV	Hepatitis A virus	Etiologic agent of "infectious" hepatitis; a picornavirus; single serotype.
	Anti-HAV	Antibody to HAV	Detectable at onset of symptoms; lifetime persistence.
	IgM anti-HAV	IgM class antibody to HAV	Indicates recent infection with hepatitis A; detectable for 4-6 months after infection.
Hepatitis B	HBV	Hepatitis B virus	Etiologic agent of "serum" hepatitis; also known as Dane particle.
	HBsAg	Hepatitis B surface antigen	Surface antigen(s) of HBV detectable in large quantity in serum; several subtypes identified.
	HBeAg	Hepatitis B e antigen	Soluble antigen; correlates with HBV replication, high titer HBV in serum, and infectivity of serum.
	HBcAg	Hepatitis B core antigen	No commercial test available
	Anti-HBs	Antibody to HBsAg	Indicates past infection with and immunity to HBV, passive antibody from HBIG, or immune response from HB vaccine.
	Anti-HBe	Antibody to HBeAg	Presence in serum of HBsAg carrier indicates lower titer of HBV.
	Anti-HBc	Antibody to HBcAg	Indicates prior infection with HBV at some undefined time.
	IgM anti-HBc	IgM class antibody to HBcAg	Indicates recent infection with HBV; detectable for 4-6 mo after infection
Delta hepatitis	HDV	Hepatitis D virus	Etiologic agent of delta hepatitis; can cause infection only in presence of HBV.
	HDAg	Delta antigen	Detectable in early acute delta infection.
	Anti-HDV	Antibody to delta antigen	Indicates present or past infection with delta virus.
Hepatitis C	HCV	Hepatitis C	Formerly parenterally transmitted non-A, non-B hepatitis (PT-NANB); shares epidemiologic features with hepatitis B.
	Anti-HCV	Antibody to HCV	Indicates past infection with HCV; usually means persistent HCV infection.
Hepatitis E	HEV	Hepatitis E	Formerly enterically transmitted non-A, non-B hepatitis (ET-NANB); shares epidemiologic features with hepatitis A.
Immune globulins	IG	Immune globulin (previously ISG, immune serum globulin, or gamma globulin)	Contains antibodies to HAV, low-titer antibodies to HBV.
	HBIG	Hepatitis B immune globulin	Contains high-titer antibodies to HBV.

INFECTIOUS DIARRHEA

A. ANTIMICROBIAL TREATMENT

Microbial Agent	Preferred	Alternative	Comment
Bacteria			
Aeromonas hydrophilia	Sulfa-trimethoprim 1 DS bid x 5 days Ciprofloxacin, 500 mg po bid x 5 days	Tetracycline, 500 mg po qid x 5 days Gentamicin, 1.7 mg/kg IV q8h x 5 days	Efficacy of treatment not established and should be reserved for patients with severe disease, immunosuppression, extraintestinal infection or prolonged diarrhea.
Campylobacter jejuni	Erythromycin, 250-500 mg po qid x 7 days Ciprofloxacin, 500 mg po bid x 7 days	Doxycycline, 100 mg po bid x 7 days Furazolidone, 100 mg po qid x 7 days	May not alter course unless given early or for severe Sx. Indications include: acutely ill, persistent fever, bloody diarrhea, > 8 stools/day, dehydration symptoms < 4 days or to prevent transmission. Resistance to erythromycin has been described. Clinical course not altered when treatment started > 4 days after onset of symptoms.
Clostridium difficile	Vancomycin, 125 mg po q6h x 10-14 days Metronidazole, 250 mg po qid x 10-14 days	Bacitracin, 25,000 units po qid x 10-14 days Cholestyramine, 4 gm packet tid	Vancomycin is preferred for severe disease. Discontinuation of implicated antibiotic is often adequate. Some strains are highly resistant to bacitracin. Relapses: Vancomycin or metronidazole x 10-14 days, then cholestyramine (4 gm po tid), vancomycin (125 mg po tid) or lactobacilli (1 gm qid) x 21 days or vancomycin + rifampin (600 mg/day). When oral treatment is not possible: metronidazole, 500 mg q8h IV.

(continued)

Microbial Agent	Preferred	Alternative	Comment
E. coli Enterotoxigenic E. coli (ETEC) Enteroadherent E. coli (EAEC)	Sulfa-trimethoprim 1 DS po bid x 3 days Ciprofloxacin, 500 mg po bid x 3 days Ofloxacin 300 mg po bid x 3 days	Trimethoprim, 200 mg po bid x 3 days Doxycycline, 100 mg po bid x 3 days Bismuth subsalicylate 60 ml quid x 5 days	Laboratory confirmation for E. coli - associated diarrhea is usually not available except for EHEC. Efficacy not established except for enterotoxin producing strains, e.g., ETEC (traveler's diarrhea). Many ETEC strains are now resistant to doxycycline and TMP-SMX
Enterohemorrhagic E. coli (EHEC)	Ciprofloxacin, 500-750 mg po bid x 5-7 days		Efficacy not established. Sulfa-trimethoprim may increase toxin production.
Enteroinvasive E. coli (EIEC)	Ampicillin, 500 mg po or 1 gm IV qid x 5 days Sulfa-trimethoprim 1 DS po bid x 5 days	Ciprofloxacin, 500 mg po bid x 5 days	Associated with hemolytic-uremic syndrome and TTP. Laboratory detection: stool culture for E. coli serotype O157:H7 or analysis for Shiga toxin
Enteropathogenic E. coli (EPEC)	Sulfa-trimethoprim 1 DS po bid x 3-5 days	Neomycin, 100 mg/kg/day po x 3-5 days Furazolidone, 100 mg po qid x 3-5 days	Presentation is dysentery as with Shigella
Food poisoning Clostridium perfringens, Staph. aureus, Bacillus cereus, Listeria	None		Self-limited and toxin mediated: antimicrobial treatment is not indicated.
Plesiomonas shigelloides	Sulfa-trimethoprim, 1 DS po bid x 5 days Ciprofloxacin, 500 mg po bid x 5 days	Tetracycline, 500 mg po x 5 days	Efficacy of treatment is not established and should be reserved for patients with extraintestinal infection, prolonged diarrhea or immunosuppression.

(continued)

Microbial Agent	Preferred	Alternative	Comment
Salmonella			Antibiotic treatment is contraindicated
Typhoid fever	Sulfa-trimethoprim 1-2	Ciprofloxacin, 500 mg po qid	in patients with uncomplicated
S. typhi	DS po bid x 14 days	x 14 days	enterocolitis; indications are typhoid
Non-typhoid	Ampicillin, 2-6 gm po or		fever, chronic bacteremia, metastatic
Salmonella)	IV/day x 14 days		infection or enterocolitis in
Enteric fever (non-	Amoxicillin, 2-4 gm po/day		compromised host (AIDS, sickle cell
typhoid Salmonella)	x 14 days		hemoglobinopathy, lymphoma, etc).
Metastatic infection	Chloramphenicol, 3-4 gm/day		AIDS patients may require long term
Chronic bacteremia	IV po x 14 days		suppressive treatment with ampicillin or
Enterocolitis in	Cefotaxime, 4-8 gm/day		ciprofloxacin.
compromised host	IV x 14 days		Patients with typhoid fever or enteric
	Cefoperazone, 1 gm bid IV		fever should receive antibiotics in high
	x 14 days		doses initially; with severe toxicity give
	Ceftriaxone, 1 gm IV bid x		dexamethasone (3 mg/kg x 1, then 1
	14 days		mg/kg q6h x 48 hr) or prednisone (60
			mg/day 20 mg/day over 3 days).
Carrier	Ampicillin, 4-6 gm/day	Ciprofloxacin, 500-750	Cholecystectomy for cholelithiasis and
	or amoxicillin, 6 gm/	mg po bid x 6 wks	carriers who relapse.
	day + probenecid, 2 gm/	Rifampin, 300 mg bid +	
	day x 6 weeks	sulfa-trimethoprim, 1 DS	
		bid x 6 wks	
Shigella	Ciprofloxacin, 500 mg po	Ampicillin, 500 mg po or	Preferred agents for empiric treatment
	bid or norfloxacin, 400	1 gm IV qid x 3-5 days	are sulfa-trimethoprim or ciprofloxacin/
	mg po bid x 3-5 days	Nalidixic acid, 1 gm po	norfloxacin.
	Sulfa-trimethoprim 1 DS	qid x 5-7 days	Ampicillin-resistant strains are common;
	po bid x 3-5 days	Cefoperazone, 1-2 gm IV	for ampicillin-susceptible strains,
		q12h x 5-7 days	amoxicillin should not be used.
			Sulfa-trimethoprim resistance is
			increasing and is common in strains
			from underdeveloped areas.

(continued)

Microbial Agent	Preferred	Alternative	Comment
Vibrio cholerae	Tetracycline, 500 mg po qid x 3-5 days Doxycycline, 300 mg po x 1	Sulfa-trimethoprim, 1 DS po bid x 3 days Furazolidine, 100 mg po qid x 3 days Erythromycin, 250 mg po qid x 3 days	
Vibrio sp. (V. parahaemolyticus, V. fluvialis, V. mimicus, V. hollisae, V. furnissii, V. vulnificus)	Tetracycline (as above - see comments)	Ciprofloxacin, 500 mg po bid x 5 days	Efficacy of treatment is not established and should be reserved for severe disease.
Yersinia enterocolitica	Sulfa-trimethoprim 1 DS po bid x 7 days Gentamicin, 1.7 mg/kg IV q8h x 7 days	Ciprofloxacin, 500-750 po bid x 7 days Doxycycline, 100 mg po bid x 7 days Chloramphenicol, 3-4 gm/ day po or IV x 7 days	Efficacy of treatment for enterocolitis or mesenteric adenitis is not established, especially when instituted late; major indications are prolonged diarrhea or generalized infection.
Parasites Cryptosporidia	Symptomatic treatment: Loparamide, lomotil etc. plus nutritional support Compromised host: Consider octretide (5-80 µg tid SC) paromomycin (500 mg po qid) or azithromycin (1500 mg/day, then 600 mg/day x 27 day, then 100 mg/day)		Consider treatment only for chronic diarrhea in compromised host. No antimicrobial agent has established efficacy
Balantidium coli	Tetracycline, 500 mg po qid x 10 days	Iodoquinol, 650 mg tid x 21 days Metronidazole, 500 mg po tid x 10 days	No antimicrobial agent has established efficacy

(continued)

Microbial Agent	Preferred	Alternative	Comment
Blastocystis hominis (see comments)	Metronidazole, 1.5-2.0 gm/day x 7 days		Role as enteric pathogen is not clear.
Entamoeba histolytica Acute dysentery	Metronidazole, 750 mg po tid x 5-10 days then diloxanide furoate, 500 mg po tid x 10 days or Iodoquinol 650 mg po tid x 21 days	Dehydroemetine, 1-1.5 mg/kg/day IM x 5 days, then diloxanide furoate	Alternatives to diloxanide furoate as oral luminal-acting drug are: iodoquinol, 650 mg po tid x 21 days, and paromomycin, 500 mg po tid x 7 days. Metronidazole may be given IV for severely ill patients (7.5 mg/kg q6h). Diloxanide furoate is available from the CDC.
Mild disease	Metronidazole, 500 mg po tid x 5-10 days, then diloxanide furoate (as above)	Paromomycin, 500 mg po tid x 7 days Metronidazole, 2.4 gm/day x 2-3 days, then diloxanide furoate Metronidazole, 50 mg/kg x 1, then diloxanide furoate	
Cyst passer	Iodoquinol, 650 mg po tid x 21 days Diloxanide furoate, 500 mg po tid x 10 days Paromomycin, 500 mg po tid x 7 days	Metronidazole, 500-750 mg po tid x 10 days	Need to treat is arbitrary, but luminal amebicides (diloxanide furoate, paromomycin or iodoquinol) are preferred. Diloxanide furoate is available from CDC 404-639-3670
Giardia lamblia	Quinacrine, 100 mg po tid x 5-7 days	Metronidazole, 250 mg po tid x 7 days Furazolidone, 8 mg/kg/day po day po x 10 days Tinidazole, 2 gm single dose	Metronidazole is less effective than quinacrine, but better tolerated. Pregnancy: Consider paromomycin, 25-30 mg/kg/day x 5-10 days.
Isospora belli	Sulfa-trimethoprim 2 DS po bid x 2-4 wks	Pyrimethamine, 25 mg + folonic acid, 5-10 mg/day x 1 month	Patients with AIDS and other immuno-suppressive disorders usually require prolonged maintenance treatment.

B. FECAL LEUKOCYTE EXAM

Often present	Variable	Not present
<u>Campylobacter jejuni</u>	<u>Salmonella</u>	Vibrio cholerae
<u>Shigella</u>	<u>Yersinia</u>	Enteroadherent
Enteroinvasive E. coli	<u>Vibrio parahaemolyticus</u>	<u>E. coli</u>
Exacerbations of	<u>C. difficile</u>	Enterotoxigenic
inflammatory bowel	<u>Aeromonas</u>	<u>E. coli</u>
disease	<u>Plesiomonas</u>	Food poisoning
	Enterohemorrhagic	<u>S. aureus</u>
	<u>E. coli</u>	<u>B. cereus</u>
		<u>C. perfringens</u>
		Viral gastroenteritis
		Adenovirus
		Rotavirus
		Norwalk agent
		Calicivirus
		Parasitic infection
		<u>Giardia</u>
		<u>E. histolytica</u>*
		Cryptosporidia
		Isospora
		Small bowel overgrowth
		"AIDS enteropathy"

* Frequently associated with blood.

C. EMPIRIC TREATMENT:

    1.   Indications (AMA's Drug Evaluation, AMA, Chicago, Vol 2, 1:20, 1991):
            Fever and acute moderate-to-severe diarrhea with dysentery (gross
            blood and mucus in stools) and/or PMN's in stool by direct exam.

    2.   Patients with acute, severe diarrhea (adults with $\geq$ 4 watery stools/day, $\leq$ 7 days)
            may be treated empirically with ciprofloxacin (500 mg po bid x 5 days) or
            norfloxacin (400 mg po bid x 5 days). (See Arch Intern Med 150:541, 1990
            and Ann Intern Med 117:202, 1992)

            <u>Alternative regimen</u>: Trimethoprim-sulfamethoxazole, 1 DS bid with or without
            erythromycin 250-500 mg po bid.

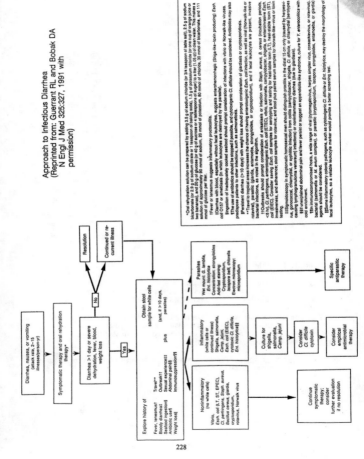

Approach to Infectious Diarrhea (Reprinted from: Guerrant RL and Bobak DA N Engl J Med 325:327, 1991 with permission)

URINARY TRACT INFECTIONS

I. Classification based on guidelines established by the Infectious Diseases Society of America and the FDA (Previewed in Clin Infect Dis 14, Suppl 2, S246, 1992)

Category	Clinical	Criteria for stated category Laboratory*	Treatment
Acute, uncomplicated UTI in women	Dysuria, urgency, frequency; no sx in last 4 wks; no fever or flank pain	> 10 WBC/mm³ > 10³ cfu/ml in MSU	All drugs active vs GNB show cure rates > 80% Single dose: TMP-SMX favored Advantages: Inexpensive, high response rates, few side effects (principally GI and Candida vaginitis) Disadvantages: Higher relapse rates due to persistence of uropathogenic E. coli in vagina and GI tract Three day treatment: Generally preferred
Acute, uncomplicated pyelonephritis	Fever chills, flank pain No urologic abnormalities	> 10 WBC/mm³ > 10⁴ cfu/ml in MSU	Mild sx: Oral TMP-SMX or fluoroquinolone x 2wk Seriously ill: Parenteral therapy until afebrile 24-48 hrs followed by oral agent x 2wks
Complicated UTI men or obstruction	Any combination of symptoms in above categories	> 10 WBC/mm³ > 10⁵ cfu/ml in MSU	UTI in men: Assure tissue invasion-renal or prostate Agents: TMP-SMX, carbenicillin, trimethoprim or fluoroquinolone Duration: 2-6 wks Obstruction: Anticipate 90% bacteriologic response rates with high frequency of relapse (same strain) or reinfection (new strain) Agents: Fluoroquinolone, 3rd generation cephalosporins
Asymptomatic**	No urinary symptoms	> 10 WBC/mm³ > 10⁵ cfu/ml x 2 separated by 24 hrs	Indications for treatment: Pregnant women, diabetic patients, immunocompromised patients and children**

* WBC = white blood cells (unspun urine); MSU = midstream urine culture
** Added by author

229

II.   Definitions of bacteriuric syndromes (Reprinted with permission from: Wilhelm MP and Edson RS, Mayo Clin Proc 62:1027,1987)*

Syndrome	Definition
Lower urinary tract infection	Lower urinary tract symptoms [T] + urine culture with $\geq 10^2$ bacteria/ml
Acute cystitis	Lower urinary tract symptoms + urine culture with $\geq 10^5$ bacteria/ml
Acute urethral syndrome	Lower urinary tract symptoms + 10^2 to 10^5 bacteria/ml or venereally transmitted agent (for example *Neisseria gonorrhoeae, Chlamydia trachomatis, Herpes simplex*) or no identifiable pathogen
Acute pyelonephritis	Upper urinary tract symptoms [TT] + urine with $\geq 10^5$ bacteria/ml
Asymptomatic bacteriuria	No symptoms + urine culture with $\geq 10^5$ bacteria/ml
Recurrent bacteriuria	Recurrent lower urinary tract symptoms[§] + urine culture with $\geq 10^2$ bacteria/ml
Relapse	Recurrent infection with same bacterial strain
Reinfection	Recurrent infection with different bacterial strain
Complicated bacteriuria	Urine culture with $\geq 10^5$ bacteria/ml with associated structural abnormality of the urinary tract[§] (for example, involvement with stones or catheter)

*   All syndromes usually associated with pyuria (≥ 8 leukocytes/mm^3 unspun urine.)
[T]   Dysuria, urgency, frequency, suprapubic pain.
[TT]   Fever, rigors, flank pain, nausea, prostration.
[§]   May be asymptomatic.

III.   **Recommendations of J. Johnson and W.E. Stamm (Urinary Tract Infections in Women: Diagnosis and Treatment. Ann Intern Med 111:906,1989)**

Cystitis: Single dose (only for uncomplicated cases)

Trimethoprim, 400 mg*	Ampicillin, 3 gm
Sulfa-trimethoprim, 320/1600 mg (2 DS)*	Cephalexin, 2 gm
Nitrofurantoin, 200 mg*	Sulfisoxazole, 2 gm
Amoxicillin, 3 gm	Ciprofloxacin, 250 mg
Amoxicillin plus clavulanate, 500 mg	Norfloxacin, 400 mg

Cystitis: Multidose regimens (3-7 days)

Trimethoprim, 100 mg q12h*	Cephalexin, 500 mg q 6 h
Sulfa-trimethoprim, 160/800 mg q12h*	Ciprofloxacin, 250 mg q12h
Nitrofurantoin, 100 mg q6h*	Norfloxacin, 400 mg q12h
Amoxicillin, 500 mg q8h	Sulfisoxazole, 500 mg q6h
Amoxicillin + clavulanate, 500 mg q8h	Tetracycline, 500 mg q6h

Pyelonephritis, oral therapy for mild pyelonephritis (treat $\geq$ 14 days)

Trimethoprim, 100 mg q12h*	Amoxicillin + clavulanate,
Sulfa-trimethoprim, 160/800 mg q12h*	500 mg q8h
Cephalexin, 500 mg q6h	Ciprofloxacin, 250 mg q12h
Amoxicillin, 500 mg q8h	Norfloxacin, 400 mg q12h

Pyelonephritis, parenteral therapy (Intravenous administration until afebrile and improved, then oral therapy to complete total of 14 days)

Gentamicin, 1.5 mg/kg q8h*	Ampicillin plus gentamicin
Ceftriaxone, 1 gm q12h*	(above doses) q8h
Sulfa-trimethoprim, 160/800 mg q12h*	Cefazolin, 1 gm (or higher) q8h
Ampicillin, 1 gm (or higher) q8h	Mezlocillin, 1 gm (or higher) q6h

* Preferred regimens

IV. **Recommendations for upper and lower urinary tract infections**
(AMA's Drug Evaluations, AMA, Chicago, Vol 2, Section 12, 1:33, 1991)

A. ASYMPTOMATIC BACTERIURIA

Indications for treatment: Pregnant women, diabetic patients, immunocompromised
   patients and children.
Regimens: Based on susceptibility tests; see cystitis for regimens.

B. ACUTE URETHRAL SYNDROME

Definition: Symptoms of acute cystitis (dysuria, frequency, urgency) without significant
   bacteriuria; most have pyuria.
Causes: Low concentrations of usual UTI pathogens or C. trachomatis (STD);
   vaginitis, N. gonorrhoeae and H. simplex may also cause symptoms of the acute
   urethral syndrome; patients with sterile urine and no pyuria have no
   demonstrable infection.
Empiric treatment: Doxycycline, 100 mg bid x 10 days
Alternative: Diagnostic evaluation and treatment for specific agents (findings
   suggesting E. coli UTI include abrupt onset of sx, symptoms < 4 days,
   hematuria, suprapubic pain, prior UTI and no recent change in sex partner;
   findings suggesting C. trachomatis are gradual onset of symptoms, symptoms
   over 7 days, no hematuria, no suprapubic pain and recent changes in sex
   partners).

C. CYSTITIS

1. Short course: Single dose therapy is considered inferior to 3 day courses and
    should be reserved for women who are not pregnant, have no evidence of
    pyelonephritis, have symptoms < 7 days and are available for follow-up.

Preferred regimens:	Single dose	3 days
TMP-SMX	2 DS	1 DS bid
Trimethoprim	400 mg	100 mg bid
Amoxicillin	3 gm	500 mg q8h
Nitrofurantoin	200 mg	100 mg q6h

Note: 1. Usual pathogens are E. coli (80%), Staph. saprophiticus (10%) and
           Enterococcus faecalis.
       2. Typical symptoms and urinalysis showing pyuria are adequate to
           initiate treatment; urine culture is optional.
       3. Must exclude vaginitis and STDs.
       4. Patients who fail to respond or relapse within 96 hrs are considered
           to have silent renal infections. These patients should have urine
           culture, and treatment 10-14 days or up to 6 wks.
       5. "Test-of-cure" urine culture at 1 week after single dose treatment is
           controversial.
2. Conventional therapy (7-14 days)
    Preferred regimens: Trimethoprim-sulfamethoxazole; ampicillin/amoxicillin,
       sulfasoxazole or nitrofurantoin.

Note: 1. Treatment is 7-14 days.
2. If relapse occurs, suspect pyelonephritis, treat for up to 6 wks and evaluate for underlying urinary tract abnormality.

D. RECURRENT UTIs

1. Relapse: Post-treatment infection caused by same organism, usually within 2 wks and usually indicates renal involvement

    Recommendations: a) Rule out structural abnormality or chronic prostatitis and b) Antibiotic treatment x 6 wks.

2. Reinfection: Recurrent infections with different organisms. This mechanism accounts for > 80% of recurrent infections in women.

    Recommendations: If > 3 episodes/yr consider long-term prophylaxis with a) trimethoprim-sulfamethoxazole, 1/2 tab daily or 3 days/wk, b) nitrofurantoin macrocrystals, 50 mg daily or c) trimethoprim, 50 mg (1/2 100 mg tab) daily.

E. PYELONEPHRITIS

1. In-patient treatment
    Preferred: Aminoglycoside + ampicillin.
    Alternatives: Trimethoprim-sulfamethoxazole, cephalosporins - 3rd generation, or aztreonam.
    Regimens: Parenteral treatment until afebrile 24-48 hr, total duration $\geq$ 14 days; relapse - treat up to 6 wks.

2. Outpatient treatment
    Preferred: Trimethoprim-sulfamethoxazole.
    Alternatives: Cephalosporin - oral, quinolone, amoxicillin-clavulanate.
    Duration: 14 days, relapse - treat up to 6 wks.

F. PROSTATITIS

1. Acute
    Bacteriology: E. coli (> 80%), other GNB
    Treatment regimens
    a) Trimethoprim-sulfamethoxazole: 160 mg/800 mg bid x 30 days.
    b) Aminoglycoside + ampicillin: Parenteral treatment until afebrile, then oral regimen based on susceptibility test of urine isolate to complete 30 days of treatment.
    c) Ciprofloxacin, lomefloxacin or ofloxacin x 30 days.

2. Chronic
    Bacteriology: E. coli (most common), other GNB, enterococcus, Ureoplasma ureolyticum (?)
    Treatment regimens
    a) Trimethoprim-sulfamethoxazole: 1 DS po bid x $\geq$ 12-24 wks.
    b) Ciprofloxacin, 500-750 mg po bid; Ofloxacin, 400 mg po bid or lomefloxacin, 400 mg po/day $\geq$ x 12.

     c)   Trimethoprim, 100 mg bid x 12 wks.
     d)   Doxycycline or erythromycin are suggested for nonbacterial prostatitis due
               possibly to <u>Ureoplasma</u> <u>urealyticum</u>.

G.   EPIDIDYMO-ORCHITIS

    1.   STD form: See <u>Neisseria</u> <u>gonorrhoeae</u> or <u>Chlamydia</u> <u>trachomatis</u> (pp 233, 236).
    2.   Non-STD form: Usual pathogens, <u>E</u>. <u>coli</u> and other GNB.
        Preferred empiric treatment
        a)   Aminoglycoside with or without ampicillin or
        b)   Trimethoprim-sulfamethoxadole
        Alternatives:
        a)   Ciprofloxacin, ofloxacin or lomefloxacin
        b)   Cephalosporin - 3rd generation

V.   Cost of oral drugs commonly used for urinary tract infections

Antimicrobial agent and regimen	Wholesale price for 10 day supply*
Ampicillin: 500 mg po tid	$ 3.90** ($ 7.50)
Amoxicillin: 250 mg po tid	$ 3.23** ($8.40)
Amoxicillin + clavulanate (Augmentin): 250 mg po tid	$51.00
Carbenicillin (Geocillin): 380 mg po qid	$64.00
Cephradine (Anspor, Velosef): 250 mg po qid	$11.36** ($32.80)
Cephalexin (Keflex): 250 mg po qid	$ 6.00** ($46.00)
Ciprofloxacin (Cipro): 500 mg po bid	$58.40
Doxycycline (Vibramycin): 100 mg po bid	$ 2.13** ($63.00)
Lomefloxacin (Maxquin): 400 mg po qd	$44.70
Methenamine mandelate: 1 gm po qid	$ 2.80
Methenamine hippurate (Hiprex): 1 gm po bid	$18.40
Nalidixic acid (NegGram): 1 gm caplet po qid	$58.60
Nitrofurantoin (Furadantin): 50 mg cap po qid	$24.00
Norfloxacin (Noroxin): 400 mg po bid	$45.00
Ofloxacin (Floxin): 400 mg po bid	$67.60
Sulfisoxazole (Gantrisin): 1 gm po qid	$ 2.80** ($16.80)
Tetracycline: 500 mg po qid	$ 2.07** ($ 4.50)
Trimethoprim: 100 mg po bid	$ 2.86
Trimethoprim-sulfa (Bactrim, Septra): 1 DS po bid	$ 1.35** ($19.80)

* Approximate wholesale prices according to Medi-Span, Hospital Formulary
   Pricing Guide, Indianapolis, May, 1992 (prices to patient will be higher).

**Price is provided for generic product if available; price in parentheses is for
   representative brand product.

SEXUALLY TRANSMITTED DISEASES

(CDC recommendations adapted from MMWR 38:S8, pp 1-43, 1989)

Revised CDC guidelines are expected in late 1992; anticipated revisions added by author in consultation with J. Zenilman are indicated by single asterisk (*)

I.   <u>Gonococcal infections</u>

    A.   Treatment recommendations are influenced by:

        1)   Spread of infections due to antibiotic-resistant <u>N</u>. <u>gonorrhoeae</u> including penicillinase-producing strains (PPNG), tetracycline-resistant strains (TRNG) and strains with chromosomally mediated resistance to multiple antibiotics.

        2)   High frequency of chlamydial infections in patients with gonorrhea.

        3)   Recognition of serious complications of chlamydial and gonococcal infection.

        4)   Absence of a rapid, inexpensive and highly accurate test for chlamydial infection.

    B.   All cases of gonorrhea should be diagnosed or confirmed by culture to enable antimicrobial susceptibility testing. (This recommendation is no longer necessary due to gonococcal surveillance and use of drugs effective for virtually all strains)*

    C.   Treatment of uncomplicated urethral, endocervical and rectal infections

        1.   <u>Recommended</u>: Cefixime, 400 mg po* x 1 <u>plus</u> doxycycline**, 100 mg po bid x 7 days or fluoroquinolone *,*** (ciprofloxacin 500 mg po x 1; ofloxacin 400 mg po x 1 or norfloxacin 800 mg po x 1) <u>plus</u> doxycycline, 100 mg po bid x 7 days or ceftriaxone, 125 mg IM* <u>plus</u> doxycycline, 100 mg po bid x 7 days.

        2.   <u>Alternative</u>:

            a.   Cefuroxime axetil, 1 gm po x 1 + probenecid, 1 gm **

            b.   Cefotaxime, 1 gm IM x 1 **

            c.   Ceftizoxime, 500 mg IM x 1 **

            d.   Spectinomycin, 2 gm IM**

        **   All regimens should include a 7 day course of doxycycline (100 mg po bid x 7 days) or tetracycline (500 mg po qid x 7 days) for presumed concurrent infection with <u>Chlamydia</u> <u>trachomatis</u>. Alternative to tetracyclines for <u>C</u>. <u>trachomatis</u> is erythromycin base or stearate (500 mg po qid x 7 days), erythromycin ethylsuccinate (800 mg po qid x 7 days) <u>or</u> azithromycin (1 gm po x 1).*

        ***   Quinolones are contraindicated in pregnant women and children < 16 yrs; activity of quinolones or spectinomycin in incubating syphilis is unknown so serology for syphilis should be obtained in 1 month.

        3.   <u>Special considerations</u>

            a.   <u>Incubating syphilis</u>: All patients with gonorrhea should have syphilis serology; patients treated with quinolones or spectinomycin should have repeat serology in 1 month to exclude incubating syphilis.

            b.   <u>Sex partners</u>: All persons exposed during preceding 30 days should be examined, cultured and treated (for gonorrhea and chlamydial infection).

            c.   <u>Follow-up</u>: Treatment failure with recommended regimen is rare so that "test-of-cure" is not essential; re-exam at 1-2 months ("re-screening") may be more cost effective.

            d.   <u>Treatment failures</u>: Culture for <u>N</u>. <u>gonorrhoeae</u> and test for antibiotic sensitivity. Many "treatment failures" are due to chlamydial infection, reinfection or non-compliance. Treat recurrent gonococcal infection with ceftriaxone, 250 mg IM x 1 plus doxycycline, 100 mg po bid x 7 days.

     e.   <u>Pregnancy</u>: Cefixime, 400 mg* po or ceftriaxone, 125 mg IM x 1 <u>plus</u> erythromycin base or stearate, 500 mg po qid x 7 days. (Quinolones and tetracyclines are contraindicated.)

D.   Gonococcal infection at other anatomical sites

    1. <u>Rectal and pharyngeal infection</u>: Cefixime, 400 mg po x 1* <u>or</u> Ciprofloxacin, 500 mg po x 1 <u>or</u> Ceftriaxone, 250 mg IM x 1 and repeat culture 4-7 days later.

    2. <u>Salpingitis</u>: See Pelvic inflammatory disease.

    3. <u>Disseminated gonococcal infection (DGI)</u>
       Hospitalize and treat with: Ceftriaxone*, 1 gm IV or IM q24h <u>or</u> Ceftizoxime*, 1 gm IV q8h <u>or</u> Ceftazidime*, 1 gm IV q8h
       Alternative to betalactams: Spectinomycin*, 2 gm IM q12h <u>or</u> IV fluoroquinolone*
       * Test for genital chlamydia or treat empirically; reliable patients with uncomplicated DGI may be discharged at 24-48 hrs after symptoms resolve and should complete 1 wk of treatment with cefixime, 400 mg po bid* <u>or</u> ciprofloxacin, 500 mg bid.

    4. <u>Gonococcal endocarditis or meningitis</u>
       IV therapy with effective agent such as ceftriaxone 1-2 gm q12h for 10-14 days (meningitis) or 4 weeks (endocarditis).

    5. <u>Gonococcal ophthalmia</u>
       Treatment of adult: Ceftriaxone, 1 gm IM x 1 <u>plus</u> ophthalmologic assessment. Antibiotic irrigation is not required.

       Prevention in newborn infants (required by law in most states, must be done within 1 hr after delivery, efficacy in preventing chlamydial infections of eye is unknown):
           Erythromycin 0.5% ophthalmic ointment x 1 <u>or</u>
           Tetracycline 1% ophthalmic ointment x 1 <u>or</u>
           Silver nitrate 1% aqueous solution

II. <u>Syphilis</u>

    A. Treatment (adult, non-pregnant)

      1. <u>Exposed</u>: Evaluate clinically and serologically; if exposure < 90 days treat presumptively (regimen for early syphilis).

      2. <u>Early syphilis</u> including primary, secondary or latent of less than 1 year duration.

        - Benzathine penicillin G, 2.4 million units IM x 1.

        - Penicillin allergy: Doxycycline, 100 mg po bid x 14 days or tetracycline, 500 mg po qid x 14 days.

        - Penicillin allergy and tetracycline contraindication or intolerance: **a)** erythromycin, 500 mg po qid x 15 days (this is acceptable only if compliance plus follow-up serology is assured); **b)** skin testing for penicillin allergy and desensitization if necessary; **c)** ceftriaxone, 250 mg IM x 1/day x 10 days with caution for sensitivity reaction.

3. Syphilis over 1 year (except neurosyphilis) including latent syphilis, cardiovascular syphilis or gummas.

   - Benzathine penicillin G, 2.4 million units q week x 3 successive weeks.

   - Penicillin allergy (efficacy of alternative regimens for neurosyphilis not established and CSF exam mandatory to exclude this complication): Doxycycline, 100 mg po bid or tetracycline, 500 mg po qid x 4 weeks.

4. Neurosyphilis

   - Aqueous penicillin G, 12-24 million units IV/day x 10-14 days, then benzathine penicillin G, 2.4 million units IM weekly x 3.

   - Procaine penicillin G, 2-4 million units IM daily plus probenecid, 500 mg po qid x 10-14 days; some recommend adding benzathine penicillin G, 2.4 million units IM weekly x 3.

   - Penicillin allergy: Confirm allergy and "consult expert"; desensitization required if truly allergic.

5. Pregnancy

   - Penicillin regimens as noted above.

   - Tetracyclines are contraindicated in pregnancy and erythromycins have a high failure rate in fetal infection. Patients with convincing histories of penicillin allergy should have skin testing and desensitization.

6. HIV infection

   a. All patients with syphilis should be counseled concerning risks of HIV and encouraged to have HIV serology.

   b. CSF from patients with HIV infection often shows mononuclear cells and increased protein. With a negative CSF VDRL there is no practical method to confirm or exclude neurosyphilis. Sensitivity of CSF VDRL is 60-70%.

B. CSF exam: Should be performed in patients with clinical symptoms or signs consistent with neurosyphilis and is desired in all persons with syphilis > 1 yr, although this decision should be individualized. Tests in CSF should include leukocyte count, protein and VDRL. A positive VDRL is diagnostic of neurosyphilis; negative VDRL does not exclude it. (Elderly patients with low titer serum VDRL probably do not require a LP.)*

C. Follow up

Form	Follow-up quantitative non-treponemal test*	Expectation	Additional comments
Early syphilis	3 & 6 months post-treatment	4-fold decrease by 3 mo. or by 6 mo. with early latent syphilis	If titer not decreased should do CSF exam and re-treat
Early syphilis + HIV infected	1, 2, 3, 6, 9 and 12 mo.		If titer does not decrease (4-fold) by 3 mo. for primary or by 6 mo. for secondary, or if titer increases (4-fold): re-evaluate for treatment failure versus reinfection, and examine CSF
Syphilis > 1 yr	6 and 12 months post-treatment	Titer declines more gradually	CSF exam if there are neurological signs or symptoms; treatment failure (titer increases 4-fold or initially high titer of ≥ 1:32 fails to decrease); non-penicillin therapy; HIV seropositive
Neurosyphilis	Six-month intervals at least 2 yrs (see comments)		Clinical evaluation and CSF analysis at 6 mo. intervals until cell count normal; if titer not decreased at 6 mo. or normal at 2 yrs, consider retreatment

* Nontreponemal tests = VDRL and RPR; treponemal tests = FTA-ABS, MHA-TP and HATTS

III. Chlamydia trachomatis

A. Treatment (urethral, endocervical and rectal infection)

- Doxycycline, 100 mg po bid x 7 days.

- Tetracycline, 500 mg po qid x 7 days.

- Azithromycin, 1 gm po x 1*.

Pregnancy: Erythromycin base or stearate, 500 mg po qid x 7 days or erythromycin ethylsuccinate, 800 mg po qid x 7 days. Women who cannot tolerate this regimen should receive half the suggested daily dose qid for at least 14 days. Alternative to erythromycin is azithromycin, 1 mg x 1 (Category II for pregnancy).

B. Sex partners: Examine for STD and treat using above regimen if contact was within 30 days.

C. Follow up: Post-treatment test-of-cure cultures are not advocated because treatment failures with recommended regimens have not been observed.

IV. Genital herpes simplex

   A. Treatment

      1. First episode (genital or rectal infection)

         Genital: Acyclovir, 200 mg po 5 x daily for 7-10 days or until clinical resolution occurs.

         Rectal: 400 mg po 5 x daily for 10 days or until clinical resolution occurs.

         Hospitalized patients: 5 mg/kg IV q8h for 5-7 days or until clinical resolution occurs.

      2. Recurrent episodes (most do not benefit from treatment unless recurrences are severe and acyclovir is started at the beginning of the prodrome or within 2 days of onset of lesions).

         - Acyclovir, 200 mg po 5 times daily x 5 days or acyclovir, 800 mg po bid x 5 days.

      3. Prophylaxis for recurrences (for patients with > 6 recurrences/yr): 200 mg po 2-5 x/day or 400 mg po bid. This suppressive regimen is contraindicated in women who become pregnant during treatment.

   B. HIV disease: The need for higher therapeutic or suppressive doses is suspected, but not established.

   C. Pregnancy: Safety of acyclovir is not established, but post-marketing surveillance shows probable safety; acyclovir is indicated during primary HSV infection during pregnancy* and for life-threatening maternal HSV disease. Major risk of neonatal HSV infection is primary infection in mother at the time of delivery (NEJM 326:916, 1992)*

V. Chancroid (Haemophilus ducreyi) infection: Recommended treatment varies by susceptibility of strains in different geographic areas.

   Recommended: Ceftriaxone, 250 mg IM x 1 or Ciprofloxacin, 500 mg po qid x 7 days.*

   Alternative regimens: Trimethoprim-sulfamethoxazole, 1 double strength tablet (160/800 mg) po bid x at least 7 days; amoxicillin, 500 mg plus clavulanic acid 125 mg po tid x 7 days or erythromycin, 500 mg po bid x 3 days

VI. Lymphogranuloma venereum treatment (genital, inguinal and anorectal)

   Recommended: Doxycycline, 100 mg po bid x 21 days.

   Alternatives: Tetracycline, 500 mg po qid x 21 days or Erythromycin, 500 mg po qid x 21 days or Sulfasoxazole, 500 mg qid x 21 days. (Azithromycin: efficacy is not established.)

VII. Pediculosis pubis

   A. Treatment

      Permethrin (1%) cream rinse applied to affected area and washed after 10 minutes or Lindane (1%) shampoo applied 4 minutes and then thoroughly washed off (not recommened for pregnant or lactating women) or Pyrethrins and piperonyl butoxide (non-prescription) applied to affected area and washed off after 10 minutes.

238

B. <u>Adjunctive:</u> Retreat after 7 days if lice or eggs are detected at hair-skin junction. Clothes and bed linen of past 2 days should be washed and dried by machine (hot cycle each) or dry cleaned.

C. <u>Sex partners:</u> Treat as above.

VIII. <u>Scabies</u>

<u>Recommended:</u> Permethrin (5% cream, 30 gm) massaged and left 8-14 hrs considered preferable drug for scabies by Medical Letter Consultants (32:21-22,1990).*

<u>Alternatives:</u> Lindane (1%) 1 oz lotion or 30 gm cream applied thinly to all areas of body below neck and washed thoroughly at 8 hr. (Not recommended for pregnant or lactating women) <u>or</u> Crotamiton (10%) applied to body below neck nightly for 2 nights and washed thoroughly 24 hr after second application.

<u>Sex partners and close household contacts:</u> Treat as above.

<u>Adjunctive:</u> Clothing or bed linen contaminated by patient should be washed and dried by machine (hot cycle) or dry cleaned.

IX. <u>Warts (Condylomata acuminata)</u> (Medical Letter 117, 1991; JAMA 265:2684, 1991)

Location	Treatment	Comment
External genital and perianal	Cryotherapy, e.g., liquid nitrogen or cryoprobe Podofilox, 0.5% bid x 3d* Podophyllin, 10%-25% applied carefully to each wart, wash at 1-4 hr, and reapply weekly; limit to < 10 cm² each session. Trichloroacetic acid (TCA) applied locally and repeat weekly; powder with talc or baking soda to remove unreacted acid Alternatives: Surgical removal electrocautery, laser therapy	All treatments show high rate of recurrence Podofilox: repeat q/wk x ≤4 Podophyllin is contra-indicated in pregnancy Women with anogenital warts should have Pap smear annually Cryotherapy is preferred because it is non-toxic, does not require anesthesia and does not cause scarring Interferon is not recommended because of low efficacy, frequent toxicity and high cost
Vaginal	Cryotherapy with liquid nitrogen Alternatives: TCA (80-90%) or podophyllin (10-25%) as above; treat < 2 cm²/session	Podophyllin is contraindicated in pregnancy Cryotherapy is preferred -- cryoprobe should not be used due to risk of vaginal perforation
Cervical	(See comment)	Must rule out dysphagia so that an expert consultant is required

(continued)

Location	Treatment	Comment
Urethral and meatal	Cryotherapy with liquid nitrogen Alternative: Podophyllin (10-25% as above)	Podophyllin is contraindicated in pregnancy
Anal	Cryotherapy with liquid nitrogen Alternative: TCA, electro- cautery, or surgical excision	Podophyllin is contraindicated

Syndromes - Female

I. Pelvic inflammatory disease (MMWR 40, RR-5:1-25, 1991)

    A. Agents

        1. Gonococcal PID: N. gonorrhoeae.

        2. Non-gonococcal PID: Chlamydia trachomatis, anaerobic bacteria ± facultative gram-negative bacilli, Actinomyces israelii, streptococci and mycoplasmas.

    B. Diagnosis

        1. Minimal criteria - lower abdominal adnexal and cervical motion tenderness.

        2. Additional criteria - oral temperature > 38.3°C, abnormal cervical or vaginal discharge, elevated ESR or creatine protein, microbial evidence of cervical infection with N. gonorrhoeae or C. trachomatis.

        3. Recommended tests - culture for N. gonorrhoeae and test for C. trachomatis.

    C. Indications for hospitalization: 1) diagnosis uncertain, 2) surgical emergencies cannot be excluded (such as appendicitis or ectopic pregnancy), 3) pelvic abscess suspected, 4) severe illness prevents outpatient management, 5) pregnancy, 6) patient unable to follow or tolerate outpatient treatment, 7) failure to respond within 72 hours to outpatient treatment, 8) clinical follow-up at 72 hours not possible, 9) patient is an adolescent (less reliable and greater long-term sequelae), 10) patient with HIV infection.*

    D. Treatment

        1. Antibiotics: Outpatient regimen - Patients treated as outpatients need to be monitored closely and re-evaluated in 72 hours.

        Recommended: Ceftriaxone, 250 mg IM x 1 dose or cefoxitin, 2 gm IM plus probenecid, 1 gm concurrently plus azithromycin, 1 gm po x 1* or doxycycline, 100 mg po bid x 10-14 days or tetracycline, 500 mg po qid for 10-14 days. Longer treatment may be necessary to prevent late sequelae.

        Alternative to tetracyclines: Erythromycin, 500 mg po qid x 10-14 days.

2. Antibiotics: <u>Inpatient regimen</u>.

Initial**	Oral follow-up***
Doxycycline, 100 mg IV bid + cefoxitin, 2 gm IV qid <u>or</u> cefotetan, 2 gm IV q12h	Doxycycline, 100 mg po bid <u>or</u> Azithromycin, 1 gm po x 1*
Clindamycin, 900 mg IV qid + gentamicin, 2.0 mg/kg IV, then 1.5 mg/kg tid	Clindamycin, 450 mg po 5x/day <u>or</u> doxycycline, 100 mg po bid (doxycycline preferred if <u>C. trachomatis</u> is suspected or confirmed)

** Parenteral treatment to continue at least 48 hrs after patient clinically improves.
*** Oral regimen to be continued to complete 10-14 days of treatment.

3. Male sex partners: Examine and treat with regimen for uncomplicated gonococcal and chlamydial infection.

4. Follow up: Outpatients should be re-evaluated within 72 hrs and patients not responding should be hospitalized.

5. Intra-uterine device: Removal is recommended soon after antimicrobial treatment is started.

II. <u>Mucopurulent cervicitis</u>

A. Diagnosis: **(1)** Mucopurulent endocervical exudate that may appear yellow or green on white cotton-tipped swab (positive swab test); **(2)** gram-stained smear of endocervical secretions shows over 10 PMN/oil immersion field; or **(3)** cervicitis documented by cervical friability (bleeding when the first swab is taken) and/or erythema or edema within a zone of cervical ectopy.

B. Laboratory evaluation: Gram stain, culture for <u>N</u>. gonorrhoeae, test for <u>Chlamydia trachomatis</u> and wet mount for <u>Trichomonas</u>.

C. Treatment

1. Gonococcal: <u>N</u>. gonorrhoeae found on gram stain or culture - treat for uncomplicated gonococcal infection and presumed chlamydial infection.

2. Non-gonococcal: <u>N</u>. gonorrhoeae not found on gram stain or culture - treat for <u>C</u>. trachomatis (pg 237).

III. <u>Vaginitis/vaginosis</u>

A. Trichomoniasis (almost always a STD)

1. Diagnosis: Wet mount or culture.

2. Usual treatment: Metronidazole, 2 gm po as single dose
Alternative: Metronidazole, 500 mg po bid x 7 days.

3. Asymptomatic women: Treat as above.

241

4. Pregnant women: Metronidazole is contraindicated in first trimester and should be avoided throughout pregnancy. For severe symptomatic disease after first trimester, give metronidazole, 2 gm x 1.

5. Lactating women: Treat with 2 gm dose of metronidazole and suspend breast feeding x 24 hours.

6. Sex partners: Treat with 2 gm dose of metronidazole or 500 mg po bid x 7 days.

7. Treatment failures: Retreat with metronidazole, 500 mg po bid x 7 days. Persistent failures: 2 gm dose daily x 3-5 days.

B. Bacterial vaginosis (non-specific vaginitis)

1. Diagnosis: Non-irritating, malodorous, thin, white vaginal discharge with pH over 4.5, elaboration of fishy odor after 10% KOH, microscopic exam showing sparse lactobacilli and numerous cocco-bacillary forms on epithelial cells ("clue cells"). Cultures for <u>Gardnerella</u> <u>vaginalis</u> are not recommended. Asymptomatic infections are common; necessity to treat asymptomatic infections is controversial.

2. Treatment
   - Metronidazole, 500 mg po bid x 7 days or 2 gm po x 1.*
   - Alternative: Clindamycin, 300 mg po bid x 7 days.* Clindamycin vaginal cream (2%), 100 mg (5g) intravaginally daily x 7*.

3. Sex partners: Treatment not indicated

4. Pregnancy: Metronidazole is contraindicated; use clindamycin regimen.

C. <u>Vulvovaginal candidiasis</u> (not considered an STD)

1. Treatment

   <u>Recommended</u>: Miconazole nitrate suppository or clotrimazole (tablet, 200 mg) intra-vaginally at bedtime x 3 days; betaconazole (2% cream, 5 g) intravaginally at bedtime x 3 days; tetaconazole (80 mg suppository or 0.4% cream) intravaginally at bedtime x 3 days.

   <u>Alternatives</u>: Miconazole nitrate vaginal suppository (100 mg or 2% cream, 5 g) intravaginally at bedtime x 7 days <u>or</u> clotrimazole (vaginal tabs, 100 mg or 1% cream, 5 gm) intravaginally at bedtime x 7 days).
   <u>Systemic</u>: Fluconazole, 150 mg po x 1 <u>or</u> ketoconazole, 200 mg po bid x 5-7 days.*

2. Sex partners: Treat only for symptomatic <u>Candida</u> <u>balanitis</u>.

3. Pregnancy: As for non-pregnant patients.

4. Prophylaxis for recurrent candida vaginitis*: Yogurt, 8oz/d po (Ann Intern Med 116:353, 1992) <u>or</u> ketoconazole (NEJM 315:1455, 1986)

I.   Urethritis

    A.   Categories

        1.   Gonococcal

        2.   Non-gonococcal: Usually caused by C. trachomatis (40-50%), other organisms (10-15%) (Ureaplasma urealyticum, T. vaginalis, herpes simplex virus); unknown cause (35-50%).

    B.   Diagnosis: Gram stain and culture of urethral discharge or urethral swab obtained with calcium amalgamate swab.

        1.   Gram negative intracellular diplococci or positive culture for N. gonorrhoeae: Treat for uncomplicated gonococci infection (pg 234).

        2.   Gram stain shows > 5 PMN/low power field plus no intracellular gram-negative intracellular diplococci: Treat for Chlamydia trachomatis (pg 237).

        3.   Stain shows < 5 PMN: Patient should return for repeat test next morning before voiding.

    C.   Persistent or recurrent NGU: Consider

        1.   Failure to treat sexual partner.

        2.   Alternative causes of discharge.

II.   Epididymitis

    A.   STD form: Usually occurs in adults < 35 yrs in association with urethritis without urinary tract infection or underlying GU pathology.

        1.   Usual agents: C. trachomatis and/or N. gonorrhoeae.

        2.   Evaluation: Urethral smear for gram stain, culture for N. gonorrhoeae and Chlamydia trachomatis and urine culture.

        3.   Treatment: Use regimens for uncomplicated N. gonorrhoeae infection.

        4.   Adjuncts: Bed rest and scrotal elevation recommended until fever and local inflammation have resolved.

    B.   Non-STD form (usually older men in association with GU pathology and/or UTI verified by positive urine gram stain and culture).

        1.   Agents: Coliforms and pseudomonads (usual agents of urinary tract infections).

        2.   Treatment: Based on severity of disease and urine culture results (pg 233).

        3.   Adjunctive treatment as above.

DURATION OF ANTIBIOTIC TREATMENT

Location	Diagnosis	Duration (days)
Actinomycosis	Cervicofacial	4-6 wks IV, then oral x 6-12 mo
Bacteremia	Gram-negative bacteremia	10-14 days
	S. aureus, portal of entry known 2 wks	
	S. aureus, no portal of entry	4 wks
	Line sepsis: Bacteria	3-5 days (post-removal)
	Candida	10 days (post-removal)
	Vascular graft	4 wks (post-removal)
Bone	Osteomyelitis, acute	4-6 wks IV
	chronic	4 wks IV, then po x 2 mo
Central nervous system	Cerebral abscess	4-6 wks, then oral
	Meningitis: H. influenzae	10 days
	Listeria	14-21 days
	N. meningitidis	7 days
	S. pneumoniae	10 days
Ear	Otitis media, acute	10 days
Gastrointestinal	Diarrhea: C. difficile	7-14 days
	C. jejuni	7 days
	E. histolytica	5-10 days
	Giardia	5-7 days
	Salmonella	14 days
	Shigella	3-5 days
	Traveler's	3-5 days
	Gastritis, H. pylori	≥ 3 wks
	Sprue	6 mo
	Whipple's disease	1 yr
Heart	Endocarditis: Pen-sensitive strep	14-28 days
	Pen-resistant strep	4-6 wks
	Staph. aureus	4 wks
	Microbes, other	4 wks
	Prosthetic valve	≥ 6 wks
Intra-abdominal	Cholecystitis	3-7 days post-cholecystectomy
	Primary peritonitis	10-14 days
	Peritonitis/intra-abdominal abscess	7-10 days after drainage
Joint	Septic arthritis, gonococcal	7 days
	Pyogenic, non-gonococcal	3 wks
	Prosthetic joint	6 wks
Liver	Pyogenic liver abscess	4-16 wks
	Amebic	10 days

(continued)

244

Location	Diagnosis	Duration (days)
Lung	Pneumonia: <u>Chlamydia pneumoniae</u>	10-14 days
	<u>Legionella</u>	21 days
	<u>Mycoplasma</u>	2-3 wks
	<u>Nocardia</u>	6-12 months
	Pneumococcal	Until febrile 3-5 days
	Pneumocystis	21 days
	Staphylococcal	≥ 21 days
	Tuberculosis	6-9 mo
	Lung abscess	Until x-ray clear or until small stable residual lesion
Nocardia	Nocardiosis	6-12 months
Pharynx	Pharyngitis - Gr A strep	10 days
	Pharyngitis, gonococcal	1 dose
	Diphtheria	14 days
Prostate	Prostatitis, acute	2 wks
	chronic	3-4 mo
Sinus	Sinusitis, acute	10 days
Sexually transmitted disease	Cervicitis, gonococcal	1 dose
	Chancroid	7 days
	<u>Chlamydia</u>	7 days (Azithromycin - 1 dose)
	Disseminated gonococcal infection	7 days
	H. simplex	7-10 days
	Lymphogranuloma venereum	21 days
	Pelvic inflammatory disease	10-14 days
	Syphilis	10-21 days
	Urethritis, gonococcal	1 dose
Systemic	Brucellosis	6 wks
	Listeria: Immunosuppressed host	3-6 wks
	Lyme disease	14-21 days
	Meningococcemia	7-10 days
	Rocky Mountain spotted fever	7 days
	Salmonellosis	
	Bacteremia	10-14 days
	AIDS patients	≥ 3-4 wks
	Localized infection	4-6 wks
	Carrier state	6 wks
	Tuberculosis, pulmonary	6-9 mo
	extrapulmonary	9 mo
	Tularemia	7-14 days
Vaginitis	Bacterial vaginosis	7 days
	<u>Candida albicans</u>	3 days
	Trichomoniasis	7 days

Index

Abscess, 31, 171, 181, 198
Absidia 117
Acanthamoeba 189
Accutane 181
Acetaminophen 165
Acetic acid 199
Achromobacter 15
Achromycin *See Tetracycline*
Acinetobacter 15
Acne 27, 181
Actinobacillus 15
Actinomyces 15, 177, 197
Actinomycosis 15, 183, 201, 244
Acyclovir (Zovirax) 1, 13, 37, 48, 53, 72, 74, 119-120, 122, 157-158, 163-164, 189, 190, 202, 238
Adenitis 32, 202
Adenovirus 189
Adriamycin 75
Adverse reactions 53-73, 145-146
Aerobes 204
Aeromonas 181
Aeromonas hydrophila 15-16, 222
Aerosporin *See Polymyxin B*
Afipia felix 16, 183
AIDS *See also HIV* 25, 245
Airway infections 171-172
Albamycin *See Novobiocin*
Albendazole (Zentel) 135-137, 139-140, 145
Alcohol 75-78, 80
Alkaloids 76
Allopurinol 78-79, 81
Alternaria 197
Amantadine (Symmetrel) 1, 13, 37, 53, 73-74, 122-123
Amcill *See Ampicillin*
Amdinocillin (Coactin) 1, 37, 48
Amebiasis 135
Amebic liver abscess 216
Amikacin (Amikin) 1, 13, 15, 20, 29-30, 35-37, 48, 53, 155, 157, 169, 193, 206, 215
Amikacin + cefoperazone 199
Amikin *See Amikacin*
Aminoglycoside(s) 15, 19-24, 27-29, 32-33, 53, 67-68,

Aminoglycoside(s) continued 74-75, 77-79, 81, 159, 168, 174, 177, 183, 186-187, 193, 195, 198, 205, 215, 233
Aminoglycoside + ampicillin 232
Aminoglycoside + anti-pseudomonad penicillin 195, 196
Aminoglycoside + aztreonam 196
Aminoglycoside + ceftazidime 15, 196, 207

Aminoglycoside + cephalosporin 200
Aminosalicylic acid (PAS) 1, 24, 53, 70, 74, 79, 104-105, 128, 155, 159
Amoxicillin (Amoxil, Polymox, Trimox, Utimox, Wymox, Larotid) 1, 13, 20, 22-23, 27, 29-31, 37, 48, 183, 199-200, 203, 205-206, 208, 217, 224, 230-231, 233
Amoxicillin + clavulanate (Augmentin) 1, 13, 17-18, 22, 24, 26, 29, 37, 48, 53, 164, 182-183, 187, 199-200, 202-203, 205, 208, 230, 232-233, 238
Amoxil *See Amoxicillin*
Amphotericin 74, 190
Amphotericin B (Fungizone) 1, 13, 37, 48, 54, 70, 74, 77, 79, 81, 111-117, 135, 137, 154-155, 184, 190-191, 216
Ampicillin, ampicillin sodium (Omnipen, Amcill, Penamp, Polycillin, Principen, Totacillin) 1, 13, 17, 20-24, 26-27, 29-32, 37, 48, 99, 105, 159, 186, 193, 195-196, 200, 203, 205-206, 215-217, 223-224, 230-231, 233
Ampicillin + clavulanate 182
Ampicillin + gentamicin 230
Ampicillin + sulbactam (Unasyn) 1, 13, 38, 48, 54, 169, 217
Anaerobes 177, 182, 200-202, 204, 206-208
Anaphylactic shock 66
Ancef *See Cefazolin*
Ancobon *See Flucocytosine*
Ancylostoma duodenale 135
Anemia 162
Angiomatosis 29
Angiostrongylus, angiostrongyliasis 135, 197
Anisakiasis 135
Anorexia 163
Anspor *See Cephradine*
Antacids 76, 78-80
Anthrax 16
Antibacterial agents 67, 68-69
Anticholinergics 74
Anticoagulants 74-75, 76-81
Antidepressants, tricyclic 80
Anti-diarrhea agents 80
Antifungal agents 70
Anti-inflammatory agents, non-steroidal 77, 165
Antimalarial agents 67
Antiminth *See Pyrantel*

247

Antimycobacterial agents 70-71
Antiparasitic agents 71
Antiparasitic agents,
  adverse effects 145-146
Antiperistaltic agents 75
Antituberculous agents 67
Antiviral agents 72-73
Anxiety 164
Apathy 165
Aphthous stomatitis 202
Aphthous ulcer 164, 172
Appendicitis 217
Ara-A See Vidarabine
Arachnia 197
Aralen HCl
  See Chloroquine HCl
Aralen phosphate
  See Chloroquine phosphate
Arsobal See Melarsoprol
Arthritis 22, 23, 26, 187-188
Ascariasis 135
Ascariasis (roundworm) 135
Aspergillus, aspergillosis 111, 172, 183, 189-191, 204
Asplenia, immunizations in 86
Atabrine See Quinacrine
Athlete's foot 118
Ativan See Lorazepam
Atovaquone (Mepron) 2, 13, 38, 48, 54, 152
  153
Atropine + corticosteroids 190
Augmentin See Amoxicillin +
  clavulanate
Azactam See Aztreonam
Azathioprine 81
Azathriaprim 77
Azithromycin (Zithromax) 2, 13, 17-18, 23-24, 26,
  38, 48, 153, 157, 200,
  203, 206-207, 225, 237,
  240
Azlin See Azlocillin
Azlocillin (Azlin) 2, 38, 174
AZT See Zidovudine
Aztreonam (Azactam) 2, 13, 20-21, 24, 27-30,
  38, 48, 52, 54, 68, 177,
  187, 196, 199, 205, 215,
  232
Aztreonam + aminoglycoside 205
Azulfidine See Sulfasalazine
Babesiosis 135
Bacampicillin (Spectrobid) 2, 38
Bacillary angiomatosis 29, 163
Bacilli, Gram-negative 187
Bacillus 16
Bacillus cereus 16, 223
Bacillus sp. 16, 190

Bacillus vaccine 82
Baci-IM See Bacitracin
Bacitracin (Baci-IM) 2, 13, 19, 54, 189-190,
  222
Bacitracin-polymyxin 189
Bacteremia 15, 17-18, 20-21, 24, 26,
  29, 168, 244-245
Bacteria 159, 197
Bacteriuric syndromes 230-231
Bacteroides fragilis 177, 198
Bacteroides sp 16, 177, 198
Bactocill See Oxacillin
Bactrim See Trimethoprim-
  sulfamethoxazole
Balantidiasis 136
Balantidium coli 136, 225
Barbiturates 78-80
Bartonella bacilliformis 17
Bartonellosis 17
Baylisascariasis 136
Beepen-VK See Phenoxyethyl
  penicillin (V)
Bejel 31
Benedryl See Diphenhydramine
Benzathine (Bicillin, Bicillin
  L-A, Permapen) 9, 13, 182
Benzathine + procaine
  (Bicillin C-R) 9
Benzathine penicillin 200, 235-236
Benznidazole (Rochagan) 140, 145
Benzodiazepines 77, 79
B-adrenergic blockers 79
Beta-betalactamase inhibitor 187
Betapen VK See
  Phenoxyethyl penicillin (V)
Biaxin See Clarithromycin
Bicillin See Benzathine
Bicillin C-R See Benzathine
  + procaine
Bicillin L-A See Benzathine
Bilharziasis 139
Biliary tract infection 169, 217
Biltricide See Praziquantel
Bipolaris 191
Bismuth subsalicylate
  (Pepto-Bismol) 23, 80, 223
Bites 18, 20, 182-183
Bithin See Bithionol
Bithionol (Bithin) 137, 145
Blastocystis hominis 136, 226
Blastomyces 111-112, 197, 204
Blastomyces dermatidis 188

Blastomycosis 184
Bone infection 186-188, 244
Bordetella pertussis 17
Boric acid 199
Borrelia bugdorferi 17, 188, 197
Borrelia recurrentis 17
Botulism 19
Brain abscess 171, 198
Branhamella catarrhalis 205
Brodie's abscess 186
Brodspec *See Tetracycline*
Bronchitis 22, 171, 208
Bronchopulmonary
   aspergillosis 172
Brucella 17, 197
Brucellosis 17, 245
Brugia malayi 136
Bumetanide 74
Buspar *See Buspirone*
Buspirone (Buspar) 164
Caffeine 76
Calymmatobacterium
   granulomatous 17
Campylobacter fetus 1
Campylobacter jejuni 17, 222, 227
Cancer chemotherapy 75
Candida 112-114, 154, 164, 182,
   184, 189-190, 204
Candida albicans 183, 202
Candida balanitis 242
Candida peritonitis 216
Candidiasis 242
Capastat *See Capreomycin*
Capillaria philippinensis 136
Capillariasis 136
Capnocytophaga 17-18
Capreomycin (Capastat) 2, 24, 38, 54, 70, 74-75,
   79, 128, 155
Capsaicin 61
Carbamazepine (Tegretol) 76-78, 80
Carbenicillin, carbenicillin
   indanyl sodium (Geocillin) 2, 38, 48, 52, 233
Cardiac conditions 103, 161, 172, 244
Cardiobacterium 18
Cardiomyopathy 161
Cardiothoracic surgery,
   antibiotic prophylaxis 98
Cat scratch disease 16, 18, 183, 202
CD4 cells 148, 150, 151
Ceclor *See Cefaclor*
Cefaclor (Ceclor) 2, 13, 38, 48, 200, 203, 208
Cefadroxil (Duricef, Ultracef) 2, 13, 38, 48
Cefadyl *See Cephapirin
   sodium*

Cefamandole, cefamandole 2, 13, 22, 30, 38, 48, 100,
   nafate (Mandol) 159
Cefanex *See Cephalexin
   monohydrate*
Cefazolin (Ancef, Kefzol, 2, 13, 38, 40, 98-102,
   Zolicef) 211, 217, 230
Cefixime (Suprax) 2, 13, 39, 48, 187, 199,
   208, 234-235
Cefizox *See Ceftizoxime
   sodium*
Cefmetazole (Zefazone) 2, 13, 39
Cefobid *See Cefoperazone*
Cefonicid (Monocid) 2, 13, 39, 48
Cefoperazone (Cefobid) 2, 13, 29-30, 39, 48, 52,
   169, 174, 177, 217, 224
Ceforanide 2, 13, 39
Ceforanide lysine (Precef) 2
Cefotan *See Cefotetan*
Cefotaxime 17, 22, 26, 29-30, 39, 49,
   101, 169, 177, 186, 193,
   195-196, 198, 201, 215,
   224, 234
Cefotaxime sodium (Claforan) 3, 13
Cefotetan (Cefotan) 3, 13, 16, 22, 39, 49, 99,
   169, 177, 240
Cefoxitin 13, 16, 22, 25-26, 39, 49,
   98-99, 101, 177, 187,
   201, 206, 215, 216,
   240-241
Cefoxitin sodium (Mefoxin) 3
Cefpodoxime 199, 200, 208
Cefpodoxime proxetil (Vantin) 3
Cefprozil (Cefzil) 3, 13, 39, 49, 193,
   199-200, 203, 208
Ceftazidime (Fortaz, 3, 13, 29, 32, 39, 49, 169,
   Tazidime, Tazicef, Ceptax) 174, 177, 193, 195-196,
   198-201, 205
Ceftin *See Cefuroxime axetil*
Ceftizoxime, ceftizoxime 3, 26, 39, 49, 169, 177,
   sodium (Cefizox) 193, 195-196, 198, 201,
   234
Ceftriaxone (Rocephin) 3, 13, 17, 22, 26, 29-31,
   40, 49, 52, 186-187, 189,
   193, 195-196, 198, 201,
   224, 230, 235, 238, 240
Cefuroxime (Zinacef) 3, 13, 22, 30, 40, 49, 98,
   159, 191, 193, 195,
   200-201, 206-208, 234
Cefuroxime axetil (Ceftin) 3, 13, 17, 26, 40,
   199-200, 203
Cefzil *See Cefprozil*
Cell-mediated immunity 173
Cellulitis 16, 19, 22, 181
Central nervous system infection 171, 192-198, 244
Cepaclor 199

Cephalexin, cephalexin mono-
hydrate (Keflex, Keftab,
Cefanex, Keflet)   3, 40, 49, 182-183, 203,
                                    217, 230, 233
Cephalosporin(s)   15, 17-24, 26-28, 30-33,
                                    55, 68, 74-75, 78, 169,
                                    174, 181-183, 187, 191,
                                    193, 195, 199-202, 205,
                                    207, 211, 217, 232-233
Cephalosporin(s), costs   203
Cephalosporin +
   aminoglycoside   22, 23
Cephalothin   40, 49, 101, 186, 211,
                                    216
Cephalothin sodium (Keflin)   3, 13
Cephapirin, cephapirin sodium
   (Cefadyl)   3, 40, 49, 186
Cephradine (Anspor, Velosef)   3, 13, 203, 233
Ceptax See Ceftazidime
Cerebral abscess   244
Cerebrospinal fluid infections   192-193
Cervical adenitis   202
Cervicitis   26, 241, 245
Chancroid   22, 238, 245
Chickenpox   120
Chlamydia   204, 245
Chlamydia pneumoniae   18, 206, 245
Chlamydia psittaci   18, 206
Chlamydia sp.   204
Chlamydia trachomatis   18, 189, 207, 234,
                                    237-238
Chloral hydrate   165
Chloramphenicol (Chloro-   3, 13, 17-22, 26-27,
   mycetin)   29-32, 40, 49, 52, 55,
                                    67-68, 75, 79, 177, 186,
                                    193, 195-196, 199,
                                    205-206, 224-225
Chloramphenicol + ampicillin   22, 201
Chloramphenicol + penicillin   198
Chloramphenicol +
   streptomycin   17, 28
Chloramphenicol palmitate
   (Chloromycetin)   4
Chloramphenicol Na
   succinate (Chloromycetin
   sodium succinate)   4
Chlorhexidine gluconate   163
Chloromycetin See Chloram-
   phenicol, Chloram-
   phenicol palmitate
Chloromycetin sodium
   succinate See Chloram-
   phenicol Na succinate
Chloropropamide   75
Chloroquine   40, 55, 67, 71, 216

Chloroquine HCl (Aralen HCl)   4, 145
Chloroquine hydroxy (Plaquenil)   4, 13
Chloroquine phosphate,
   chloroquine PO_4 (Aralen
   phosphate)   110, 135, 137-138, 145
Chlorpromazine   79
Cholecystitis   217, 244
Cholera   32, 108
Cholera vaccine   87
Cholestyramine   19, 222
Chromoblastomycosis   114
Ciclopirox   182
Cimetidine   78
Cinobac See Cinoxacin
Cinoxacin (Cinobac)   4, 41
Cipro See Ciprofloxacin
Ciprofloxacin (Cipro, Cipro   4, 13, 19, 22, 24-26,
   IV)   29-30, 32, 41, 49, 55,
                                    75-76, 157, 159, 183,
                                    187, 199, 201, 205, 208,
                                    222-225, 230, 232-234,
                                    238
Ciprofloxacin + rifampin   206
Cisplatin   74, 81
Citrobacter   18-19
Cladosporium   197
Claforan See Ceftaxime sodium
Clarithromycin (Biaxin)   4, 13, 18, 23-26, 31, 41,
                                    155, 157, 200, 203, 207
Clarithromycin + ethambutol   25
Clarithromycin + rifampin   206
Clavulanate   183
Cleocin HCl See Clindamycin HCl
Cleocin pediatric See Clindamycin
   palmitate HCl
Cleocin PO_4 See Clindamycin PO_4
Cleocin VC See Clindamycin
   vaginal cream
Clindamycin, Clindamycin HCl   4, 13, 15-19, 21-22, 27,
   (Cleocin HCl)   30-31, 41, 49, 52, 55, 68,
                                    75, 98-101, 135,
                                    138-139, 152, 169, 177,
                                    181-183, 186-187,
                                    200-203, 205-206, 208,
                                    215-216, 240, 242
Clindamycin + gentamicin   240
Clindamycin palmitate HCl
   (Cleocin pediatric)   4
Clindamycin PO_4 (Cleocin PO_4)   4
Clindamycin vaginal cream
   (Cleocin VC)   4
Clofazimine (Lamprene)   4, 13, 25, 41, 50, 79,
                                    155, 157
Clofibrate   79
Clonorchis sinensis   137

Clostridia 19, 177
Clostridium difficile 222, 244
Clostridium jejuni 244
Clostridium perfringens 177, 223
Clostridium trachomatis 240-241
Clotrimazole 13, 112, 154, 163, 182, 202
Cloxacillin (Tegopen, Cloxapen) 4, 13, 41, 49, 182, 186
Cloxapen See Cloxacillin
CMV 204 Coactin See Amdinocillin
Coccidioides 114, 197
Coccidioides immitis 188
Coccidioides sp. 204
Codeine 165
Coliforms 199, 200, 205, 215
Colistimethate 56, 79
Colistin (Coly-Mycin M, Coly-Mycin S) 4, 41
Colitis 19, 30, 121
Coly-Mycin M See Colistin
Coly-Mycin S See Colistin
Complement deficiencies 173
Condylomata acuminata 239-240
Conjunctivitis 18, 189
Contraceptives 78-80
Corticosteroids 74, 76, 78-79, 111, 163, 189, 190, 202
Corynebacterium diphtheriae 19, 200
Corynebacterium Jk strain 19
Corynebacterium hemolyticum 200
Corynebacterium minitissimum 19
Corynebacterium pneumoniae 200
Corynebacterium ulcerans 19
Costs of oral drugs 203, 233
Cotrim See Trimethoprim-sulfamethoxazole
Coumadin 75-77
Coxiella burnetii 19, 207
Crotamiton (Eurax) 145, 239
Cryptococcal meningitis 154
Cryptococcus 115, 184, 195, 197, 204
Cryptosporidia 136, 153, 225
Crystallin See Procaine
Crystalline G sodium (Penicillin G sodium) 9
Curvularia 191
Cutaneous larva migrans 136
Cyanotic heart disease 198
Cyclacillin 41
Cyclacillin (Cyclapen-W) 4
Cyclapen-W See Cyclacillin
Cycloserine (Seromycin) 4, 13, 24-26, 41, 56, 75-77, 128, 155
Cyclosporine 74, 76-81, 157

Ciprofloxacin 25
Cysticercus 197
Cysticercus cellulosae 139
Cyst(s) 139
Cystitis 230-232
Cytomegalovirus 121-122, 158, 164
Cytovene See Ganciclovir
Dapsone 4, 13, 41, 55, 67-68, 75-76, 79, 81, 139, 152
Daraprim See Pyrimethamine
ddC (dideoxycytidine, HIVID, Zalcitabine) 5, 13, 42, 56, 76, 124, 150-151
ddI (Videx, Dideoxyinosine, didanosine) 5, 13, 42, 56, 75, 76, 124, 150-151
Declomycin See Demeclocycline
Dehydroemetine 135, 145, 226
Delirium 164
Delta hepatitis virus 219-220, 221
Demeclocycline (Declomycin) 5, 11
Dental infections 16, 202
Depression 164
Dermatologic diseases 25, 26, 163
Dermatophytes 182
Dermis infections 181
Desyrel See Trazodone
DFMO See Eflornithine
DHPG 58
Diabetes, innoculations in 87
Diabetic foot 184
Dialysis 216
Dialysis, dose regimens for 48-51
Diarrhea 15, 17, 27, 106-108, 164, 222-228, 244
Dibromopropamide isethionate 189
Dicloxacillin (Dycil, Dynapen, Pathocil) 5, 13, 41, 50, 203
Dicumarol 75
Didanosine See ddI
Dideoxyinosine See ddI
Dientamoeba fragilis 136
Diethylcarbamazine, diethylcarbamazine citrate (Hetrazan) 5, 136, 160, 145
Diflucan See Fluconazole
Difluoromethylomithine See Eflornithine
Digitalis 74, 79, 161
Digoxin 76-77, 80-81
Dilaudid 165
Diloxanide, diloxanide furoate (Furamide) 5, 56, 135, 216, 226
Diphenhydramine (Benedryl) 163, 165
Diphtheria 19
Diphtheria vaccine 82, 88
Diphyllobothrium latum 139

Dipylidium caninum 139
Diquinol See Iodoquinol
Disopyramide 76, 79
Disulfiram 77-78
Diuretics 74, 161
Diverticulitis 217
Doxy caps See Doxycycline
Doxycycline (Vibramycin, 5, 11, 25-26, 42, 50, 79,
    Doxy caps, Doxy tabs, 99-100, 110, 128, 164, 181,
    Vibra-tabs, Doxy-100,200) 203, 206, 222-223, 231,
                            233-235, 237, 240-241
Doxycycline + gentamicin 17
Doxycycline + rifampin 17, 206
Dracunculus medinensis 136
Dramamine 163
Drechslera 191
Drug abuse 149, 186
Drug abusers, immunizations
    for 86
Drug interactions 74-81
DT 82
DTP 82
Duodenal ulcer 23
Duration of antibiotic
    treatment 244-245
Duricef See Cefadroxil
Dycil See Dicloxacillin
Dyclone 163
Dynapen See Dicloxacillin
Dysgammaglobulinemia 173
Dysgonic fermenter
    type 2 (DF₂) 19, 182
E-Base See Erythromycin
E-mycin See Erythromycin
E. coli 21, 196, 223, 227, 232
E.E.S. See Erythromycin
    ethylsuccinate
Ear infections 199, 244
Echinococcus (tapeworm) 139
Echovirus 197
Econazole 182
Edwardsiella tarda 20
Eflornithine (Difluoromethyl-
    ornithine, DFMO, Ornidyl) 5, 140, 145
Ehrlichia, Ehrlichiosis 20
Eikenella corrodens 20, 183
Elimite See Permethrin
Emetine, emetine HCl 5, 57, 216
Encephalitis 121
Encephalitis vaccine 88
Endocarditis 15, 18, 20-23, 31, 198,
                            235, 244
Endocarditis prevention 103-105
Endocarditis treatment 209-214
Endocervicitis 18, 32

Endophthalmitis 172, 189-190
Enflurane 74, 77
Enoxacin (Penetrex) 5, 42
Entamoeba histolytica 226, 244
Entamoeba polecki 136
Enteric fever 30, 224
Enteritis 121
Enterobacter 20
Enterobacteriaceae 195, 198, 205
Enterobius vermicularis (pinworm) 136
Enterococcus 20-21, 232
Enterocolitis 32, 224
Environmental settings,
    immunizations 85
Eosinophilia 136
Epidermis infections 181
Epidermophyton 182
Epididymitis 18, 243
Epididymo-orchitis 233
Epiglottitis 22, 171, 201
Epinephrine 66
Epstein-Barr virus (EBV) 122, 171, 200-201
Eramycin See Erythromycin
    stearate
Ergot alkaloids 76
Erwinia 21
ERYC See Erythromycin
Erypar See Erythromycin
    stearate
EryPed See Erythromycin
    ethylsuccinate
Erysipelas 181
Erysipelothrix rhusiopathiae 21
Ery-Tab See Erythromycin
Erythematous lesions 181
Erythrasma 19
Erythrocin lactobionate See
    Erythromycin lactobionate
Erythrocin stearate See
    Erythromycin stearate
Erythromycin (E-mycin, 5, 13, 15-19, 21-22,
    ERYC, Ery-Tab, E-Base, 24-27, 29-32, 42, 50, 57,
    Erythromycin Base, 68, 76, 99, 159, 163, 177,
    Ilotycin, PCE, RP-Mycin, 181- 182, 189-203,
    Robimycin) 205-207, 222, 225, 227,
                            233-235, 237-238, 240
Erythromycin + defuroxime 207
Erythromycin + rifampin 23
Erythromycin + sulfa-
    methoxazole 199
Erythromycin Base
    See Erythromycin
Erythromycin estolate
    (Ilosone) 5

Erythromycin ethylsuccinate
(E.E.S, EryPed)   5, 237
Erythromycin gluceptate
(Ilotycin gluceptate)   5
Erythromycin lactobionate
(Erythrocin lactobionate)   5
Erythromycin stearate
(Eramycin, Erypar, Ethril,
Wyamycin S, SK-
erythromycin)   6
Erythropoietin   13
Esophageal disease   121, 164
Estrogens   79
Ethacrynic acid   74-75
Ethambutol (Myambutol)   6, 13, 24-25, 42, 57, 70,
127, 157
Ethionamide (Protionamide,
Trecator-SC)   6, 24-25, 42, 57, 70,
75-77, 128, 155, 157
Ethril *See Erythromycin
stearate*
Eurax *See Crotamiton*
Extra-intestinal infection   27
Eye infections   24, 172, 189-191
Fansidar *See Pyrimethamine +
sulfadoxine*
Faran *See Nitrofurantoin*
Fasciola hepatica   137
Fasigyn *See Tinidazole*
Fecal leukocyte exam   227
Fever, of unknown origin   174, 178
Fever, relapsing   17
Filiaris   136
Finger infections   182
Flagyl *See Metronidazole*
Flavobacterium   21
Floxin *See Ofloxacin*
Flubendazole   145
Fluconazole (Diflucan)   6, 13, 42, 50, 57, 70, 76,
112, 113, 115, 154-155,
184, 202, 242
Flucytosine (Ancobon)   6, 13, 42, 50, 70, 75,
113-115, 189
Fluke   137
Fluoroquinolone(s)   15-21, 23-24, 26-33, 76,
155, 205, 234
Fluorouracil   78
Fluoxetine (Prozac)   164
Folinic acid   139
Folliculitis   181
Food poisoning   16, 223
Fortaz *See Ceftazidime*
Foscarnet (Foscavir)   6, 13, 42, 58, 73, 77, 79,
119-121, 157-158, 164
Foscavir *See Foscarnet*
Francisella   22

Fulvicin *See Griseofulvin*
Fungal infections   111-118, 154, 163, 182,
184,188, 190-191, 197,
204
Fungizone
See Amphotericin B
Furadantin *See Nitrofurantoin*
Furalan *See Nitrofurantoin*
Furamide *See Diloxanidine*
Furaton *See Nitrofurantoin*
Furazolidone (Furoxone)   6, 17, 32, 58, 137, 145,
222-223, 225-226
Furosemide   74, 75
Furoxone *See Furazolidone*
Furunculosis   181-182
Fusaria   197
Fusarium solani   189
Fusobacteria   22, 177
G-CSF   13
Gamimmune   13
Ganciclovir (DHPG, Cytovene)   6, 13, 43, 50, 58, 73, 75,
77, 121-222, 158, 164
Gantonol
See Sulfamethoxazole
Gantrisin *See Sulfisoxazole*
Garamycin *See Gentamicin*
Gardnerella   22
Gas gangrene   19
Gastritis   23, 244
Gastroenteritis   20
Gastrointestinal diseases   163, 244
Gastrointestinal surgery,
antibiotic prophylaxis   98-99
Genital herpes simplex   238
Genital tract infection   16, 26
Genitourinary surgery,
endocarditis prevention   105
Gentamicin (Garamycin,
Gentamicin SO$_4$,
Add-Vantage, Gentamicin
SO$_4$ in 5% dextrose
piggyback, Gentamicin SO$_4$
Injection, Gentamicin SO$_4$
Isotonic)   6, 13, 17-18, 20-22, 24,
30-32, 35-36, 43, 50, 98,
100-101, 168, 174, 193,
196, 205, 215-217, 222,
225, 230
Gentamicin SO$_4$ Add-Vantage,
See Gentamicin
Gentamicin SO$_4$ in 5% dextrose
piggyback *See Gentamicin*
Gentamicin SO$_4$ Injection
See Gentamicin
Gentamicin SO$_4$ Isotonic
See Gentamicin
Geocillin *See Carbenicillin*
Germanin *See Suramin sodium*
Giardia   244

Giardia intestinalis	137
Giardia lamblia	226
Giardiasis	137
Gingivitis	202
Glanders	28
Glucantime See Meglumine antimoniate	
Glucocorticosteroids	170-172
GM-CSF	34
Gnathostoma spinerum	137
Gnathostomiasis	137
Gonococcal infection	234, 245
Gramicidin	101
Granuloma inguinale	17
Grifulvin V See Griseofulvin	
Gris-PEG See Griseofulvin	
Grisactin See Griseofulvin	
Grisactin Ultra See Griseofulvin	
Griseofulvin (Grisactin, Fulvicin, Grifulvin V, Gris-PEG, Grisacin Ultra, Fulvicin P/G)	6, 13, 43, 58, 70, 77, 163, 182
Gynecologic and obstetric surgery, antibiotic prophylaxis in	99-100
H_2 antagonists	77, 78
Haemophilus ducreyi	238
Haemophilus influenzae	22, 86, 159, 196, 199-201, 206-208, 244
Haemophilus influenzae b vaccine	82, 84
Hafnia alvei	22
Haldol	164
Halfan See Halofantrine	
Halofantrine (Halfan)	138, 145
Haloperidol	79, 163
Hantaan virus	171
Haverhill fever	31
Head and neck surgery, antibiotic prophylaxis	100- 101
Health care workers, immunizations for	85-86
Helicobacter pylori	23, 244
Hematologic diseases	161
Hemodialysis	161, 186
Hemodialysis, dose regimens	48-51
Hemophilia	149
Hepatitis	124, 172
Hepatitis A	218, 221
Hepatitis A vaccine	84, 87, 93
Hepatitis B	125, 172, 188, 218, 221
Hepatitis B postexposure prophylaxis	96-97
Hepatitis B serologic markers	94-96
Hepatitis B vaccine	82, 84-88, 93
Hepatitis C	172, 219, 221
Hepatitis delta virus	219-220
Hepatitis E virus	220, 221
Hepatitis nomenclature	221
Hepatitis types	218-220
Hermaphroditic infection	137
Herpes simplex	119, 157, 164, 182-183, 189, 190, 202, 238, 245
Herpes zoster	158, 170, 189, 190
Herpetiform ulcers	202
Heterophyes heterophyes	137
Hetrazan See Diethyl-carbamazine	
Hiprex See Methenamine hippurate	
Histoplasma	115, 197, 204
Histoplasmosis	190
HIV See also AIDS	86, 124, 126, 147-148, 197, 202, 236, 238
HIV, care plan	150-151
HIV, complications	160-165
HIV, occupational exposure	166
HIV, opportunistic infections in	152-160
HIV, seroprevalence rates	149
HIVID See ddC	
Homosexuals	149
Homosexuals, immunizations for	86
Hookworm	137
Humatin See Paromomycin	
Hydatid cyst	139
Hydroxychloroquine sulfate (Plaquenil)	110
Hymenolepsis nana	139
Hypogammaglobulinemia	173
Hypoglycemics	77-80
Hyposplenism	173
Hypoxia	170
Ilosone See Erythromycin estolate	
Ilotycin See Erythromycin	
Ilotycin gluceptate See Erythromycin gluceptate	
Imipenem	15, 17-31, 43, 58, 68, 77, 155, 159, 169, 177, 187, 196, 199-200, 205-206, 215
Imipenem + aminoglycoside	169, 205
Imipenem aztreonam	207
Imipenem/Cilastin (Primaxin)	6, 13
Immune globulins	221
Immunizations	83-88
Immunodeficiency	173-176
Immunodeficiency, vaccines for	86-87
Impetigo	182
Inflammatory bowel disease	227
Influenza	122-123, 204

Influenza vaccine | 82, 83, 84, 85, 86, 87, 89-90
INH | 25, 77, 124, 156-157, 202, 216
Insomnia | 165
Interferon | 75
Interferon alfa | 58-59
Interferon alfa-nl | 125
Interferon alpha 2a (Roferon A) | 6, 13, 125
Interferon alpha 2b (Intron A) | 7, 124-125
Intra-abdominal infection | 16, 20-21, 23, 27-28, 169, 215-221, 244
Intron A See Interferon Alpha 2b
Iodoquinol (Yodoxin, Diquinol, Yodoquinal) | 7, 135- 136, 145, 216, 225-226
IPV | 82
Iron | 76, 80
Isethionate | 189
Isoniazid (Laniazid, Tubizid, Nydrazid) | 7, 13, 43, 50, 52, 59, 67, 70, 75-76, 78-79, 127
Isospora | 154
Isospora belli | 137, 226
Isosporiasis | 137
Itraconazole (Sporanox) | 7, 13, 43, 50, 59, 70, 77, 111, 114, 116-117, 154, 155
Ivermectin (Mectizan) | 136, 139, 145
Joint infections | 186-188, 244
Kanamycin (Kantrex, Klebcil) | 7, 24-25, 24-26, 35-36, 43, 50, 53, 128, 155
Kantrex See Kanamycin
Kaolin | 79
Kaposi's sarcoma | 162
Keflet See Cephalexin monohydrate
Keflex See Cephalexin monohydrate
Keflin See Cephalothin sodium
Keftab See Cephalexin monohydrate
Kefzol See Cefazolin
Keratitis | 189
Ketoconazole (Nizoral) | 7, 13, 43, 50, 59, 70, 76- 79, 111-112, 114, 116-117, 154-155, 163, 182, 184, 202, 242
Kingella sp. | 23
Klebcil See Kanamycin
Klebsiella pneumoniae | 23
Klebsiella sp. | 23
Kwell See Lindane
Lactobacilli | 19

Lampit See Nifurtimox
Lamprene See Clofazimine
Laniazid See Isoniazid
Lariam See Mefloquine
Larotid See Amoxicillin
Larva migrans | 136, 140
Laryngitis | 201
Laxatives | 80
Ledercillin VK See Phenoxyethyl penicillin (V)
Legatrin See Quinine
Legionella | 23, 204, 206-207, 245
Legionnaire's disease | 23
Leishmaniasia | 137
Leprosy | 25
Leptospira | 23, 197
Leptotrichia buccalis | 23
Leukoplakia | 163
Leukovorin | 13, 146
Lice | 137
Lidocaine | 161, 163
Lincocin See Lincomycin
Lincomycin (Lincocin) | 7
Lindane (Kwell) | 137, 145, 239
Listeria | 195, 197, 223, 244, 245
Listeria monocytogenes | 24, 196
Lithium | 78, 80
Liver disease | 20, 172, 216, 244
Liver disease, dose regimens for | 52
Loa loa | 136
Lodoquinol | 71
Lomefloxin | 13
Lomefloxacin (Maxaquin) | 7, 43, 76, 232, 233
Lomotil | 75, 164, 225
Loparamide | 75, 164, 225
Lorabid See Loracarbef
Loracarbef (Lorabid) | 7, 43, 199-200, 208
Lorazepam (Ativan) | 163-164
Lung infection | 16-17, 22, 24-27, 29, 161, 179-180, 204-208, 245
Lymphadenitis | 133, 183
Lymphangitis | 181
Lymphogranuloma venereum | 18, 245
Lymphoma | 162
Lyphocin See Vancomycin
M-cresyl acetic otic drops | 199
Macrodantin See Nitrofurantoin
Madura foot | 184
Madurella mycetomatis | 184
Malaria | 171
Malaria prophylaxis and treatment | 108-110, 137-138
Malassezia furfur | 182
Malathion (Ovide) | 137, 145

Mandelamine *See*
  Methenamine mandelate
Mandol *See Cefamandole*
  nafate
Mansonella — 136
Marrow transplantation — 176
Mastoiditis — 200
Maxaquin *See Lomefloxacin*
Mazlocillin — 196
Measles vaccine — 82-86, 88, 90
Mebendazole (Vermox) — 7, 71, 78, 135-137, 140, 145
Mectizan *See Ivermectin*
Mefloquine (Lariam) — 7, 43, 59, 71, 110, 138, 145
Mefoxin *See Cefoxitin sodium*
Megace — 163
Meglumine antimoniate
  (Glucantime) — 137, 145
Melarsoprol (Arsobal) — 140, 145
Melioidosis — 29
Meningitis — 15, 16, 18, 22, 24, 26, 31, 170-171, 194-198, 235, 244
Meningococcal vaccine — 82, 84, 88
Meningococcemia — 245
Meningoencephalitis — 135
Meperidine — 165
Mepron *See Atovaquone*
Mercaptopurine — 81
Mesenteric adenitis — 32
Metagonimus yokogawai — 137
Methacycline (Rondomycin) — 7
Methadone — 80, 165
Methenamine — 13, 59, 68
Methenamine hippurate
  (Hiprex) — 7, 44, 233
Methenamine mandelate
  (Mandelamine) — 7, 44, 233
Methicillin (Staphcillin) — 7, 30, 44, 169
Methotrexate — 74, 79-81
Methoxyflurane (Penthrane) — 74, 80
Metizol *See Metronidazole*
Metric 21 *See Metronidazole*
Metronidazole (Flagyl, Metryl, — 7, 13, 16, 19, 22, 27, 44,
  Metizol, Protostat, — 50, 52, 59, 67-68, 78, 99,
  Metric 21, Satric) — 100, 135-137, 140, 145,
    163-164, 169-170, 177, 181,
    187, 201, 203, 215- 216,
    222, 225-226, 242
Metronidazole + penicillin — 198, 202, 208
Metryl *See Metronidazole*
Mexiletine — 80
Mezlin *See Mezlocillin*
Mezlocillin, mezlocillin Na — 8, 13, 23, 44, 50, 52,
  (Mezlin) — 169, 174, 199, 230
MgSO₄ — 74
Miconazole (Monistat) — 8, 14, 44, 60, 70, 78,

Miconazole (Monistat) — 112, 154, 163, 182, 189, 242
Microspordiosis — 138
Microsporin — 182
Microsulfon *See Sulfadiazine*
Mile's solution — 163
Milk — 80
Minocin *See Minocycline*
Minocycline (Minocin) — 8, 11, 14, 25-26, 30, 44, 50, 184
Mintezol *See Thiabendazole*
MMR — 82
Molindone — 80
Molluscum contagiosum — 163
Moniliformis — 138
Monistat *See Miconazole*
Monoamine oxidase inhibitors — 80
Monocid *See Cefonicid*
Moraxella — 24, 207, 189
Moraxella catarrhalis — 24, 199-201, 205
Moraxella scrofulaceum — 202
Morganella — 24
Motrin — 165
Mouth diseases — 163
Moxalactam (Moxam) — 8, 44, 50, 177
Moxam *See Moxalactam*
Mucor — 117
Mumps vaccines — 82-86
Mupirocin — 182
Myambutol *See Ethambutol*
Mycifradin *See Neomycin*
Mycobacteria (scrofula) — 126-134, 183, 197, 202, 204
Mycobacterium avium complex
  (MAC) — 133
Mycobacterium avium-
  intracellulare — 133
Mycobacterium bovis — 133
Mycobacterium chelonae — 25, 134
Mycobacterium fortuitum — 25, 133, 188
Mycobacterium haemophilum — 134
Mycobacterium kansasii — 24, 157, 133, 188
Mycobacterium leprae — 25
Mycobacterium malmoense — 133
Mycobacterium marinum — 25, 133, 188
Mycobacterium morganii — 24
Mycobacterium scrofulaceum — 133
Mycobacterium simiae — 133
Mycobacterium smegmatis — 134
Mycobacterium szulgai — 133
Mycobacterium tuberculosis — 24, 188, 197
Mycobacterium ulcerans — 25
Mycobacterium xenopi — 133
Mycobutin, *See Rifabutin*
Mycoplasma — 200, 245

Mycoplasma fermentans 26
Mycoplasma pneumoniae 26, 206-207
Mycoplasma sp. 204
Mycostatin *See Nystatin*
Mycotic aneurysm 30
Myocarditis 172
Myositis 16
Nafcil *See Nafcillin*
Nafcillin (Unipen, Nafcil, Nallpen) 8, 14, 44, 50, 52, 101, 159, 182-183, 186, 205, 211, 216
Naftidine 182
Nail fold infection 182
Nalidixic acid (NegGram) 8, 14, 30, 44, 60, 78, 224, 233
Nallpen *See Nafcillin*
Nanophyetus salmincola 137
Naprosyn 165
Narcotics 74
Natamycin 189, 190
Nausea/vomiting 163
Nebcin *See Tobramycin*
Nebu Pent *See Pentamidine*
Necator americanus 137
NegGram *See Nalidixic acid*
Neisseria gonorrhoeae 26, 187-201, 240-241
Neisseria meningitidis 26, 188, 190, 195, 244
Neomycin (Mycifradin) 8, 99, 101, 199
Neomycin-bacitracin 189
Neotrizidine *See Trisulfapyrimidines*
Netilmicin (Netromycin) 8, 14, 35-36, 44, 50, 53, 169
Netromycin *See Netilmicin*
Neupogen 162
Neuritis 121
Neuroborreliosis 171
Neurocysticercosis 171
Neurologic diseases 161
Neuromuscular blocking agents 79
Neurospora 190
Neurosyphilis 236, 237
Neutropenia 162, 169, 173-175
Niclocide *See Niclosamine*
Niclosamine (Niclocide) 8, 71, 137, 139, 145
Nifurtimox (Lampit) 140, 145
Nilstat *See Nystatin*
Nitrofurantoin (Macrodantin, Furadantin, Furaton, Furalan, Faran) 8, 14, 44, 60, 67, 69, 78, 230-233
Nix *See Permethrin*
Nizoral *See Ketoconazole*
Nocardia 159, 184, 197, 206, 245
Nocardia asteroides 26
Nocardia sp. 204
Nocardiosis 26
Nodules 184

Norfloxacin (Noroxin) 8, 14, 45, 76, 223-224, 230, 233, 234
Noroxin *See Norfloxacin*
Nortriptyline 161, 164
Novobiocin (Albamycin) 8
Nursing homes, vaccines for 85
Nydrazid *See Isoniazid*
Nystatin (Mycostatin, Nystex, Nilstat) 8, 14, 45, 70, 70, 112, 154, 202
Nystex *See Nystatin*
Occupational exposure, HIV 166
Occupational groups, immunizations 85-86
Octreotide (Sandostatin) 153, 225
Octreotide 225
Ocular infections *See Eye infections*
Ofloxacillin 223
Ofloxacin (Floxin) 8, 14, 18, 24-25, 45, 51, 60, 76, 205, 207, 232-234
Omeprazole + amoxicillin 23
Omnipen *See Ampicillin*
Onchocerca volvulus 136
Ondansetron (Zofran) 163
Ophthalmia 235
Opisthorchis viverrini 137
OPV 82
Oral drugs, costs of 203, 233
Oral infection 20, 22-23, 27
Ornidazole (Tiberal) 145
Ornidyl *See Eflornithine*
Osteomyelitis 16, 26, 133, 183, 187, 244
Otitis 22, 24, 198
Otitis externa 199
Otitis media 199, 244
Otomycosis 199
Ovide *See Malathion*
Oxacillin (Bactocill, Prostaphlin) 8, 14, 45, 51, 159, 186, 205, 211
Oxamniquine (Vansil) 9, 71, 139, 145
Oxytetracycline (Terramycin, Uri-Tet) 11
Paludrine *See Proguanil*
Pancreatitis 76
Panmycin *See Tetracycline*
Paracoccidioides 117
Paraflu 204
Paragonimus westermani 137
Parasitic infections 135-144, 197
Paregoric 164
Paromomycin (Humatin) 9, 71, 81, 135-137, 145, 153, 216, 225-226
Paronychia 182
Parotitis 201

PAS *See Aminosalicylic acid*
Pasteurella multicoda 26, 182
Pathocil *See Dicloxacillin*
PCE *See Erythromycin*
Pediculosis pubis 238-239
Pediculus capitus 137
Pediculus humanus 137
Pelvic inflammatory disease 18, 32, 240-241, 245
Penamp *See Ampicillin*
Penetrex *See Enoxacin*
Penicillin(s) 15, 17-22, 24, 27-28, 30-31, 33, 60, 69, 78-79, 159, 177, 181-183, 187, 190, 193, 195-196, 198, 200-202, 205, 207-209

Penicillin(s), costs of 203
Penicillin + aminoglycoside 15, 18, 20, 23, 211
Penicillin + streptomycin 16, 209
Penicillin + vancomycin 21
Penicillin allergy 64-67, 104-105, 210-212
Penicillin desensitization 65-66
Penicillin G (Pentids) 9, 14-17, 19-20, 22-23, 26-27, 30-32, 51-52, 182-183, 193, 195, 201, 203, 205, 216, 235-236

Penicillin G + aminoglycoside 22
Penicillin G benzathine 45
Penicillin G crystalline 45
Penicillin G procaine 45
Penicillin V 9, 14, 31, 45, 51, 66, 182-183, 201, 203, 205

Pentam 300 *See Pentamidine*
Pentamidine, pentamidine isethionate (Pentam 300, NebuPent) 9, 14, 45, 51, 60, 71, 76-77, 79, 137, 139-140, 145, 152
Penthrane *See Methoxyflurane*
Pentids *See Penicillin G*
Pentostam *See Stibogluconate sodium*
Pen-Vee K *See Phenoxyethyl penicillin (V)*
Pepto-Bismol *See Bismuth subsalicylate*
Peptostreptococci 17, 201
Pericarditis 26, 170, 172
Perimandibular infections 201
Periocular infections 189-191
Periodontal disease 17
Peripheral neuropathy 76
Peritoneal dialysis 216
Peritoneal dialysis dose regimens 48-51
Peritonitis 170, 215-216, 244
Peritonsillar abscess 201

Permapen *See Benzathine*
Permethrin (Nix, Elimite) 137, 146, 238-239
Pertussis 17
Pertussis vaccine 82
Petriellidium boydii 184
Pfizerpen *See Procaine*
Phacomycetes 117
Pharyngitis 19, 31, 200-201
Pharynx disease 245
Phenformin 80
Phenobarbital 75
Phenothiazines 79
Phenoxyethyl penicillin (V) (Beepen-VK, Betapen VK, Pen-Vee, V-Cillin K, Veetids, Ledercillin VK, Robicillin VK) 9
Phenytoin 75-78, 80-81
Phialophora verrucosa 184
Phthirus pubis 137
Phycomycosis 191
Pinta 31
Pinworm 136
Piperacillin (Pipracil) 9, 14, 18, 23, 45, 51, 169, 174, 177, 196, 216-217
Piperazine 9, 72, 79
Piperonyl butoxide (RID) 146, 238
Pipracil *See Piperacillin*
Plague 32
Plague vaccine 82
Plaquenil *See Chloroquine hydroxy; Hydroxychloroquine sulfate*
Plasmodium falciparum 109, 110
Plesiomonas 227
Plesiomonas shigelloides 223
Plesiomonas shigellosis 27
Pleurisy 170
Pneumococcal penumonia 245
Pneumococcal vaccines 82-87, 92
Pneumocystis 245
Pneumocystis carinii 139, 152, 171
Pneumocystis sp. 204
Pneumonia 15, 18-24, 26, 28-32, 139, 139, 171, 245
Pneumonitis 24, 121-122, 205-207
Podofilox 14, 239
Podophyllin 239, 240
Poliovirus vaccines 82, 84, 86, 88
Polycillin *See Ampicillin*
Polymox *See Amoxicillin*
Polymyxin(s) 61, 81, 199
Polymyxin B (Aerosporin) 10, 45, 79, 101
Praziquantel (Biltricide) 10, 14, 46, 72, 137, 139, 146

Precef *See Ceforanide lysine*
Prednisone   161, 163-164, 189, 202
Pregnancy, adverse reactions to
  antimicrobial agents during   67
Pregnancy, immunization   83-84
Pregnancy, safety of
  antimicrobial agents during   68
Preventive medicine   82-110
Primaquine   10, 61, 72, 75, 110
Primaquine + clindamycin   139
Primaquine phosphate   138, 146
Primaxin *See Imipenem/*
  Cilastin
Principen *See Ampicillin*
Prisons, immunizations   85
Providencia stuartii   28
Probenecid   74-75, 77-79, 186, 224
Procainamide   81
Procaine (Crystallin, Pfizerpen,
  Wycillin)   9
Progestins   80
Proguanil (Paludrine)   110, 138, 146
Prokine   162
Proloprim *See Trimethoprim*
Propamadine   189
Propionibacterium acnes   27, 181
Prostaphlin, *See Oxacillin*
Prostatitis   232-233, 245
Proteus indole positive   27
Proteus mirabilis   27
Protionamide *See Ethionamide*
Protostat *See Metronidazole*
Protozoa   152
Providencia rettgeri   28
Prozac *See Fluoxetine*
Pseudoallescheria   117, 197
Pseudoallescheria boydii   188
Pseudomonas   190, 199-200
Pseudomonas aeruginosa   28, 159, 181, 189, 195-196,
                                       198-199, 205
Pseudomonas cepacia   28
Pseudomonas mallei   28
Pseudomonas maltophilia
  (Xanthomonas maltophilia)   28
Pseudomonas pseudomallei   29
Pseudomonas putida   29
Psittacosis   18
Psychiatric disorders   164-165
Pulmonary infections
  See Lung infections
Pyelonephritis   229, 230, 232
Pyogenic liver disease   216, 244
Pyorrhea   202
Pyrantel, pyrantel pamoate   10, 72, 136-137, 140, 146
  (Antiminth)

Pyrazinamide   10, 14, 25, 46, 51, 61, 71,
                                       79, 127, 216
Pyrethrins   137, 146, 238
Pyrimethamine (Daraprim)   10, 14, 46, 61, 72, 75, 79,
                                       146, 153, 154, 190
Pyrimethamine + folonic acid   226
Pyrimethamine + sulfadiazine   139
Pyrimethamine + sulfadoxine
  (Fansidar)   10, 14, 110, 138-139, 152
Q fever   19, 29, 207
Quin-260 *See Quinine*
Quinacrine (Atabrine)   10, 14, 46, 72, 146, 226
Quine 200, 300 *See Quinine*
Quinidine   80
Quinidine dihydrochloride   137, 138
Quinidine gluconate   137, 138
Quinidine sulfate   138
Quinine (Legatrin, Quine 200,300,
  Quin-260)   10, 14, 46, 61, 67,
                                       72, 135
Quinine dihydrochloride   10, 146
Quinine sulfate   146
Quinolone(s)   61, 69, 76, 177, 187, 196,
                                       232, 234

Rabies vaccine   82, 88, 91
Rat bite fever   30, 31
Renal diseases   161
Renal failure, dosing regimens   34-51
Retinitis   121
Retrovir *See Zidovudine*
Rhodococcus equi   29, 159
Rickettsia   29
RID *See Piperonyl butoxide*
Rifabutin (Mycobutin)   10, 157
Rifadin *See Rifampin*
Rifamate *See Rifampin*
Rifampin (Rifadin, Rifamate)   10, 14, 19, 21, 25-26,
                                       30-31, 46, 51-52, 62, 67,
                                       71, 74-75, 77-80, 101,
                                       127, 156-157, 159, 169,
                                       182, 184, 186, 195-196,
                                       198-199, 205-206, 216,
                                       224
Rifampin + ethambutol   25
Rifampin + pyrazinamide   202
Ringworm   118, 182
Ritalin   165
Rivabutin   25
Robicillin VK *See Phenoxyethyl*
  penicillin (V)
Robimycin *See Erythromycin*
Robitet *See Tetracycline*
Rocephin *See Ceftriaxone*
Rochagan *See Benznidazole*
Rochalimaea henselae   29, 183

Rochalimaea quintana 29, 159
Rocky Mountain spotted fever 29, 245
Roferon A *See Interferon*
   Alpha 2a
Rondomycin *See Methacycline*
Roundworm 135
Rovamycine *See Spiramycin*
RP-Mycin *See Erythromycin*
RSV 204
Rubella vaccine 82-86
Salmonella 159, 224, 227, 244
Salmonella sp. 30
Salmonella typhi 29, 224
Salmonellosis 245
Salpingitis 26
Sandostatin *See Ocreotide*
Sarcoptes scabiei 139
Satric *See Metronidazole*
Scabies 139, 239
Schistosoma 197
Schistsomiasis 139
Seborrhea 163, 190
Seldane 76, 78
Selenium sulfide 182
Sepsis 19, 20, 22, 168-169
Sepsis, gram-negative 170
Septic shock 168
Septicemia 15-17, 19, 21, 23-24,
   26-32

Septra *See Trimethoprim-*
   sulfamethoxazole
Serratia 189
Serratia marcescens 30
Sexually transmitted diseases 234-243, 245
Shigella 30, 224, 227, 244
Shock 170
Sickle cell disease 186
Silver nitrate 202, 235
Sinus tract infections 183
Sinusitis 22, 24, 198, 200, 245
SK-erythromycin *See*
   Erythromycin stearate
Skeletal muscle relaxants 74
Skin infection 25
Skin testing 64
Soft tissue infection 25, 31, 185
Spectinomycin (Trobicin) 10, 26, 46, 62, 69, 80, 234
Spectrobid *See Bacampicillin*
Spinegerum 197
Spiramycin (Rovamycine) 139, 146
Spirillum minus 30, 183
Sporanox *See Itraconazole*
Sporothrix 117
Sporothrix schenckii (thorns) 184, 188
Sporotrichum 197

Sprue 244
SSKI 117
Staphcillin *See Methicillin*
Staphylococcus aureus 30, 169, 181, 182, 184,
   187, 189-191, 195-196,
   198-202, 205, 207,
   211-212, 223, 244
Staphylococcus epidermidis 31, 183, 195-196,
   211- 212
Staphylococcus pyogenes 191
Staphylococcus aureus 184
Staphylococcus saprophyticus 31
Steroids 140
Stibogluconate sodium
   (Pentostam) 137, 146
Stomatitis 202
Streptobacillus moniliformis 31, 183
Streptobacillus moniliformis 31, 183
Streptococci 31, 187, 198, 202,
   209-210
Streptococcus, Gram A 181-184
Streptococcus pneumoniae 31, 159, 184, 189-191,
   194-195, 199-200, 205,
   207-208, 244-245
Streptococcus sp. 198
Streptomyces pyogenes 200-202
Streptomycin 14, 17, 20, 22, 24, 30-32,
   46, 51, 67, 127, 157
Streptomycin + tetracycline 28
Strongyloides stercoralis 139
Strongyloidiasis 139
Subcutaneous tissue infections 181
Sulfa 26, 206
Sulfacetamide 189
Sulfadiazine (Microsulfon) 10, 26, 46, 139, 159, 190
Sulfamethoxazole (Gantonol) 11, 14, 18, 101
Sulfamethoxazole-trimethoprim 67
Sulfapyridine 11
Sulfasalazine (Azulfidine) 11, 13
Sulfa-trimethoprim 15-18, 19-24, 25-32, 183,
   196, 205-208, 222-226,
   230
Sulfa-trimethoprim + rifampin 206
Sulfisoxazole (Gantrisin) 11, 14, 18, 26, 46,
   230-231, 233
Sulfonamide(s) 10-11, 18, 21, 25-26, 62,
   67, 80, 184, 206
Sulfonylureas 76
Sumycin *See Tetracycline*
Suprax *See Cefixime*
Suramin, suramin sodium
   (Germanin) 140, 146
Surgery, prophylactic antibiotics in 98-102
Swimmer's ear 199
Symmetrel *See Amantidine*

Taenia	139
Tapeworm	139
Targocid *See Teicoplanin*	
Tazicef *See Ceftazidime*	
Tazidime *See Ceftazidime*	
Td	82-85, 88
Tegopen *See Cloxacillin*	
Tegretol *See Carbamazepine*	
Teicoplanin (Targocid)	11, 21, 30, 46, 196, 205
Terfenadine	77
Terfonyl	
See Trisulfapyrimidines	
Terramycin *See Oxytetracycline*	
Tetanus	19
Tetanus immune globulin	19
Tetanus vaccine	82, 88, 92
Tetra	177
Tetracycline(s) (Achromycin,	11, 14-15, 17-24, 26-27,
Tetralan, Brodspec,	29-33, 47, 51, 62, 67, 69, 76,
Panmycin, Robitet,	80, 136, 138, 181-183, 199,
Sumycin)	202-203, 205-208, 217,
	222-223, 225, 230, 233, 235,
	237, 240
Tetracycline +	
chloramphenicol	29
Tetracycline + streptomycin	17
Tetralan *See Tetracycline*	
Theophylline(s)	75-78, 80-81
Thiabendazole (Mintezol)	11, 72, 81, 135-136, 139-140,
	146
Thiazide diuretics	74, 81
Thrombocytopenia	161-162
Tiberal *See Ornidazole*	
Ticar *See Ticarcillin*	
Ticarcillin (Ticar)	11, 14, 47, 51-52, 169, 174,
	183, 196, 199, 215-216
Ticarcillin + clavulanic acid	11, 14-15, 28, 47, 51-52, 63,
(Timentin)	169, 174, 177, 217
Tick bite fever	29
Timentin *See Ticarcillin +*	
clavulanic acid	
Tinea capitis (ringworm)	118
Tinea corporis (ringworm)	118
Tinea cruris (jock itch)	118
Tinea pedis (athletes foot)	118
Tinea versicolar	182
Tinea versicolor	118
Tinidazole (Fasigyn)	135, 137, 140, 146, 226
TMP-SMX	184, 231
Tobramycin (Nebcin)	11, 14-15, 28, 35-36, 47, 51,
	53, 101, 168, 174, 193, 199,
	215-217
Tolbutamide	75
Tonsillar abscess	201
Tonsillitis	17
Totacillin *See Ampicillin*	
Toxic shock syndrome	170, 176
Toxocara	190
Toxoplasma encephalitis	153
Toxoplasma gondii	139-140, 197
Toxoplasmosis	139-140, 190, 202
Trachoma	18
Transplantation	121, 176
Travel, disease prevention	87-88, 106-110
Traveler's diarrhea	106-108, 244
Trazodone (Desyrel)	165
Trecator-S *See Ethionamide*	
Trench fever	29
Treponema carateum	31
Treponema pallidum	31, 197
Treponema pallidum ss endemicum	31
Treponema pallidum ss pertenue	32
Triazolam	76
Trichinosis	171
Trichloroacetic acid	239
Trichomonas vaginalis	140
Trichomoniasis	140, 241-242, 245
Trichophyton	182
Trichostrongylus	140
Trichuriasis	140
Trichuris trichiura (whipworm)	140
Tricyclic antidepressants	80
Trifluridine	119, 189
Trimethoprim (Proloprim,	11, 14, 47, 63, 69, 75,
Trimpex)	80-81, 101, 152, 223,
	230-233
Trimethoprim-sulfamethoxazole	12, 14, 47, 51, 63, 69, 81,
(Bactrim, Septra, Cotrim)	137, 139, 153-154, 177,
	193, 196, 199-200, 203,
	205, 227, 231-233, 238
Trimetrexate + folinic acid	139
Trimetrexate + leucovorin rescue	146
Trimox *See Amoxicillin*	
Trimpex *See Trimethoprim*	
Triple sulfa *See*	
Trisulfapyrimidines	
Trisulfapyrimidines (Triple sulfa,	
Neotrizine, Terfonyl)	10
Trivalent equine antitoxin	19
Trobicin *See Spectinomycin*	
Trypanosoma, Trypanosomiasis	140
Tryparsamide	146
Tuberculosis	24, 170, 186, 245
Tuberculosis prevention	131-132
Tuberculosis screening	132-133
Tuberculosis treatment	126-130
Tuberculous peritonitis	216
Tubizid *See Isoniazid*	
Tularemia	22, 245
Tumors	162

TWAR agent 206
Typhoid fever 29, 170, 224
Typhoid fever vaccine 82, 87
Typhus 29
Tyramine 77
Ultracef *See Cefadroxil*
Unasyn *See Ampicillin + sulbactam*
Unipen *See Nafcillin*
Upper respiratory infections 199-203
Ureaplasma urealyticum 32, 232-233
Ureidopenicillin 174
Urethral syndrome 18, 231
Urethritis 18, 26, 32, 243, 245
Urinary tract infection 18-20, 21-24, 27-32, 229-233
Uri-Tet *See Oxytetracycline*
Utimox *See Amoxicillin*
Vaccines 82-97
Vaginitis/vaginosis 241-242, 245
Vancocin HCl *See Vancomycin*
Vancocin pulvules
    See Vancomycin
Vancomycin (Vancocin 12, 14, 16, 18-21, 27, 29-31,
    pulvules, Vancocin HCl, 47, 51, 63, 69, 74, 79, 81, 98,
    Vancocin HCl IV, 101, 100-102, 105, 159, 169,
    Lyphocin) 174, 177, 181, 183, 187, 193,
    195, 198, 201, 205, 207,
    211-212, 216, 222
Vancomycin + aminoglycoside 211
Vancomycin + gentamicin 20
Vancomycin + rifampin 19, 196
Vansil *See Oxamniquine*
Vantin *See Cefpodoxime proxetil*
Varicella vaccine 84, 85
Varicella-zoster 120
Vasodilators 161
V-Cillin *See Phenoxyethyl penicillin (V)*
Veetids *See Phenoxyethyl penicillin (V)*
Velosef *See Cephradine*
Verapamil 80
Vermox *See Mebendazole*
Vibramycin *See Doxycycline*
Vibrio cholerae 32, 225
Vibrio parahaemolyticus 227

Vibrio sp. 181, 225
Vibrio vulnificus 32
Vidarabine (Vira-A, Ara-A) 12, 47, 51, 63, 73, 81,
    189
Vinblastin 75, 162
Vincent's infection 23, 201-202
Vincristine 75
Vira-A *See Vidarabine*
Viremia 121
Viruses 157-158, 171, 190, 197,
    200-202, 204, 207- 208
Vivonex TEN 14
Vulvovaginal candidiasis 242
Warts (Condylomata acuminata) 239-240
Wasting 164
Whipple's disease 244
Whipworm 140
Whitlow 182
Wound infection 19-22, 24, 25, 27, 30, 32
Wuchereria bancrofti 136
Wyamycin S *See Erythromycin stearate*
Wycillin *See Procaine*
Wymox *See Amoxicillin*
Xanthomonas maltophilia 28, 32
Yaws 32
Yellow fever vaccine 82, 87
Yersinia 227
Yersinia enterocolitica 32, 225
Yersinia pestis 32
Yersinia pseudotuberculosis 32
Yodoquinal *See Iodoquinol*
Yodoxin *See Iodoquinol*
Zalcitabine *See ddC*
Zefazone *See Cefmetazole*
Zentel *See Albendazole*
Zidovudine (Retrovir, AZT) 2, 12, 14, 47, 51, 63,
    73-74, 77, 124, 150, 151,
    161
Ziduvidine, prophylactic 166-167
Zinacef *See Cefuroxime*
Zinc 77, 80
Zithromax *See Azithromycin*
Zofran *See Ondansetron*
Zolicef *See Cefazolin*
Zovirax *See Acyclovir*
Zygomycetes 197, 204